Patient Education

ISSUES, PRINCIPLES, PRACTICES

Patient Education

ISSUES, PRINCIPLES, PRACTICES

Third Edition

Sally H. Rankin, Ph.D, R.N., C.R.N.P., F.A.A.N.
Associate Professor
Boston College School of Nursing
Boston College
Chestnut Hill, Massachusetts

Karen Duffy Stallings, R.N., M.Ed.
Associate Director for Program Activities
North Carolina AHEC Program
The University of North Carolina at Chapel Hill
School of Medicine
Chapel Hill, North Carolina

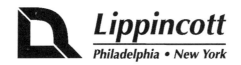

Lippincott
Philadelphia • New York

Acquisitions Editor: *Margaret Belcher*
Coordinating Editorial Assistant: *Emily Cotlier*
Project Editor: *Ellen M. Campbell*
Indexer: *Kathy Pitcoff*
Design Coordinator: *Melissa Olson*
Interior Designer: *William T. Donnelly*
Cover Designer: *Ilene Griff*
Production Manager: *Caren Erlichman*
Production Coordinator: *Kevin P. Johnson*
Printer/Binder: *R.R. Donnelley & Sons Company/Crawfordsville*

Third Edition

6 5 4 3 2 1

Library of Congress Cataloging-in-Pubiication Data

Rankin, Sally H.
    Patient education: issues, principles, practices / Sally H. Rankin, Karen Duffy Stallings. -- 3rd. ed.
      p.   cm.
    Includes bibliographical references and index.
    ISBN 0-397-55194-0
    1. Patient education. 2. Nurse and patient. I. Stallings, Karen Duffy. II. Title.
  RT90.R35   1995
  615.5'07--dc20   95-10728
                                                 CIP

Dedication

To the real heroes of patient education—
those nurses and other health care providers
who are on the front lines educating
and empowering patients and their families

Authors

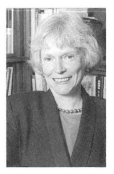

Sally Heller Rankin began her career in social work in the 1960s and became convinced while making home visits that clients needed more than she could offer as a caseworker. She noted their needs for health education at that time and decided to pursue nursing. She received her BSN from California State University, Los Angeles.

After working as a staff nurse at Duke University Medical Center and in inservice education, she obtained her MSN from Duke University where she taught for two years. During her years at Duke she began work on the first edition of *Patient Education: Issues, Principles, and Practices*. Returning to California in the early 80s, she taught at Mt. St. Mary's College and the University of Southern California and then moved to the San Francisco area. Sally completed her Ph.D. at UCSF in 1988, and then went on the faculty, receiving her certificate from Sonoma State University as a Family Nurse Practitioner in 1991. In 1993, she moved with her family and became an Associate Professor at Boston College School of Nursing. Her clinical practice areas have included cardiac nursing, diabetes education, and primary care practice in student health. Recently, Sally received the Distinguished Alumna award from Duke University School of Nursing, and in 1989 she received the Carol Lindeman New Investigator Award from the Western Institute of Nursing.

Her work in the area of patient education has been informed by her research interests in the area of chronic illness, especially coronary artery disease and diabetes mellitus, both diseases that take a tremendous toll on the individual and family members. Dr. Rankin is currently completing a study of women recovering from myocardial infarction that is funded by the National Institute of Nursing Research.

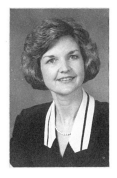

Karen Duffy Stallings received her BSN from Boston College and her Masters in Adult Education from The University of North Carolina at Chapel Hill. She is Associate Director for the North Carolina Area Health Education Centers Program (AHEC), an educational partnership linking the university health science centers and the state's communities to help meet the primary health care needs of North Carolinians. She provides leadership and administrative support for nursing, mental health, aging, health promotion, and interdisciplinary initiatives. She is an adjunct instructor for The University of North Carolina at Chapel Hill School of Nursing. Previously, she held numerous positions in staff nursing, management, staff development, and community-based nursing education. Her clinical practice areas have included acute care inpatient psychiatry and community and family medicine. Her diverse background has also included directing a refresher program for inactive RNs who wished to resume their clinical practice.

Throughout her career, patient education has been an area of concentration. Karen is actively involved as a teacher and consultant, in North Carolina and nationally, with special interests in the promotion of interdisciplinary models and the role of staff development in patient education.

Contributors

Rae L. Jayne is a Certified Diabetes Educator who has practiced as a clinical nurse specialist at the Diabetes Center at the University of California, San Francisco for the past 12 years. She completed her Ph.D. in Nursing at UCSF in 1993, having previously finished the BS to MS program there. Her A.D. in Nursing was earned at Pasadena City College. In addition to teaching classes to patients, Dr. Jayne lectures to medical and nursing students at UCSF and currently serves as Associate Director of the Diabetes Center. She contributed a chapter on diabetes education to the second edition of this book.

Ronna E. Krozy received her basic nursing education at Beth Israel Hospital School of Nursing, Boston, MA, her B.S. and M.S. in Community Health Nursing from Boston College, and her Ed.D. in Health Education, with a subspecialty in sex education, from Boston University. She has been teaching Community Health Nursing since 1973 and has served as Department Chair. Dr. Krozy has developed numerous community-based programs on health promotion, sexuality, and aging, with particular emphasis on incorporating cultural competence. She created and serves as faculty coordinator for the Por Cristo-BSCON Health Project, teaching community health nursing through an overseas immersion experience in Ecuador.

Ellen M. Robinson is currently a doctoral candidate at Boston College School of Nursing, Chestnut Hill, MA, and a Clinical Nurse Specialist in direct patient care on the Cardiac Access Unit at Massachusetts General Hospital, Boston, MA. She obtained her bachelor's degree in nursing from Salem State College and her M.S. from Boston College. Ms. Robinson is a member of both the Nursing Ethics and Optimum Care Committees at Mass General. She has taken advanced coursework in ethics, including the Intensive Bioethics course at the Kennedy Institute of Georgetown University in 1993. Her dissertation research will focus on the experience of surrogate decision makers in living through end-of-life decisions for their loved ones with dementia of the Alzheimer's type.

Preface

Thirteen years ago when the first edition of *Patient Education: Issues, Principles, Practices* was written, we were certain that patient education was the panacea for frustrated patients and dissatisfied nurses. While we continue to believe in patient education as a vehicle for empowering patients and enhancing job satisfaction for nurses, we have extensively revised the original work to reflect the increasing complexity of health care and the growth of nursing as a discipline.

Changes in staffing patterns and personnel, utilization of health care as mandated by federal regulations, increasing patient acuity, and movement of technology-based nursing care into the home have necessitated new approaches to patient education. Patient teaching is now occurring in a plethora of settings that were not considered possible when the first edition of the book was written. For example, the increasing demands on family members to manage complex care in the home requires sophisticated patient education practices by home care nurses, a topic that was not even considered in the first edition.

In response to nursing educators' requests, the third edition of this book includes more theory-based chapters as well as more "how-to's" for patient teaching. For example, theories pertaining to life-span development, immigration stressors, health promotion, stress and coping, and self-regulation have been added. The role of staff development in supporting patient education efforts is a new feature that many practicing nurses will find helpful in preparing for JCAHO accreditation. Other special features include a spotlight on Benner's work to promote the development of expertise in patient education. A chapter on case management is also new to this edition. It stresses the integration of patient education into all aspects of case management and offers change-agentry skills essential to these efforts. Readers of the previous editions will also note the addition of learning objectives and strategies for critical analysis and application to each chapter.

The text is designed to be helpful to both generic and advanced practice nursing programs. Additionally, practicing nurses will find this edition even more useful than previous editions in terms of dealing with systemwide issues that affect the delivery of patient education. We believe that members of all health care disciplines will find the book valuable, but because the authors are themselves nurses practicing in nursing arenas, the work draws heavily on nursing examples and the science and research of our discipline. Since all health care providers share a central interest in the welfare of patients, readers from other disciplines will appreciate the patient-centered approach. The authors apologize for their gender stereotyped language—we have referred to nurses as women and patients as men, a convention that does not adequately recognize the male portion of our profession.

As in the previous editions, the third edition is organized in terms of issues, principles, and practices. The first section of the book, *issues* (Chapters 1–5), addresses such changes in the health care system that have influenced patient teaching (Chapter 1) and the critical need to prepare *all* nurses as patient teachers (Chapter 2). Chapter 3, Patient Education as a Tool for Normalization and Self-Regulation, is a totally new chapter that arose from important theory generating research on the importance of self-regulating one's therapeutic regimen so that life can be lived normally. The implications for patient education are discussed in terms of the health care provider's tailoring of teaching to needs for normalization. The issue of providing patient education for special groups who present a particular challenge is addressed from various theoretical perspectives that suggest directions for practice. The last chapter in the issues section, Informed Consent: An Important Concept in Patient Education, presents informed consent as the nexus of legal and ethical issues pertaining to patient education. A theoretical framework that addresses the relationship of patient education to informed consent is presented.

The second section of the book, *principles* (Chapter 6–11), encompasses theoretical approaches to teaching and motivating patients as well as the five extremely useful chapters on the nursing process and patient education. Nursing students in the past have found these chapters very helpful as they endeavor to furnish skills for critical thinking that are so important to the process of patient education and clinical judgment. Case studies are used liberally to illustrate the different facets of the nursing process: nursing assessment and diagnosis, planning, implementation, and evaluation. The reader will note the authors' belief in the importance of involving the entire family in the process of patient education. Family involvement is another avenue to enhance nurses' job satisfaction and to fortify therapeutic patient/family relationships. We believe that the family should be assessed from a systems perspective and, therefore, that goals, interventions, and evaluations should include the entire family. In the process of refining these chapters, additional material has been added in the areas of implementation of patient education interventions and the area of designing patient education applicable to family and home constraints.

The third section, *practices* (Chapters 12–15), has been augmented by an excellent new chapter that applies health education concepts to the practice of improving health for aggregates, an important precept of community health nursing. The entirely new chapter on case management, Chapter 13, and the importance of tailoring patient education across various product lines (e.g., surgery, ambulatory care settings) will particularly enhance the practice of those health care providers involved in the administration of various services and programs. Chapter 14, a popular roundtable on dealing with problems in practice settings, has been expanded with the addition of information on teaching children with learning disabilities, nurse practitioners and patient education, patient education under difficult conditions such as homelessness, patient teaching with persons with AIDS, and an international comparison of patient education. Chapter 15, the last chapter in the book, has been enhanced by a section on writing research proposals.

Our commitment to patient education has not changed, as we continue to view it as an essential patient empowerment tool, even though our own practice settings have changed since we wrote the first edition of this book. The first author's involvement as a family nurse practitioner in the education of students in primary care has enhanced her appreciation of the need for patient education on health promotion and disease prevention. The second author's work in the provision of continuing education to health care providers in the state of North Carolina has increased her awareness of wider system issues that affect the provision of patient education in diverse settings. Feeling powerless is perhaps the most devastating aspect of illness for a patient. Patient education can be implemented by the nurse as the most effective means of returning control to the patient. Patient education can reduce feelings of helplessness and enhance the patient's ability to be the chief decision maker in the management of health and illness problems. We view patient education as the *essence* of nursing practice. In today's tumultuous health care climate created by changing mandates for health care reform, the growing presence of uninsured people with little or no access to health care, and the increased acuity of patients, confident and competent nurses are even more important in the delivery of quality patient care and patient education than when this book was first written.

Sally H. Rankin, Ph.D., R.N., C.R.N.P., F.A.A.N.

Karen Duffy Stallings, R.N., M.Ed.

Acknowledgments

Without the questions of our students, the exemplary practice of our colleagues, and the inspiration of dedicated nurses who make us proud of our profession, we would not have persevered in the revisions of this text. As we speak to audiences on the topic of patient education, we are encouraged by the comments of staff nurses who are working across all health care settings. In particular, we recognize the expertise of nurses who assume leadership roles in managed care, making patient education its centerpiece, we are awed by the dedication of nurses working in acute and ambulatory care settings who struggle to clarify the intricacies of complex medical regimen, and we appreciate the educators who speak to the utility of our textbook.

We would like to express our appreciation to Lin Mitchell, Care Coordinator at Duke University Medical Center in Durham, North Carolina, and to Cindy Stewart, RNC, BSN, CCRN, Patient Care Coordinator for Cardiovascular Surgery at High Point Regional Hospital in North Carolina for sharing their experiences and thoughts with us regarding patient education and case management. We are grateful to the late Eugene S. Mayer, MD, MPH, Director of the North Carolina AHEC Program, whose pioneering spirit, dedication, and leadership in health sciences education included strong support for nursing and for this project. We acknowledge Jon Haycock, Media Specialist at Boston College School of Nursing, and the lively photographs that illustrate the various facets of patient education. We appreciate the guidance offered by nursing editors at Lippincott during the various revisions of this book; in particular, we recognize Emily Cotlier and Margaret Belcher for their help and encouragement with the third edition. Lastly, we gratefully acknowledge the love and support of our families which is visible to us between the lines of the text. A special note of gratitude goes to Amy Rankin-Williams, Bill and Rob Rankin, and Frank, Sarah, and Emily Stallings.

Contents

CHAPTER 10

Designing Patient Education Programs in the Community and in the Home, 201

CHAPTER 11

Evaluation: Determining and Documenting Patient Learning Outcomes, 219

CHAPTER 12

Community Health Promotion: Assessment and Intervention, 245

RONNA E. KROZY

CHAPTER 13

Case Management, Critical Paths, and Patient Education, 273

CHAPTER 14

Patient Education

ISSUES, PRINCIPLES, PRACTICES

CHAPTER

1

The Nurse as Patient Teacher: Changing Needs and Mandates

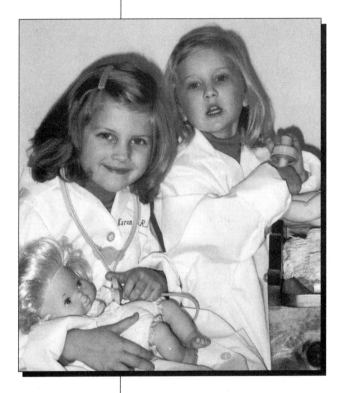

OBJECTIVES FOR CHAPTER 1

After reading this chapter, the nurse or student nurse should be able to:

1 Define "patient education."

2 Describe the relationship between patient education and discharge planning.

3 Discuss the important role of patient education in a reformed health care system.

4 Describe patient education as a dimension of nurse caring.

Feeling powerless is perhaps the most devastating aspect of illness for a patient. Patient education is the most effective means of returning control to the patient by reducing feelings of helplessness and enhancing the ability to be the chief decision maker in the management of one's health and illness problems.

SALLY RANKIN AND KAREN STALLINGS, 1990

Nurses clearly see themselves as advocates, as persons who stand along side of and empower patients and their families to have a voice when they are weak and vulnerable.

PATRICIA BENNER, 1984

The goal of educating the patient and family is to improve patient health outcomes by promoting recovery, speeding return to function, promoting health behavior, and appropriately involving the patient in his or her own care decisions.

JOINT COMMISSION ON THE ACCREDITATION
OF HEALTHCARE ORGANIZATIONS, 1994

Patient Education as a Dimension of Nurse Caring

Caring is assumed as an integral part of nursing practice, but studies show that this "hidden work" may go unrecognized by patients and their families, except when the behaviors and attitudes associated with nurse caring are missed. Caring is viewed as the essence of nursing, which helps to heal, cure, and improve patients' health. In several studies describing the process of nurse caring, shared vulnerability between nurse and patient and activities directed toward the welfare of the patient are identified. Nurse caring includes such behaviors as active listening, comforting, knowing the patient as a person, respecting the patient, touching the patient, providing information for decision-making, realizing that patients know themselves best, being perceptive of patient needs, and giving good physical care (Wolf,

Giardino, Osborne, & Ambrose, 1994). Caring includes being an advocate, empowering the patient to make informed decisions, and promoting autonomy. At the same time it includes making the patient feel safe, comforted, and valued (Tanner, Benner, Chesla, & Gordon, 1993).

Patient education is a dimension of nurse caring when it considers the best interests of the patient, knowing that the best case manager for a patient is ultimately the patient himself. Nurse caring is a delicate balance of comfort and challenge, a creative ability to maximize resources for the patient's benefit. Dr. Patricia Benner's research (1982, 1984) and research with her colleagues (Benner & Wrubel, 1989; Benner, Tanner, & Chesla, 1992) reveals that as novice nurses move through the developmental stages of advanced beginner, competent, proficient, and expert practice, patient education becomes an integral part of nurse caring.

> Nurses become experts in coaching a patient through an illness. They take what is foreign and fearful to the patient and make it familiar and thus less frightening. Expert nurses have learned to communicate and teach in extreme situations. And in this teaching they are forced to use themselves, their attitudes, tone of voice, humor, skill, and a variety of approaches to the patient. (Benner, 1984)

We hope that the combination of issues, principles, and practices addressed in this text will help nursing students and novice nurses to develop "survival skills" for teaching. For nurses working toward expert practice, we hope the text will promote an integration of patient education in creative ways with an endless variety of practice and patient populations. Furthermore, we hope expert nurses will discover validation for their teaching efforts and a call to provide leadership in research, education, and practice arenas.

The images of a "caring nurse" developed early in childhood can influence the willingness and effectiveness of nurses to become patient teachers.

How Does Patient Education Begin?

It was a rainy Saturday. In an upstairs bedroom four sisters opened a doll hospital. Dolls of various sizes were placed carefully in shoe boxes, and the end of each box was labeled with the patient's name. The patients were all sick; it didn't much matter with what. The four little nurses scurried busily among the patients, giving baths, administering shots with straight pins from their mother's sewing basket, and applying scarf bandages, Band-Aids, and plasters of baking soda with water or toothpaste. While doing so, the four nurses reassured their patients they would take care of everything and make them better soon. Eventually, their mother's voice at the bottom of the stairs called the sisters down to lunch. This completed the recoveries of all the patients. The sisters dressed the dolls, put them back in their usual places, and cleaned up the messy bandages to prevent discovery of their magic treatments.

Years later, the four sisters went off to college. One chose to study nursing, and her first day of clinical was, in many ways, as full of adventure as that rainy Saturday.

Those of us who became nursing students walked onto the floors of hospitals with excitement, fear, and a certain reverence. We watched the nurses rush about, answering calls and caring for sick patients. Each of us was assigned a patient, and we reached anxiously for the chart. We hoped for a patient who needed dressing changes, injections, or treatments we had never performed. We hoped we would be able to decipher the doctor's handwriting and understand the medical jargon. Would we have to make an occupied bed? Would there be an intravenous or central venous pressure line?

Many of us were first attracted to the nursing profession during our childhoods. We were prompted by the desire to help people become healthier and happier and to take away their pain. We viewed the fields of medicine and nursing as enveloped in mystery, and we hoped to be able to evoke cures. We

discovered, during nursing school or early in our first jobs, that we could not fix everything or take away all the pain. No easy cure, panacea, or magic remedy existed. We came to terms with our own strengths and limitations. Our effectiveness was determined more by our ability to influence people than by our ability to control them. We found out that the control we exercised in the hospital did not necessarily help patients, or their families, to survive at home after they were discharged. Despite our well-meaning and knowledgeable advice, patients did not always follow our directions.

We learned that the patients in our care often have many health problems, are sicker than we imagine, and are discharged from the hospital earlier than we wish. Nurses, we discovered, must provide care in a variety of settings, including ambulatory care, acute care, home care, and long-term care. Educating patients is part of the care nurses provide in all these settings. But rarely is there enough time to teach the patient and family all they need to know, and often patients are too sick to participate. As nurses we must be skilled in assessing each patient's needs and setting priorities to meet the most critical of these needs before the patient's discharge from our care (see Chaps. 7 and 8).

Moreover, our patients are influenced by beliefs and values often different from our own. Many have limited ability to read or write; others are not fluent in the English language. We must be open, flexible, and creative (see Chaps. 4 and 8).

The health care delivery system is driven by economic reality, and nursing care must be defined, qualified, and quantified. Nurses must be able to relate to administrators as well as patients and learn to provide effective interventions and quality, cost-effective care through nursing case management systems (see Chap. 13).

Thus, we have learned that nurses do not interact with patients in a vacuum. Rather, nurses are members of a larger team, which includes a variety of health care professionals. Each team member has a special expertise or contribution that should not be ignored.

Learning to work in harmony with other team members is much more difficult than learning technical skills. Also difficult is changing our view of patients: they are not just recipients of the care we give, but rather, they and their families are at the head of the health care team. We develop this shift in focus by recognizing their right to choose their own futures and by willingly sharing our knowledge with them. This is known as *patient education*, a practice based on influence, not control. We also learn to appreciate the roles of the other team members and to find ways to articulate the contributions of each team member in helping patients and their families.

Overview of Nursing and Patient Education

During the past three decades, patient education has become widely recognized as a professional role of nurses. The growth of consumerism and the self-help movement has alerted people to take responsibility for their own health, while simultaneously nudging nurses and other health care professionals to actively pursue patient education as an important aspect of patient care. Providing patient education is central to the role of every nurse providing patient care, regardless of job title or clinical setting. Advanced education provides expanded career options for today's nurses, including the roles of nurse practitioner, clinical nurse specialist, and nurse midwife.

Due to the changing environments for delivering health and illness care, today's nurses are found in acute care hospitals, subacute settings, rehabilitation and long-term care facilities, retirement communities, health maintenance organizations, preferred provider organizations, specialized inpatient and outpatient settings (including ambulatory care, urgent care, birthing centers, and day care centers), schools, mental health centers, rural health centers, and home health and hospice agencies. Knowledge and skills to provide patient education, and the ability

to work as a member of an interdisciplinary team, are critical to nurses' effectiveness in these settings. Nurses describe patient education as a key to enhancing job satisfaction because it creates greater patient and nurse autonomy. In addition, nurses in advanced practice attribute success in competing for new employment positions to possessing skills and experience in patient education.

Teaching was recognized as a function of nursing when Florence Nightingale wrote her significant treatises on nursing (Nightingale, 1860). In fact, throughout the history of nursing, whenever nurses have acted as agents in empowering patients to take responsibility for their own health, some of the power has been reflected back to nursing, thus increasing the profession's credibility and viability.

In the words of Virginia Henderson, "The unique function of the nurse is to assist the individual, sick or well, in the performance of those activities contributing to health or its recovery (or to a peaceful death) that he would perform unaided if he had the necessary strength, will or knowledge. And to do this in such a way as to help him gain independence as rapidly as possible" (Henderson & Nite, 1960). Patient education is key to ensuring such individualized care.

Although teaching has always been an integral part of nursing practice, nursing education has not always prepared nurses for the teaching role. In the early part of this century, the National League for Nursing (NLN) voiced concern that nursing education dealt only with disease and not with preparation for teaching (National League for Nursing Education, 1918). The NLN has continued to speak out on the importance of educating nurses to teach. In 1993, Redman pointed to the concern that graduate education in nursing has not yet made a commitment to prepare nurses for patient education as a specialty, based on the absence of master's level courses in patient education (Redman, 1993a; Redman & Braun, 1991).

In 1975, the American Nurses Association (ANA) published a document entitled *The Professional Nurse and Health Education*. It stated that the professional nurse's responsibility includes "teaching the patient and family relevant facts about specific health-care needs and supporting appropriate modification of behavior." The ANA's *Model Nurse Practice Act* (1979) defines patient education as a component of the RN's practice. LPNs are responsible for reinforcing what is taught. References to patient education are found in health care agency policies, nursing job descriptions, and the ethics codes of nursing organizations. Furthermore, the courts have consistently upheld the rights of patients to know about their health problems and treatments. Patient education has become a professional expectation and a legal duty of nurses.

Patient Compliance Issues

A recent nursing graduate shared the following story:

> I think that patient education is an important part of the care patients receive. We should be willing to share what we know with patients and help them understand what choices they have.
>
> Sometimes I feel that it really makes a difference and I can tell that the patient understands. But my experiences are not all positive ones and I end up feeling frustrated and angry. After all, patient education takes time out of an already busy schedule of patient care. It requires patience and extra effort to explain procedures and answer questions. I usually have to repeat the information several times or try to explain it in a different way so he can understand. After all my effort, some patients still don't take medications or treatments as they should. I end up wondering if they just don't want to be well or if they would have taken the information more seriously if it came from a doctor. Then I ask myself, "What did I do wrong?"

Physicians express similar feelings of anger and frustration when patient education fails. Although we all recognize that patients have the right and free will to make choices, we also question our own skills in teaching our patients. We wonder, "Should I have done things differently?"

Patient Partnership Versus Compliance

Many health care professionals describe patient education as giving patients information about their problems and treatments. The quality of patient education is perceived to have a direct correlation with the availability of audiovisual programs, well-equipped file drawers, and the presence of informative posters in the physician's office. When patients fail to perform the desired behaviors, we assume that they were not given enough information or that they failed to assimilate it. We respond by repeating the information or giving it in a different form. When the behaviors of patients fail to change, can we assume that they have not learned the facts we have tried to impress on them? Godfrey Hochbaum (1980) suggests that the temptation to give more (or more forceful) information to drive home to patients possible dire consequences when they do not exhibit desired behaviors comes from our own assumptions that human behavior is shaped by rationality and sufficient motivation. When health professionals examine their own health behaviors and note that they often fail to "practice what they preach," the challenge of lifelong behavior change is better appreciated. The health behaviors nurses prescribe for patients involve not a single decision, but many difficult daily decisions that often involve pain, expense, social isolation, a perceived loss of independence, and the difficulty of breaking old habits. Changing a single behavior pattern, such as what one eats, is difficult. We frequently ask patients to change two or more behaviors simultaneously (such as diet, exercise, and smoking cessation). The term compliance not only oversimplifies the way patients are educated, but also overlooks the needed negotiation, coaching, and integration of health practices in the patient's and family's daily life.

When nurses discuss obstacles in their experiences with patient education, they often identify problems motivating patients to change current behaviors to improve the patient's health status. When asked to elaborate, it becomes evident that nurses see motivation and compliance as closely related. The implication is that a sufficiently motivated patient will comply with the doctor's or nurse's instructions.

Many health professionals have justified their involvement in patient education by asserting that it would increase patient compliance; in other words, it would convince patients to follow our instructions. It is apparent that, despite teaching, patients frequently do not make the choices recommended to them by nurses, physicians, and other health care professionals. This is often termed as *noncompliance*.

The term compliance implies that we may dictate to the patient what is to be done or changed and the patient must obey us. We are often uncomfortable with the patient's right to choose not to follow our advice or to change his or her mind. We should strive to enlist the patient's partnership, rather than compliance, and look on patient education as a process of influencing behavior in ways acceptable to the patient. An orientation toward cooperation causes us to think about our own effectiveness in patient education in a different light. Patient education successes have more to do with the patient's preparation to make informed choices than with acts of compliance. In fact, if patient education acknowledges the patient's free will to make choices, it must afford understanding of the importance of his values and wishes and his ability to participate in decision-making. Chapter 3 provides an in-depth discussion of the issues surrounding patient decision-making.

The notion of compliance with a medical regimen is an important goal of patient education, but it is not the only goal. A significant process occurs between education and compliance, one in which the client internalizes the teaching and then makes informed choices about applying the teaching to his life. Indeed, compliance is a product not only of learning about the medical regimen but also of the patient's life-style, a complex group of behaviors including social and family patterns, activities of daily living, and dietary, exercise, and sleep patterns.

Although the term compliance is so ingrained in discussions of patient education that it is difficult to replace it with another term that reflects mutuality, we would like to suggest the use of the terms *adherence*, *concurrence*, and *cooperation* as alternatives to compliance. All three terms suggest choice, mutuality of goals, and a patient-provider relationship based on respect and trust.

Reforming Health Care: A Central Role for Patient Education

An intense debate about health care delivery in the United States is certain to continue on both the state and national levels. Questions about how to provide universal access to basic health services and how to finance rising health care costs are central to the debate. With millions of Americans having no health care insurance, appropriate and early medical treatment is often avoided or deferred. When patients present themselves for treatment only in the event of acute episodes or, as they often do, with exacerbation of chronic illness, costs, complications, disability, and mortality rise. The hopes for a reformed health care system hold promise of the availability and access to early detection and improved management of chronic health conditions, with lower cost and better outcomes. Nursing views itself as a valuable and visible contributor to managed health care systems of the present and future. In addition, the ANA is a voice for nursing in the United States, promoting a changed delivery system featuring consumer responsibility for self-care, informed decision-making, and choices in the selection of health care providers and services (American Nurses Association, 1991). In his 1993 address to the nation, President Clinton emphasized that a comprehensive, high quality, and affordable national health care system for all Americans would be categorized by the following "guiding stars":

1. Security: benefits could not be taken away because of loss of employment or health status
2. Simplicity: less paperwork for providers and a simpler system for consumers
3. Savings: simplified insurance system and incentives to provide cost-effective care
4. Increased choices: consumers choose their health plans
5. Improved quality of health care
6. Increased individual responsibility: individuals promote their own health and providers use the system prudently.

The image of a reformed system calls for increasing patient involvement in the health care team and increasing emphasis on the patient's role in improving health status. Patient education is the vital link for patient empowerment to assume these responsibilities.

A national initiative to improve the health of all Americans through prevention is entitled *Healthy People 2000* (U.S. Department of Health and Human Services, 1990). Its overall goals are to increase healthy life span, reduce health disparities, and achieve access to preventive health services for all Americans. Three hundred specific health promotion and disease prevention objectives are targeted to be met by the year 2000 through the partnership of government agencies, health professionals, and private partners. Nurses have assumed leadership in many activities associated with *Healthy People 2000* and are using their expertise in patient education to encourage health promotion.

Although a national consensus on a basic health care benefits package and how to finance a comprehensive system is difficult to achieve, health care reforms are sweeping across traditional settings where nurses are employed and are influencing nursing education. The downsizing or "right sizing" of hospitals is moving nurses into community-based practice. The delivery of patient care continues to move closer to home. In schools of nursing, increasing emphasis is placed on preparing students for public, community, and home health settings and for delivering preventive health services in the context of managed care. Nursing school curricula emphasize patient education as an integral part of nursing practice. RNs returning to school to pursue BSN degrees gain new knowledge of patient education based in a wide variety of practice settings. In addition, nurses enrolled in nurse practitioner and advanced degree programs should refine patient education skills needed for practice. In efforts to meet the public's needs for primary care, the expanded training of medical students for generalist roles is accompanied by an increased amount of training in rural, underserved, and community-based sites. Nursing programs are expanding student exposure to include similar clinical training sites. A growing demand for nurse practitioners, nurse midwives, and physician's assistants is also related to improving the access and cost of primary care services to meet the public's needs. Patient education is a critical component of graduate nursing education programs that prepare nurses to assume advanced practice roles.

Marc Rivo, MD, MPH, Division Director of the U.S. Department of Health and Human Services states: "Regardless of the direction and pace of our journey towards health care reform, it seems self-evident that relentless changes in the health marketplace inexorably will influence the mission, structure, and function of our Nation's health professions education system." He offers the growth and popularity of managed care networks as one of the major forces driving these changes (Rivo, 1994).

Beyond Informed Consent

Nurses who were prepared to practice in the 1970s witnessed the importance of providing for the *informed consent* of the patient. The patient's right to know includes the right to know what is wrong, the right to know what diagnostic and therapeutic processes will be used, and the right to know what the prospects are for physical recovery (Regan, 1975). The patient has a right to refuse treatment and to be informed of the consequences of those actions (American Hospital Association, 1975). The nature of this contractual agreement guarantees a patient's right to know what he can do to effect his physical recovery and, thus, would include necessary patient education. Nursing education and literature addressing informed consent stressed the importance of providing information on diagnosis, prognosis, and proposed treatments or procedures to all patients. Redman notes that until the late 1960s, health care professionals shared with patients information that they perceived to be useful. Information thought to be harmful or upsetting was withheld. Presently, health care providers consider the ethical dilemmas of withholding information, and many providers feel obligated to share information in a complete way (Redman, 1993a,1993b). Chapter 5 provides a further discussion of informed consent as a special case of patient education, considering its legal and ethical considerations.

By the end of the 1970s, the focus of patient teaching witnessed a shifting and expanding list of priorities. No longer were new nurses educated solely for hospital-based practice. Practice in ambulatory care, long-term care, and home care settings helped nurses gain greater appreciation for the vital link between patient education, discharge planning, and continuity of care. Patients were discharged from hospitals to other settings "sicker and quicker."

Discharge Planning and Patient Education

"Discharge planning begins on the day of admission." Every nurse was taught this golden rule during nursing education. Up until the past decade, however, the number of days a patient stayed in the hospital was flexible and often could be extended to prepare patients and families to assume self-care. As health care costs continued to rise, fingers were pointed at hospitals, claiming inefficiency and financial rewards for the amount of money they spent to care for patients. American industry and government agencies pressed for changes in health care reimbursement that would build in incentives for efficiency and hold the line on costs to third-party payers.

A major new trend in reimbursement became law in 1983. Medicare began using a prospective payment system called diagnosis-related groups (DRGs). Payments were no longer made to hospitals based on the costs of services or the number of days of care provided to a patient. Instead, a predetermined payment was assigned to each of the DRGs. Each DRG has an assigned mean "length of stay," the number of days Medicare would pay for services. An "outlier cutoff," the maximum number of days for which a hospital can bill Medicare, was set; to negotiate payment the hospital must prove that the client's condition was complicated. Many health care analysts predicted that major insurance companies would adopt similar prospective-pricing payment systems (Vestal, 1995; Malloy & Hartshorn, 1989) Since then, the health insurance industry has introduced sweeping changes, and new alliances for managed health care evolve daily. Cost and quality are the key components of managed health care.

With the advent of DRGs, the golden rule of discharge planning took on a new meaning. Financial incentives were now tied to the discharge date because hospitals were reimbursed fixed amounts based on these DRGs. The strategies developed for fiscally managing patient care range from new approaches to preadmission screening to inpatient case management, and from outpatient specialty clinics to high-technology home care. Health care systems emerged, linking providers across a continuum of health care settings. Case management involves ensuring continuity of patient care services and maximizing the quality of care while minimizing the costs. With the advent of each new approach, patient education has taken center stage. Discharge planning in most cases implies patient education.

The primary focus of patient education in the 1980s shifted from provider outcomes to patient and family outcomes. Successful patient education could not be guaranteed based solely on the ability and willingness of health care providers to deliver understandable information about diagnosis, prognosis, and treatment. The goals for education of all patients must include learning survival skills, recognizing problems after discharge, and making decisions that contribute to self-care management. The American Hospital Association published *Guidelines for Discharge Planning* (1984) to assist hospitals in evaluating and improving their discharge planning functions, stressing that each hospital should develop a system based on its own requirements and resources and the needs of its patients. Discharge planning is viewed as part of routine patient care, an interdisciplinary process to help patients and their families develop and implement a feasible posthospital plan of care. Special discharge-planning services are warranted when posthospital needs are expected to be complex. The same guidelines can be applied to other settings.

Guidelines and methods for integrating discharge planning and patient education planning are covered in Chapter 7.

Growing Needs of the Elderly Population and Persons With Chronic Health Conditions

The fastest growing segment of our society is our elderly population. Health care advances and medical technology have helped older citizens to live longer; nevertheless, they continue to suffer from chronic health conditions, physical disabilities, and functional limitations and, therefore, depend heavily on health care services, particularly nursing care. Together with increases in the number of elderly and the arrival of prospective payment has come a boom in the home health care industry and rehabilitative programs of long-term care institutions. Many treatments and technologies now used in the home were unimaginable a decade ago. More acute care is being provided in the home, and nurses realize that the trend to discharge patients from the hospital "sicker and quicker" places

heavy demands on them to provide patient and family teaching and continuity with caretakers in the home.

Recognizing the growing threats of acquired immunodeficiency syndrome (AIDS) and tuberculosis, nurses employed in public health departments have assumed an active role in new prevention and detection programs for high-risk populations. Patient education for prevention is targeted to the homeless, migrant farm workers, and prison populations. Nurses have augmented their skills in patient education with a new understanding of how culture and poverty can influence patient behavior.

Another priority for nursing's involvement in health promotion and disease prevention is in the area of substance abuse, now the nation's number one health problem (U.S. Department of Health and Human Services, 1994). Substance abuse involving tobacco, alcohol, and drugs is the primary cause of preventable illness, injury, and death in the United States. Efforts in prevention and early intervention are enhanced by the involvement of school health nurses. Nurses in all settings should know how to counsel patients about smoking and how to refer patients to smoking cessation programs in the community.

A Gallup poll funded by the Robert Wood Johnson Foundation revealed that although one in seven Americans faces major limitations from chronic illness, one third do not seek routine or preventive health care; they receive care only for acute problems. The exacerbation of chronic illness is the only time they may access the health care system. Without patient education and patient involvement in care to prevent acute episodes, health care is costlier and quality of life suffers. Chronic disorders account for a large portion of U.S. expenditures on health care, in a health care system geared to cure acute diseases. The number of Americans living with chronic health conditions—diabetes, cancer, emphysema, heart disease, muscular dystrophy, spina bifida, AIDS, chronic mental illness, dementia, disabling injuries, alcoholism, blindness, and disabling arthritis— is currently estimated at 35 million (Schroeder, 1993). "Virtually everyone with a chronic illness has the same desire—to live as independently and with as much dignity as possible, with minimum pain, disability, and social stigma. Too much money is spent on services that are inappropriate, while many service needs go unattended" (Schroeder, 1993).

The following problems, for which the elderly and persons with chronic health conditions are especially at risk, are priorities in discharge planning and patient teaching:

• Medications
• Nutrition and hydration
• Unintentional injury
• Mobility and transportation
• Support services needed at home
• When and how to seek appropriate treatment

JCAHO Standards: Mandates for Education of Patients and Families

In 1993, new hospital accreditation standards published by the Joint Commission on the Accreditation of Healthcare Organizations (JCAHO) made patient and family education outcomes a high priority and a focus survey area. Meeting this requirement to achieve accreditation placed heightened emphasis on patient education activities within hospitals and in their relationships with other posthospitalization health care providers.

The JCAHO standards and scoring guidelines for education of patient and family have brought renewed interest, accountability, and leadership for patient education, which has ultimately benefited both nurses and patients. Staff nurses who are committed to the importance of patient education have long struggled to gain recognition for the skill, time, and resources needed to succeed. Patient education often competes with high-technology nursing skills for recognition. JCAHO supports and requires for accreditation an accountability for all health care providers

to show evidence of patient learning outcomes. This provides important reinforcement of nursing's long-standing commitment to teach.

The JCAHO upholds the concept of patient-centered care, with patient and family education viewed as a centerpiece for involving patients as members of the health care team. Patient education is also seen as central to processes for quality management. Health care organizations are expected to show evidence of patient learning outcomes, focus on discharge and continuity of care, and coordinate patient teaching across disciplines. The development of patient-centered care guidelines requires renewed attention to the ways patients and families are educated and innovative approaches to achieve patient outcomes appropriate to the patient's length of stay. Nurses must turn their attention to what the patient and family can "do" rather than what the nurse has "taught."

The JCAHO identifies the goals of patient education (Box 1-1): "to improve patient health outcomes by promoting recovery, speeding return to function, promoting health behavior, and appropriately involving the patient in his or her care decisions" (JCAHO, 1994).

These education standards call for a systematic approach to patient education. Scoring guidelines reflect the expectations that all patients will benefit from appropriate education. The accountability for patient teaching lies within the scope of practice of every nurse. Accountability must also be assumed by nurses in management, staff development, and clinical specialist roles to ensure that staff nurses develop the necessary skills as patient educators. Novice nurses bring enthusiasm and knowledge about patient education to practice, but they look for coaching and modeling to make patient teaching purposeful (Boswell, Pichert, Lorenz, & Schlundt, 1990). Experienced nurses frequently struggle with implementing outdated protocols that are nurse centered and based on outcomes unrealistic for current lengths of stay. Involvement of nurse managers and educators is needed to promote patient education in the following ways:

As outlined in the 1995 JCAHO Standards, patient education should:

- Facilitate the patient and family's understanding of the patient's health status, health care options, and consequences of options selected
- Encourage patient and family participation in the decision-making process about health care options
- Increase the patient and family's potential to follow the therapeutic health care plan
- Maximize patient and family care skills
- Increase the patient and family's ability to cope with the patient's health status and prognosis and outcome
- Enhance the patient and family's role in continuing care
- Promote a healthy patient life-style

JCAHO defines "family" as the person(s) who play a significant role in the patient's life. This includes an individual who may or may not be legally related to the patient (JCAHO, 1994).

- Helping nurses define patient learning outcomes
- Aiding in the identification of critical learning needs and teaching priorities
- Assisting nurses with the evaluation of patient learning outcomes
- Promoting innovative programs that ensure continuity of patient education
- Reflecting the value of patient education in the nursing performance appraisal system

Our suggestions for continuing education that aids skill acquisition in patient education are based on Benner's four stages of development: advanced beginner, competent, proficient, and expert. The JCAHO standards and scoring guidelines and the role of staff development in promoting patient education are more thoroughly discussed in Chapter 2.

Integrating Patient Education in Nursing Practice: Nursing Process Revisited

Nurses' Concerns in Providing Patient Education

As nurse educators, we are aware that a great deal of literature is available on patient education. When we first planned this book, we felt strongly that another how-to approach to patient education was not needed. Instead, our commitment was to examine issues arising in our own practice environments, as well as issues suggested by our colleagues that posed challenges not dealt with by other texts. The first six chapters, dealing with issues, were thus born. Nurses identified pressing concerns that centered around issues of leadership and administrative support for patient education, influencing and understanding patient decisions, effective work with high-risk populations, legal and ethical concerns related to patient education, and motivational theories.

As we designed the remaining chapters, we responded to nurses' questions about the principles of patient education. Nursing faculty also identified specific needs of their students in the implementation of patient education. In summarizing these evaluations we became convinced that the section of our book dealing with principles of patient education, Chapters 6 through 11, was also needed. We discovered that nurses from all types of practice settings were looking for practical guidance in integrating patient education into the nursing process. We found that nurses wanted realistic approaches that consider the pressures of time, extensive patient care responsibilities, and paperwork overloads. Staff nurses find they must possess teaching skills, astutely define patient learning needs, and know how to involve patients' families. In addition, they want reassurance that patient education can be an integral part of patient care. We have attempted throughout the text to offer practical, realistic approaches.

How patient education is actually accomplished does vary from setting to setting. Nurses in outpatient clinics, who have a short time with each patient, find they must teach throughout the encounter, set priorities, and rely on educational materials appropriate for the patient. Nurses in acute care settings, facing shortened lengths of patient stay, are refining skills at setting priorities and realistic goals, making referrals, and evaluating a patient's ability to perform survival skills. They must also be able to evaluate the patient's readiness and ability to learn and incorporate patient education literature (Doak, Doak, & Root, 1995). Nurses in home care are sharing more high-technology care with the family and coordinating community resources in the patient education role. Nurses in long-term care are also relying on their skilled assessments to set priorities and develop meaningful plans of care by valuing the input of patients and families; they use patient education as a way to involve the patient and family in restorative care.

The same process for patient education is used by nurses in all settings and with all types of patients. It is our hope that both students and experienced nurses will find the text helpful by applying the principles of patient education described in the following chapters to daily practice. The principles of patient education are also illustrated by case studies throughout this text to provide practical examples of how to perform various steps of the process. According to Benner, much can be learned from the wisdom of nurses who are expert teachers and coaches. Teaching and coaching are embedded in nursing care and vary based on demands, resources, and constraints of the situation. Yet she cautions us that learning from experts requires attention to the context and avoidance of hasty generalizations (Benner, 1984).

Community assessment and health promotion, the role of patient education in case management, patient education research, and a "roundtable" discussion comprise the remaining chapters of this text, addressing applications beyond individual patients and families.

The Nursing Process Includes Patient Education

Nurses provide patient care through the application of the nursing process, a problem-solving method designed to meet client needs in a systematic way. The process has four steps. First, the nurse gathers information about patient needs and formulates a list of nursing diagnoses. *Nursing diagnoses* are statements of human responses to actual or potential health problems, which the nurse can legally identify and for which the nurse can intervene (Carpenito, 1992). Many nursing diagnoses relate to patient and family learning needs. The nurse focuses on functional problems and daily management. In the second step the nurse develops the plan for patient care, outlining priorities and client goals (both short-term and long-term ones). Specific learning objectives are part of the patient care plan. The third step spells out how the plan will be implemented, outlining specific nursing interventions including patient teaching targeted to meet client goals. Finally, in the fourth step, evaluation provides information about how well goals were met. During the process of evaluation, nursing diagnoses are either resolved or referred for continuing care. Thus, implementing the nursing process entails more than a cognitive, four-step procedure.

Clinical decision-making based on clinical judgments arises from the expert nurse's grasp of qualitative distinctions in individual cases. The nurse must be attuned to each patient situation, with a sense of what is salient and the confidence to set priorities. Clinical judgment is learned through experience: a combination of hands-on care, mentoring, and continuing education with a case study approach. Expert nurses learn to notice patients and families in new ways and adapt agency patient education resources to culture, beliefs, context, and environment (Benner, Tanner, and Chesla, 1992). A faculty member teaching BSN students shared with us one of the difficulties teaching patient education skills in the undergraduate program. "Students see only a small proportion of the hospital episode. They are not prepared to teach patients over the long run." Thus, it is critical that undergraduate education use case study approaches that encourage students to develop critical thinking. Chapters 7 through 11 in this text are dedicated to the nursing process as it is applied to patient education and include case studies that "bring the content to life" for students.

The nurse must recognize significant others, especially the family, who have a direct influence on the client. When patient education is incorporated throughout the nursing process, it is a tool to empower clients, enabling them to assume an active role in their care and providing a safer transition on the day of discharge. The client who can recognize symptoms and ask for help, who can cope effectively with the exacerbations of chronic illness, and who can prevent injury, accident, and illness has an autonomy that will help in negotiating an increasingly complex health care system.

Patient education plans are part of the total plan for patient care and are targeted to priorities for each patient. Patient education begins with early screening on admission to determine what is likely to cause trouble for this patient and to anticipate functional problems rather than with a preset teaching plan for all patients with a common medical diagnosis (e.g., diabetes). It also looks realistically at anticipated length of stay and determines how much to teach and when to teach. For example, nurses report that they must modify standardized teaching plans for diabetic patients when patients' needs vary due to age, complications, experience, presenting problem, and other simultaneous health issues. Thus, patient education cannot be accomplished with a cookbook approach and should not be delegated to inexperienced or unlicensed personnel. Effective patient education requires critical thinking and clinical judgments that allow nurses to plan individualized approaches for patient care.

Patient education is not accomplished by simply tucking a list of instructions or a booklet into the patient's hand or instructing him or her to turn on the television to the "patient education channel." It is a *therapeutic relation-ship* providing an individualized response to patient needs (rather than to a broad medical diagnosis) and bringing in whatever resources are available to meet those needs.

Clinical Judgment, Patient Education, and the Nurse Practitioner

Since the publication of the second edition of *Patient Education: Issues, Principles, and Practices*, the nurse practitioner movement has grown exponentially. Additionally, one of the authors has become a Family Nurse Practitioner and has developed an appreciation for the importance of patient education to primary care providers.

The process of making primary care clinical judgments and performing diagnostic reasoning is similar to the nursing process. The nurse practitioner uses SOAP note recording in much the same way as the staff nurse does. Just as the staff nurse collects subjective and objective data so does the nurse practitioner derive a differential diagnosis based on the subjective and objective findings. Once these data have been reduced to the differential diagnosis, also referred to as assessment in problem-oriented recording, the practitioner is ready to derive a treatment plan. The staff nurse does not generate a differential diagnosis; instead he or she is likely to choose a nursing diagnosis from a taxonomy that best describes the patient's problem. The treatment plan constituted by the nurse practitioner consists of:

Dx: Diagnostic tests and consultation
Rx: Pharmacologic and other therapeutic interventions
Pt Ed: Patient education
F/U: Follow-up

Thus, the nurse practitioner is constantly reminded that patient education is one of the four important parts of the treatment plan that should always be considered and charted. The follow-up portion of the treatment plan is the opportunity for the nurse practitioner to chart how he or she will evaluate the patient's response to treatment, for example, using a telephone call or return visit.

Satisfaction on the part of the public with nurse practitioner care is high (Office of Technology Assessment, 1986). Indeed, double blind comparisons of physician-nurse practitioner practice indicate that management of uncomplicated, primary care problems has the same, if not better, outcomes for nurse practitioners (Mundinger, 1994). One of the reasons cited for public approbation of the nurse practitioner role is the amount of patient teaching performed by nurse practitioners. One physician explained his preference to hire nurse practitioners rather than physician assistants because he is aware of the preparation in patient education that nurses have in their generic educational programs. One nurse practitioner in describing her collaborative practice with a physician at a large, university medical center said:

> We work very well together and we co-manage all of the prenatal patients. She sends the client for her first prenatal visit to me because she knows I will do the physical exam and prenatal work-up as well as all of the necessary teaching related to diet, physical and environmental factors associated with pregnancy, guidelines for management of common problems, and instructions related to subsequent visits. She's more interested in the problems and pathology while I'm more interested in day-to-day management of the prenatal patient.

Certified nurse midwives also bring a nursing background and preparation to advanced clinical practice. Patients frequently state that they chose midwifery services because of excellent patient education and patient empowerment to participate in preventive care, prenatal care, and the delivery experience.

Anticipating Patient Needs and Problems

Knowledge of the nursing process itself is not assurance that nurses are fully prepared to deliver patient education. Nurses must also have knowledge about the health problems faced by their clients and anticipate the needs the client typically exhibits. To be a capable patient teacher, nurses must assess their own learning needs, as well as those of their patients, and find resources to meet them. For example, a community health nurse received the referral of a new client who was discharged from a nearby medical center with a rare diagnosis. She was unfamiliar with the diagnosis, the prognosis, the functional problems typically affecting the patient, and the learning needs of the patient and family. She went to the medical center library and found a recent article from a nursing journal describing the disease, epidemiology, clinical characteristics, medical management, and nursing management. Fortunately, the article also outlined nursing diagnoses applicable to patients with this diagnosis, suggested actions, and reviewed infection control guidelines. This prepared the nurse to make an individual assessment of the patient and family and anticipate their needs and priorities.

Nurses also understand that cultural factors have a profound effect on patient education. Nursing care and the teaching-learning process must consider the cultural diversity of patients and their families (Leininger, 1970). For example, patient education for chronic diseases such as hypertension and diabetes targets life-style changes (dietary habits and daily activities) related to cultural patterns and traditions. Nurses recognize the need to learn about religions and cultures and the need to incorporate cultural assessment in the process of patient teaching. To design effective patient teaching interventions, nurses need information about how to work with clients from culturally diverse backgrounds. Providing culturally relevant nursing care (Andrews & Boyle, 1995) requires that the nurse use transcultural concepts in the application of the nursing process, including identifying cultural needs, understanding the cultural context of patient and family, using culturally sensitive nursing strategies to meet mutual goals, using resources from a variety of cultural subsystems in the community, and learning from and responding to culturally diverse situations. Chapter 4 addresses special challenges involved in teaching patients from a different ethnocultural group.

Interdisciplinary Collaboration for Patient Education

The importance of interdisciplinary involvement by the total health care team is central to effective patient care. Yet lack of good communication between disciplines often leads individuals to feel they are not valued as patient teachers. Lack of communication can lead to battles over "turf" and inability to collaborate, both one-on-one and in team conferences.

Understanding the contributions that other health care professionals can make to patient teaching increases the effectiveness of patient education and improves attempts to develop collegiality and collaboration of the health care team.

We have found that members of other health care professions tend to be as involved as nurses in patient teaching, particularly those who are recent graduates and those who actively pursue their own continuing education. However, we have often heard nurses generalize that because they have received opposition or lack of cooperation in the past, most physicians, for example, are not supportive of patient education. Such assumptions thwart collaboration and the delivery of patient education. During the last three decades, the emphasis of nursing education and practice has reflected an expanded focus for interdisciplinary patient teaching efforts. Furthermore, because of nursing's continuous and visible presence at the patient's side, nurses are in the unique position to provide leadership for patient education and to capitalize on the strengths of each discipline for the patient's ultimate benefit. The need to coordinate teaching efforts is especially critical for patients who are acutely ill and unable to absorb ambitious teaching activities. Nursing involvement is key to ensuring effective patient education with appropriate learning outcomes in mind to empower rather than overcome the patient.

Case management involves leadership from a nurse or other health professional to oversee the process of providing care, with the goal of improving efficiency, increasing effectiveness of interventions, and containing costs. Critical paths, care maps, and other case management tools incorporate patient and family education consistently across the plan of care. This plan for patient learning involves the input of the health care team and a focus on patient learning outcomes. When nurses assume the role of case manager or care coordinator, they must be especially committed to interdisciplinary planning and team building. Chapter 13 addresses in greater detail how patient education is provided in the context of case management.

Staff development and continuing education targeted to helping health care professionals increase skills in patient education must also address the health care team approach. This is accomplished most effectively when members of the health care team engage in the learning experience together. Chapter 2 explores the role of staff development in patient education and offers suggestions for organizing such continuing education programs.

Nurses gain valuable insights that promote the work of the health care team by talking with other health care professionals who are interested in patient teaching. We have initiated such conversations with physicians, dietitians, physical therapists, pharmacists, and hospital social workers. We asked them to tell us how they see their patient teaching roles and how they perceive the nurse's role. Each suggested ways to increase collaboration. These "interviews" were also an opportunity to teach other health care professionals about the nurse's involvement in patient education and generate ideas for new teaching programs. Some comments from these interviews are given in the Table 1-1.

TABLE 1–1. Comments on Patient Education From Health Care Professionals

Physicians	Dietitians	Physical Therapists	Pharmacists	Hospital Social Workers
What is your involvement in patient education?				
"I teach patients one-on-one. I try to tell them what they want and need to know in language they understand. I want them to understand and agree with the treatment plan, to know what the goals are, and to participate in decision-making." "I try to incorporate patient education into my inter-action with the patient. I think you need to be consciously aware of patient education, and you have to have a good feeling that your patients are understanding and doing what you, together, agree is appropriate. I think we assume more than we should."	"We educate patients about the diets they need to follow at home. We try to find out what the patient usually eats and how we need to modify this. Sometimes we have to discuss the diet with the doctor because what he orders is inappropriate. We make the necessary changes and teach the patient."	"We inform patients about their disease, about what to expect, and about any procedures that are done. We teach them about ambulation, functional activities, and safety, especially postsurgically. Physical therapists have a large role in educating patients about rheumatic diseases and how to deal with and prevent flare-ups. We also teach patients about prostheses and help patients with them."	"The pharmacist is often the first person to see patients when they have problems. When patients ask for advice, the pharmacist must know if a referral to other health care providers is needed. The pharmacist also has to teach about how a drug works in the body. If the patient knows the reason for taking the drug, he's more likely to take it as he should. A lot of patients know nothing about their medication. They don't know what it is or how to store it. Some times they don't even take it, depending on how they feel. This is especially true for hypertensive patients."	"Our biggest role is as a hospital, staff, and community liaison. If the patient cannot take care of himself when he leaves the hospital, we talk with the patient, doctor, and family about agencies or resources that can help and coordinate the plans. Many families have problems before they even come into the hospital. We help with these too. We give emotional support and answer questions about things patients are really afraid of. Patients tend to tell things to social workers that they are embarrassed to tell doctors and nurses."
How do you see the nurse's role in patient education?				
"I see it as necessary and important. Nurses have a different perspective from mine. The doctor teaches about diagnosis and prognosis; the nurse teaches daily management. There is combined strength. Patients tend to confide different information to nurses. For example, patients are more open about fear of cancer with the nurse, and talk with me about stomach pain. Nurses clarify and	"Nurses reinforce what the dietitian tells the patient and emphasize the importance of following the diet plan. Nurses let us know what is going on with the patient, and this helps us to evaluate whether the patient understands the diet plan. Nurses also teach medications, treatments, and basic survival skills. They explain what the doctor has said to the	"The role of the nurse is educating and orienting the patient about the disease and reinforcing the teaching of other health care personnel. Nurses give patients emotional support, teach them about activities of daily living, and give general instructions about medications. Nurses reinforce precautions in transfer and positioning. This is extremely	"All patients have a right to know what medications they are taking, how much, and why. Nurses can teach this when they administer medications. There are so many new drugs. For nurses to teach patients, we need to collaborate. The nurse can reinforce the teaching done by the team and communicate with other team members to meet the patient's learning needs.	"The nurses do a tremendous amount of patient teaching, especially with surgical patients. They answer questions patients never ask their doctors. I get my best referrals from nurses. There's something about hanging an IV bag, giving a shot, washing hair, giving a bath—patients tell things to nurses at these times. Some nurses are very aware of the situation a patient is going home to

"and they involve us when we are better able to handle certain kinds of crises."

Nurses have a big job to do, and patients expect a lot of them."

"Nurses need to know where their limits are. The patient needs follow-up after discharge to learn and to reinforce teaching. Social workers can help by making referrals that go beyond discharge, but we have to work together and focus less narrowly on rescuing."

"Good notes in the patient record are very important. I read all the notes, especially the patient's response to the nurses. Details help me assist the family in planning for discharge, such as whether the patient is incontinent or nonambulatory. Notes from the health care team validate what I see. Patient care rounds are also a good opportunity to collaborate."

patient after the doctor leaves."

important. They can help to motivate the patient and coordinate pain medications with the treatments."

"Nurses make valuable assessments about the patient and family and what their supports are like. The nursing assessment should be shared more, especially in the progress notes."

"There should be continuing education for health care professionals. Pharmacists could teach nurses about new drugs coming out, making nurses better able to teach patients. Pharmacists should be more open to nurses' questions and encourage their calls."

What increases your collaboration with the nurse and other members of the health care team in patient education?

"We should acknowledge that we have the same goal: getting the patient ready to handle discharge. We should plan teaching together and construct teaching programs where we reinforce teaching and give emotional support from admission to discharge."

"Nursing shifts change frequently. Therefore, we often have no consistency and have little interaction. Frequent team meetings and good verbal and written communication would increase collaboration in patient education. This would promote mutual respect among the disciplines, cooperation, and knowing how to use other's expertise in different cases."

"We need planning meetings. We need to know what other people are teaching the patient. The patient should not have to hear things over and over, in different ways. Protocols for teaching help. You know what other people are teaching, although you don't always know at what level the patient is understanding."

"Documentation! The nurse's assessment of the patient's readiness to learn is especially helpful. For team work, people must go out of their way to communicate with one another."

reinforce what I teach. Nurses teach patients and families, especially in dealing with chronic diseases."

"Patient education is often left to the nurse. Yet, nurses often lack confidence in their ability to teach."

"Personal knowledge and trust. Having time to get to know other members of the health care team. Asking the patient who is teaching him. The patient is really the center of the team and can help me work with the team. Writing and reading interdisciplinary progress notes is extremely important. One of the most crucial things you do for the patient is document how you educate him."

"The most important thing is discussion. There has to be a desire on all parts. People can find the time to do it. Take a half hour to discuss a difficult patient and bring in everyone who is involved in the care. You formulate an approach and cross-educate one another. It optimizes patient care for that particular patient, but it also teaches people how to deal with difficult patients."

A Health Care Team Approach

Although those health care team members we interviewed stressed the importance of protocols and organization (such as the development of critical pathways and teaching protocols), they frequently stated that attitudes and skills of individuals directly influenced the success of teamwork in patient education. They emphasized the following criteria for successful teamwork:

- Communication (verbal and written), facilitated by planning meetings, care conferences, telephone consultation, good documentation, and "the willingness to go out of our way to communicate with one another"
- Mutual respect among disciplines, recognizing respective areas of expertise, knowing one's limits, and teaching each other
- Desire to work as a team and recognition of a common goal.

Summary

The profession of nursing has embraced the role of patient education as central to the nursing process and as a dimension of nurse caring. During the past three decades, changing needs and mandates have increased the visibility, involvement, and expertise of nurses as patient teachers. We have described informed consent, discharge planning, the prevalence of chronic health problems, and patient compliance as issues that require nursing's leadership in patient education. Mandates from JCAHO, debate about the need to reform health care delivery, the emergence of managed care, and the growth of the nurse practitioner movement are also addressed as they relate to patient education.

Clearly, every nurse, regardless of title, setting, or specialty, is called on to provide patients and families with an opportunity to learn in their health care encounters. Patient education reduces feelings of helplessness, empowers patients, and promotes continuity of care.

In providing care that is truly patient centered, nurses acknowledge that the key is to merge into a health care team approach. Nurses must reflect on their roles and the roles of others, and the respective strengths that each brings to patient care. Patient education is built on the foundations of respecting one another, caring, and communicating, not just between the nurse and patient and family, but among all members of the health care team.

Strategies for Critical Analysis and Application

1. Review the seven objectives of patient and family education as stated by JCAHO. Provide examples of how the nurse might meet these objectives when caring for a patient and family.

2. Identify a patient, friend, or family member who has a chronic health problem. Ask this individual to describe what knowledge and skills are needed to care for himself or herself. What resources has this person found helpful for learning to manage care?

3. Interview members of other health care disciplines about their involvement in patient education. Then summarize what you learn and discuss how nurses and other health professionals might promote teamwork in providing patient education. You might pose the following questions to physicians, dietitians, occupational and physical therapists, pharmacists, dentists, and hospital social workers:

   - How are you involved in patient education?

   - How do you see the nurse's role in patient education?

   - How does your role interface with the nurse's role?

   - How can members of the health care team increase their collaboration in patient education?

REFERENCES

American Hospital Association. (1975). *A patient's bill of rights*. Chicago: Author.

American Hospital Association. (1984). *Guidelines for discharge planning*. Chicago: Author.

American Nurses Association. (1975). *The professional nurse and health education*. Kansas City, MO: Author.

American Nurses Association. (1979). *Model nurse practice act*. Kansas City, MO: Author.

American Nurses Association. (1991). *Nursing's agenda for health care reform*. Washington, DC: Author.

Andrews, M., & Boyle, J. (1995). *Transcultural concepts in nursing care*. Philadelphia: J. B. Lippincott.

Benner, P. (1982). From novice to expert. *American Journal of Nursing, 82,* 402-407.

Benner, P. (1984). *From novice to expert*. Menlo Park, CA: Addison-Wesley.

Benner, C., Tanner, C., & Chesla, C. (1992). *From beginner to expert: Clinical knowledge in critical care nursing* [Video]. Athens, OH: Fuld Institute for Technology in Nursing Education.

Benner, P., & Wrubel, J. (1989). *The primacy of caring: Stress and coping in health and illness*. Menlo Park, CA: Addison-Wesley.

Boswell, E., Pichert, J., Lorenz, R., & Schlundt, D. (1993). Training health care professionals to enhance their patient teaching skills. *Journal of Nursing Staff Development, 6(5),* 233–239.

Carpenito, L. (1992). *Nursing diagnosis: Application to clinical practice* (4th ed.). Philadelphia: J. B. Lippincott.

Doak, C., Doak, L., & Root J. (1995). *Teaching patients with low literacy skills* (2nd ed.). Philadelphia: J. B. Lippincott.

Henderson, V., & Nite, G. (1960). *Principles and practice of nursing*. New York: MacMillan.

Hochbaum, G. (1980). Patient counseling versus patient teaching. *Topics in Clinical Nursing, 2,* 1-8.

Joint Commission on the Accreditation of Healthcare Organizations. (1993, 1994). Education of the patient: Standards and scoring guidelines. In *1995 comprehensive accreditation manual for hospitals* (pp. 190-206). Chicago: Author.

Leininger, M. (1970). *Nursing and anthropology: Two worlds to blend*. New York: John Wiley & Sons.

Malloy, C., & Hartshorn, J. (1989). *Acute care nursing in the home*. Philadelphia: J. B. Lippincott.

Mundinger, M. (1994). Sounding board: advanced-practice nursing—good medicine for physicians? *New England Journal of Medicine, 330,* 211-214.

National League for Nursing Education. (1918). *Standard curriculum for schools of nursing*. Baltimore: Waverly Press.

Nightingale, F. (1860/1992). *Notes on nursing: What it is and what it is not*. Philadelphia: J. B. Lippincott.

Office of Technology Assessment. (1986). *Nurse practitioners, physicians assistants, and certified nurse-midwives: A policy analysis*. Washington, DC: U.S. Government Printing Office (Health Technology Case Study #37-OTA-HCS-37).

Rankin, S., & Stallings, K. (1990). *Patient education: Issues, principles, and practices* (2nd ed.). Philadelphia: J. B. Lippincott.

Redman, B. (1993a). Patient education at 25 years; where have we been and where are we going? *Journal of Advanced Nursing, 18,* 725-730.

Redman, B. (1993b). *The process of patient education* (7th ed.). St. Louis: Mosby-Year Book.

Redman, B., & Braun, R. (1991). Courses in patient education in masters programs in nursing. *Journal of Nursing Education, 30,* 42-43.

Regan, W. (1975). The patient's right to know. *Regan Report of Nursing Law, 16,* 1.

Rivo, M. (1994). *Update: Division of Medicine, Winter 1994*. Washington, DC: U.S. Department of Health and Human Services, Health Resources and Services Administration, Bureau of Health Professions.

Schroeder, S.A. (1993). Chronic health conditions. *Annual Report 1993*. Princeton, NJ: The Robert Wood Johnson Foundation.

Tanner, C., Benner, P., Chesla, C., & Gordon, D. (1993). The phenomenology of knowing the patient. *Image - The Journal of Nursing Scholarship, 25,* 273-280.

U.S. Department of Health and Human Services. (1990). *Healthy people 2000*. Washington, DC: Author.

U.S. Department of Health and Human Services. (1994). *Update: Healthy People 2000*. June–July, 1994. Washington, DC: Author.

Vestal, K. (1995). *Nursing management concepts and issues* (2nd ed.). Philadelphia: J. B. Lippincott.

Wolf, Z., Giardino, E., Osborne, P., & Ambrose, M. (1994). Dimensions of nurse caring. *Image - The Journal of Nursing Scholarship, 26(2),* 107-112.

CHAPTER

2

The Role of Staff Development in Patient Education: Meeting JCAHO Standards and Beyond

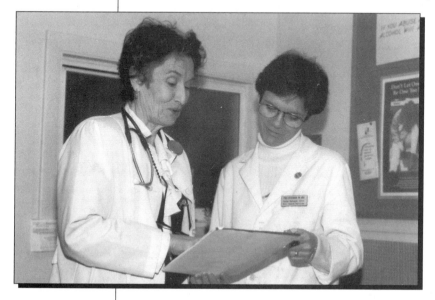

OBJECTIVES FOR CHAPTER 2

After reading this chapter, the nurse or student nurse should be able to:

1 Discuss the potential role for staff development in planning organizational approaches to patient education in light of JCAHO standards.

2 Outline the four key JCAHO standards for patient and family education, the corresponding teaching targets, and examples of patient learning outcomes that should be documented.

3 Describe continuing education needs of staff to fulfill JCAHO standards.

4 Identify four barriers perceived by staff nurses in the provision of patient education.

5 Provide examples of educational and institutional support to promote patient education expertise for nurses identified in Benner's four stages of skill acquisition: advanced beginner, competent, proficient, and expert.

JCAHO's Focus on Patient and Family Education: Implications for Staff Development

Standards for patient and family education developed by the Joint Commission on the Accreditation of Hospitals (JCAHO) made patient learning outcomes a special focus in survey visits beginning in 1993. To achieve JCAHO accreditation, health care organizations must show evidence that all patients receive teaching and that health care providers can demonstrate patient learning. In addition to individualized teaching, there must be an organization-wide patient and family education focus and evidence of the direct impact of education on the patient and family (JCAHO, 1994).

These standards have placed renewed emphasis on the need for all nurses to provide education to all patients as an integral part of care. In addition, they call for coordinated interdisciplinary approaches. Many staff development specialists with whom we are familiar have been challenged to develop the staff, through continuing education, to be skilled as patient teachers and to demonstrate patient learning outcomes.

One of the purposes of this chapter is to review JCAHO Standards and Scoring Guidelines for Patient and Family Education and to consider how staff development can provide support and leadership in achieving successful JCAHO accreditation surveys. We will review key elements of individual and organization-wide teaching and address the valuable leadership provided by staff development to promote patient education within an organization. Also offered in this chapter is the plan for a full-day workshop for nurses and interested members of other disciplines addressing patient-centered approaches to patient education. Complete with objectives, agenda, content outline, and teaching methodologies, the workshop plan illustrates how the content in Chapters 7 through 11 of the text can be incorporated in a continuing education offering.

The chapter also examines how nurses develop clinical expertise in patient teaching,

based on the work of Benner (1984) and Benner and her colleagues (Benner & Tanner, 1987; Benner, Tanner, & Chesla, 1992). This discussion will help the reader to discover answers to pressing issues and questions posed by staff development and continuing education professionals around the following topics:

- How to motivate staff nurses to teach
- How to best use the roles of clinical nurse specialist and patient education specialist within an organization
- How to promote the recognition and charting of patient learning outcomes
- How to streamline outdated teaching protocols
- How to promote a health care team approach
- How to determine what types of education and training are needed for staff

A Need for Innovation

From our experience as health care professionals as well as patients, most of us recognize that innovation is needed for the ways patients are currently taught to participate in their care. There are several reasons for this pressing need. The most obvious explanation is that rapidly changing models of health care delivery are characterized by short hospital stays and care provided across multiple settings. Most patient education programs developed during the past decade are outdated due to lengths of stays that do not accommodate ambitious learning activities. In fact, teaching programs often become outdated within a year of their creation. Continuing education and coaching, which helps staff revise teaching to focus on survival skills and patient outcomes, is often neglected. Staff become frustrated with the difficulty of trying to teach too much in too short a time, and do not know how to go about streamlining teaching. To accommodate patients' need to learn how to manage their care in a limited time, hospitals must refine existing patient education programs and devise teaching interventions that reach homes and outpatient clinics. A strong component of education has become a necessity in all clinical services (Wasson & Anderson, 1994). Patient education has become an integral component of case management efforts, and critical pathways and existing programs must be revised to coincide with carefully tracked outcomes. Chapter 13 provides guidance in dealing with patient education issues as they relate to case management.

Depending on their educational preparation and practice experiences, individual health care professionals may assign different priorities to the various facets of patient education. For example, graduates of nursing schools in the 1970s were taught that an anatomy and physiology lesson was the way that patient education always begins and that informed consent is a primary aim. In the 1980s, basic nursing education stressed discharge planning for high-risk patients but offered less emphasis on individualized teaching for low-risk patients. Nurses who have had the advantage of education in the 1990s, as well as nurses who have assumed new roles as case managers, have a heightened awareness of the need to streamline teaching in favor of survival skills. From their colleagues who were taught to teach patients only for informed consent, these nurses may encounter resistance to redesigning teaching programs with less anatomy and more problem-solving skills.

In every practice setting, we discover a community of professionals reflecting a variety of preparation and approaches. This often causes them to disagree on priorities for patient teaching and on how to provide teaching interventions (Lipetz, Bussiget, & Risley, 1990). Many are attempting to follow patient education programs and standards developed in the 1970s based on drastically different lengths of hospital stay. Many nurses have practiced at a time when all patient teaching for specific health problems (diabetes, cardiac, prenatal) was delegated to a patient education specialist. They may not accept that their role includes teaching and may have had no formal training in how to teach. In addition, few health care professionals have benefited from continuing education oppor-

tunities aimed at developing interdisciplinary approaches. Continuing education provides an avenue for bringing together practitioners with differing perspectives and centralizing efforts to provide innovative new approaches to patient education.

The Challenges for Staff Development

Staff development is defined as employer-sponsored professional development activities aimed at expanding and improving competencies of health care professionals (Kelly, 1992). These activities can help to bridge the gaps between education and practice in the following ways:

- Formal, ongoing, and immediate training related to responsibilities in the work setting, for example, knowledge of JCAHO standards
- Socialization into the work setting to increase competence and excellence, for example, coaching, feedback, and mentoring for staff by patient education experts
- Emphasis on improvement of group performance in the work setting to achieve quality and excellence, for example, making patient education programs visible and valued

Staff development relates to patient education in many critical ways to bridge gaps between education and practice and to improve the competencies of health care professionals to provide patient teaching in a rapidly changing health care delivery system. Examples of the powerful role staff development activities can play include:

- Providing leadership, oversight, or coordination of organization-wide approaches to patient education
- Providing formal, ongoing, and immediate training about JCAHO Standards and Scoring Guidelines for Patient and Family Education
- Teaching managers, supervisors, staff nurses, and other providers how to meet the standards and show evidence of patient learning

- Helping the organization to develop specialized patient education programs and educational interventions that are realistic for the patient's length of stay, interdisciplinary in their approach, and focused on patient survival skills
- Identifying barriers that nurses and other providers perceive in the delivery of patient education and designing strategies in partnership with agency management to break down the barriers
- Raising awareness of the need for new, innovative approaches to patient education based on the patient's needs, as opposed to the provider's determination for achieving compliance. These new models for patient teaching span both inpatient and outpatient settings and involve patients in prioritizing learning needs along a continuum of care.

In summary, organizations cannot afford for staff development to stand on the sidelines of patient education efforts. In the context of JCAHO standards, this chapter outlines the developmental needs of an organization and its staff relative to patient education and offers suggestions for staff development interventions.

JCAHO Standards for Patient Education

In 1993, stimulus for innovation in patient education came to hospitals in the form of new JCAHO standards and focus surveys addressing patient teaching and discharge planning. The new standards prompted administrators to look at organization-wide approaches and individual patient experiences and ask the question "What's wrong with our patient education?" The total organization was forced to acknowledge the priority of educating patients, the ways education is delivered, and the resources allocated to patient and family education. "How do we currently teach patients?" and "Where do we document it?" were asked in every department. The planned process for patient educa-

tion was often lacking structure, function, goals, objectives, and most important, the tracking of outcomes. As members of the management team, staff development professionals have valuable skills needed by the organization to interpret an overall approach and to ensure that quality patient education services are provided.

Table 2-1 outlines the JCAHO 1995 standards related to goals, objectives, and applications of a patient education program in the organization. Staff developers will find this table useful in teaching managers and staff about JCAHO's expectations for patient and family outcomes. This underscores that evaluation of patient education must provide evidence that the organization assesses the need for focused programs and allocates resources to accomplish them. The most important resource is staff who have the skills, interest, and time to teach. The JCAHO education standards address that a systematic approach to education should be demonstrated throughout the organization, but JCAHO does not describe specific structures or titles of personnel. The organization is encouraged to focus on its current processes and how continuity of care can be best accomplished.

The JCAHO standards address patient-focused care, including organizational approaches and individualized patient and family activities. Comparing patient and family activities to the organization's goals is a key component of quality performance (JCAHO, 1994). Four standards that relate to specific educational needs of patients and families are defined with "targets" or outcomes for patient-centered interventions (Table 2-2).

Implementing an Organization-wide Approach

Implementation is the act of fulfilling or accomplishing. Before the process of patient education is completed, a number of steps that we refer to as the *implementation process* must be accomplished. An example of an orderly process for implementing patient education follows, along with a discussion of the issues

TABLE 2-1. Organizational Approach to Patient Education

Goal of patient/family education:	Organizational approach: impact areas
To improve patient health outcomes by promoting recovery, speeding return to function, promoting healthy behavior, and appropriately involving the patient in his or her care decisions.	1. Organization's focus on education 2. Direct impact of education on the patient and family 3. Evaluation of the program of patient and family education relative to goal achievement
Education should:	**Practical application**
• facilitate patient's (family's) understanding of patient's health status, health care options, and consequences of options selected • encourage patient (family) participation in the decision-making process about health care options • increase patient's (family's) potential to follow the therapeutic health care plan • maximize patient (family) care skills • increase patient's (family's) ability to cope with the patient's health status/prognosis/outcome • enhance patient's (family's) role in continuing care • promote a healthy patient life-style	1. Assess organization-wide patient and family education programs and activities. 2. Organization establishes goals of patient and family education program. 3. Organization allocates resources for patient and family education. 4. Determine specific educational needs of patient and family. 5. Prioritize and sequence educational needs. 6. Present information to patient/family and determine appropriate follow-up. 7. Evaluate whether needs met. 8. Compare patient and family activities to organizational goals for quality improvement.

Adapted from *1995 Comprehensive Accreditation Manual for Hospitals*. Chicago: JCAHO.

confronted during implementation. The organization must assign responsibility for overseeing or directing the implementation of patient education. This responsible party may be a "patient education coordinator" or a director of a department such as education or clinical services. We refer to this individual as the "coordinator" although we recognize that responsibility for patient education activities is shared throughout an organization and across disciplines. We are familiar with many staff development directors who have been assigned responsibilities as "coordinator" of the organization-wide approach.

Although we have instituted individual patient education programs to meet the needs of particular client groups, we do not recommend this single-shot approach to implementing patient education at the organization level. This approach tends to be hurried and crisis motivated, in that staff efforts are directed toward assuaging the needs of the most obviously needy group. Instead, we suggest using the approach validated by JCAHO: conducting a systematic patient education needs assessment.

Conducting a Needs Assessment for the Organization

A needs assessment requires about 6 months to complete, but it is the cornerstone for planning and implementing patient education. Such a needs assessment will allow for long-range planning and direction, so that continuity of program planning is ensured, independent of changes in leadership or personnel.

The American Hospital Association developed a comprehensive "Institutional Assessment Guide," published in 1979, that is useful for assessing various aspects of the hospital environment to implement a comprehensive patient education program (American Hospital Association, 1979). The guide can also be modified for use in assessing out-

TABLE 2-2. JCAHO Standards for Patient/Family Education

Standard	Targets	Evidence*
Standard PF.1 Patient and family provided with appropriate education and training to increase knowledge of illness and treatment needs, and skills/behaviors to promote recovery and improve function.	• Patient and family understanding of current health problem and reason for admission • Patient informed consent re: treatment • Patient and family understanding of treatment plan and the role they will play • Overview of survival skills needed for safe discharge	• All patients receive instruction. • Priorities for education are identified by the organization.
Standard PF.2 Patient and family receive education specific to patient's assessed needs, abilities, readiness, and appropriate to length of stay.	• Safe and effective use of medications • Medical equipment • Potential drug-food interactions, modified diets • Rehab techniques • Community resources • How to obtain further treatment • Ongoing health care needs	• Patient assessment • Information understandable to patient • Teaching is culturally appropriate.
Standard PF.3 Any discharge instructions given to the patient and family are provided to the organization responsible for patient's continuing care.	• Written discharge instructions, understandable to patient, include targets for PF.2. • Continuing care provider identified • Instructions provided to continuing care providers	• Discharge planning involves patient and family. • Discharge instructions clear: who is to do what
Standard PF.4 The organization plans and supports the provision and coordination of patient and family education activities and resources.	• Classes • Community resources access • Closed circuit TV • Multimedia library • Patient education materials data base • One-on-one presentations • Interdisciplinary educational process	• Provision and coordination of patient education activities and resources • Resources selected based on patient needs • Health care team involvement • Educational formats based on specific needs

Adapted from *1995 Comprehensive Accreditation Manual for Hospitals*. Chicago: JCAHO.
*Policies and procedures, progress notes, flowsheets, referral and consultation notes, interviews with staff, written information given to patients and families.

patient educational needs. The assessment guide is in chart format and suggests assessment tasks and questions as well as sources and methods of data collection in answer to the questions. The guide is divided into 10 areas. Box 2-1 lists the 10 targeted areas, types of questions asked in each area, and suggested sources of data.

Appointing a Steering or Advisory Committee

A patient education steering committee should be appointed early in the implementation process. The steering committee acts in an advisory fashion and should include physicians, nurses, members of other health

BOX 2–1. Areas of Institutional Review

1. Hospital philosophy, goals, and policies

What is the philosophy of the hospital and what are the goals for patient care? Do these goals require the implementation of patient education? The sources of information include documents that can be obtained from administrators or the board of trustees.

2. Organization of the hospital staff

What types of staff are employed?

3. Patient care support staff

Who is responsible for orientation of all new hospital patient care staff? Data pertaining to this question can be obtained by contacting department heads or sending them a questionnaire.

4. Characteristics of the patient population

What are the most common diagnoses, diagnosis-related groups (DRGs), and surgical procedures for the various hospital units? Answers to this question can be procured from the admitting office and their computerized data banks as well as from medical records. Interviews of various nursing and medical personnel may also be helpful. What are the "high risk" or "high volume" diagnoses, patient groups, or product lines that are commonly identified by staff in various departments? For example, due to discharge of newly delivered prenatal patients less that 48 hours after admission, this population may be targeted as high risk.

5. Patient admission

What information is made available to patients *before* admission to inpatient services, short-stay surgery, or outpatient services? Answers to this question should be obtained from a number of sources. Interviews can be conducted or questionnaires can be sent to admitting and short-stay surgery as well as outpatient services. Additionally, the public relations department, admitting staff physicians, and community referral agencies should be contacted.

6. Patient care process

How are patient care goals determined and revised? Do the medical, nursing, dietary, and other staff groups use a team planning method to assist in determining goals? Are patients included in the goal planning process? Answers to these questions can be acquired by interviewing head nurses and other unit managers involved in patient care services. Consider mailing questionnaires to patients who have been recently discharged.

7. Staff perceptions of current and needed patient education programs

What patient education programs or activities are currently being implemented? Are they conducted on each shift? What resources in terms of audiovisual, printed, and other media are being used in these efforts? Interview or send questionnaires to head nurses, appropriate department heads, and supervisors who may be involved with patient teaching.

8. Adequacy of existing patient education programs for specific populations

Are there written goals and objectives for each patient education activity and are they evaluated after the patient completes the activity? Answers to these questions should be obtained for all programs or activities presently being conducted in the institution. Sources of information include extensive interviews with the staff responsible for the programs, review of written program materials, and participation in a program.

(continued)

BOX 2–1. *(Continued)*

9. Patient education resources within the hospital

What types of media are available within the hospital for patient teaching? What types of appropriations have been made for the purchase of audiovisual media, closed circuit television, and software? Where are patient education materials located, catalogued, and reviewed? Do staff use the materials? Are materials up to date? The questions can be answered by contacting department managers and hospital administrators and by talking with staff on the units. Chapter 9 in this text offers information about the many types of educational media that can be used to enhance patient learning and how they can be developed and evaluated.

10. Patient education resources in the community

Which community patient care agencies provide follow-up care on discharge from the hospital? How do they interpret their role in patient education? Is there a feedback mechanism between the community agency and the hospital? Answers to these questions can be obtained by contacting the community agencies that have been identified by staff as being involved in follow-up care. The discharge planning nurse or social worker should also be contacted. The needs assessment does not have to be conducted in a vacuum; other patient education activities can be taking place while the needs assessment data is being gathered.

care disciplines, administrators, and others having an active interest in patient education. A patient education coordinator, hospital education director, or clinical specialist is usually the person responsible for initiating the committee and should judiciously gather recommendations for committee members. Appointment of physicians should be made by the medical staff although the coordinator can attempt to have physicians appointed who are known proponents of patient education. Nurses at the decision-making level should be appointed to the steering committee with the input of the nursing service coordinator. The historical involvement of such health professionals as dietitians, pharmacists, and physical therapists makes their membership valued in many institutions. Efforts should be made to include other health professionals because their cooperation can enhance patient education programs.

After the assessment guide has been completed, the patient coordinator will have a data base that will aid the advisory committee in organizing and directing the organization's efforts. While the needs assessment is being conducted and the advisory committee is being appointed, the committee coordinator should review the literature to discover what

types of programs have worked, why they have been successful, and where they have been located. We can gather a great deal of information from the successes and mistakes of others, and it is limiting to ignore the ever-increasing quantity of material about diverse patient education programs. This is also a propitious time to make contacts with patient education efforts in other community and inpatient settings. These individuals will be able to share ideas about the needs of the community, as well as help prevent a duplication of efforts.

Establishing Goals and Priorities

Once the patient education needs assessment is completed, it is time to set goals and priorities for the development of programs. The advisory committee should be aware of the importance of wisely choosing the first specific patient education programs to be implemented. Especially when attempting to forge new alliances in interdisciplinary patient education programs, it is helpful to focus the coordinator's attention and the organization's resources on one or two major start-up programs at a time.

Creating Task Forces for Specific Programs

After priorities and goals have been established, a task force willing and able to establish a specific patient education program should be appointed (Marchiondo & Kipp, 1987). If, for example, the highest priority is to establish or institute a new education program for patients with chronic obstructive pulmonary disease (COPD), then the committee should consist of health professionals involved in caring for COPD patients in all departments of the organization. It is essential that a physician be a member of this committee because approval must be gained from the medical staff to implement the teaching program. It should be recognized, however, that including physicians on such task forces does not always guarantee wide medical staff approval. It is also essential that providers who care for patients in the community (doctor's office and home health) be included in planning the program so that it will promote continuity of care.

Evaluating the Program

Evaluation of patient education programs presents some of the most difficult problems encountered in the entire patient teaching venture. Chapter 11 provides a lengthy discussion of the many aspects and issues associated with the evaluation of patient learning. We believe that evaluation should be an integral part of program planning. A means of evaluation should be built into the original program design. The inclusion of a design for evaluation in any proposal for funding will make health care administrators more likely to approve the proposed program. Evaluation frequently occurs after a program has been operational for a while. This type of evaluation procedure should augment a formative evaluation procedure which aids refinement of the educational interventions.

Outcomes To Be Evaluated

When the program is being formulated, it is important to decide which outcomes are to be evaluated. There are many different outcomes and it is impossible, if not inappropriate, to evaluate all of them.

As discussed in Chapter 1, many of the more traditional nurses and physicians view the outcome of patient education in terms of desired *patient compliance*. Although it is true that compliance is desirable, many other positive outcomes can accrue as a result of patient education. Therefore, one of the issues in evaluation becomes how to decide which outcome should be evaluated and whether this outcome indicates that the program is, indeed, beneficial.

The desired outcome must be related to the type of intervention. For example, the desired outcome of educating a group of 13-year-olds on the relationship of cigarette smoking to cardiovascular disease and lung cancer is *prevention* of smoking. The desired effect of such education with a group of the teenagers' smoking parents, however, is *cessation* of smoking.

As more research is done on the relationship of *knowledge acquisition* to behavioral change, we realize that acquisition of knowledge does not always guarantee the desired change. When we apply this to our group of cigarette-smoking parents, we may decide that a more realistic immediate outcome is simply knowledge about the effects of smoking. Perhaps later a behavioral change (cessation of smoking) will occur; this may or may not be related to the knowledge acquisition. In any case, an argument can be made for improving and increasing the patient's knowledge and understanding of his health status even if it does not lead to improved adherence to and cooperation with the medical regimen. Increasing the patient's understanding of his health can be interpreted as part of the patient's legal right to know. We believe he deserves the information even if he does not choose to act on it.

Other outcomes defined as important by JCAHO, and summarized in Table 2-1, are patient participation in decision-making about health care options, the increased potential to follow the health care plan, the development of self-care skills, increased patient and family coping, enhanced participation in continuing care, and healthy life-style.

Evaluating the costs of patient education is imperative. Hospital administrators must calculate staff time, materials, and education equipment as part of the cost of care. In many cases, well-planned and executed education can be shown to decrease length of stay and costs of hospitalization. This can be used to justify the professional staff time needed to accomplish teaching before discharge. This information can also be used to determine the efficacy of specialized outpatient teaching programs versus inpatient teaching.

Staffing for Patient Education

Perhaps the thorniest issue around implementation, involving types of staffing for patient education, must be faced straightforwardly. It does require more RN hours to accomplish high-quality patient education. Most LPNs have not been taught the fundamentals of patient teaching during their educational programs nor is teaching defined as being within their scope of practice. A hospital heavily staffed with LPNs and aides will not be able to deliver as much high-quality patient education as will the larger or more professionally staffed institution. We found LPNs involved in prenatal education in an outpatient setting to be willing and enthusiastic about attending classes but unprepared and unable to lead patient discussions or teach didactic or lecture components of the class. LPNs are frequently excellent reinforcers of patient education performed initially by RNs, but they should not be delegated the primary responsibility for teaching. The debate about the appropriateness of delegating patient teaching to multiskilled workers or other unlicensed (less expensive) staff is often encountered by staff development professionals. It is important to remember that patient teaching is not a procedure, but rather it involves assessment, critical thinking, and negotiation in addition to knowledge of the topic to be taught. Professional staff nursing time is required to accomplish patient education. The amount of staff time needed for pa-

tient education will vary with the number of disease processes covered, the sophistication and experience of the nurses and other involved personnel such as dietitians, the usefulness of the patient teaching protocols or care maps, and the amount of preparation the staff has had in teaching/learning theory. Documenting the number of hours required for patient education can be combined with documenting the patients' responses to education; this eventually helps in evaluating the overall effectiveness of the patient education program. It is also important to use staff time as a measure of the practicality of a teaching plan in relation to the patient's length of stay. Are nurses able to allocate time for patient teaching during short lengths of stay in the hospital? How well are they prepared to implement standardized teaching plans and individualize them based on patient needs and length of stay?

It is important to assess whether the staff who are to provide patient teaching have received formal preparation in how to use standardized teaching plans, what teaching resources are provided in the organization, and where to get assistance with teaching for difficult patient situations. In short, one hospital discovered in its organizational assessment that the success of its programs hinged on staff development. The majority of nurses indicated that they had received no formal training in how to develop teaching plans (Goldrick, Jablonski, & Wolf, 1994). In other studies, nurses stated that even when recognizing their need to learn how to teach, training was not readily available. Nurses also identified the need to learn teaching skills, not just concepts and theories (Boswell, Pichert, Lorenz, & Schlundt, 1990).

Interface of Political and Financial Issues Affecting Patient Education in Organizations

The connection between power and political and financial issues should not be overlooked because it is often encountered in the planning of organizational approaches to patient education. If the people who control a budget are opposed to patient education, it will be much more difficult to implement a program. Our experience in hospitals has been that if hospital administrators and key physicians believe in the efficacy of patient education, then implementation is fairly straightforward and simple. On the other hand, if these people feel that patient education is a "frill" and not beneficial in terms of cost, it is extremely difficult to initiate patient education programs.

In the latter situation, it is sometimes possible to sell the notion of patient education as an image maker to the reluctant administrative and medical staff. In other words, patient education becomes more appealing when it is marketed to the community as an agency attempt to reduce the high cost of health care through prevention, as a purveyor of better patient services, and as a way of securing more consumer participation. In some communities with many medical facilities, patient education has been used as an advertising come-on. Although this marketing is often effective, it has also meant that a proliferation of mediocre patient teaching programs have developed in metropolitan areas with a plethora of hospitals. Especially popular in the late 1980s and 1990s have been the programs that have sought the interest of the middle-class, well-educated client, such as programs in cholesterol reduction, stress abatement, parenting, and women's health issues. Efforts to address health education issues related to social problems such as homelessness, teenage pregnancies, and the crack cocaine epidemic have been largely ignored by both proprietary and nonprofit hospitals.

In this era of rising health care costs caused by the technology explosion, decisions about the expenditure of increasingly tight funds must be made. Most hospitals will choose to spend funds on magnetic resonance imaging and the establishment of rehabilitation and heart centers for wealthy and middle-class clients before they will budget funds for patient education. The public, urged on in many instances by health profes-

sionals, is demanding greater technocracy and more lifesaving assistance devices, which cause the costs of health care to skyrocket. The high costs of technologic advances, therefore, demand that patient education be marketed in increasingly clever ways.

In addition to the influence of decisions made by hospital administrators and political influence on financial issues, we must also consider the power exerted by physicians in setting priorities for patient education. The power and influence of certain physicians will frequently dictate which programs are implemented first. If the chief of staff decides that cardiac education is the most important priority in the hospital, it would not be surprising if the initial output of funds was directed toward cardiac education. Ideally, an assessment of patient education needs should be conducted first; however, this frequently does not occur. In such a situation the nurse who desires a strong patient education program would be well advised to support the chief of staff's plan and implement a vigorous patient education program in cardiac teaching, which then could serve to garner support for other patient education programming.

To nurses, physicians, and other health care professionals who have been historically committed to patient education and actively promoting it in their organizations, the JCAHO standards and focus surveys for patient and family education provide important support and ammunition for the effort. The mandates and priorities of JCAHO have required new attention to assessing the learning needs of patients and families and evidence of effective responses to these needs.

JCAHO Standards and Scoring Guidelines: Individual Patient Focus

Just as staff nurses must find a way to teach complex information to patients in practical, usable ways, so must staff development present JCAHO standards to staff nurses and members of other disciplines. We have summarized 14 pages of the JCAHO standards and scoring guidelines in Table 2-2. This table, along with Table 2-1, is a valuable teaching tool that can be duplicated for inservice classes and preparation for surveys. A theme seen throughout the scoring guidelines applies to all four standards: patient education outcomes should be evident in 90% to 100% of patients' records. To score well in a survey, the organization strives to demonstrate that patient education is an integral part of care for every patient, not just patients who receive a specialized teaching protocol. Hospitalization is a learning experience for every patient and family. Patient outcomes include evidence of the patient's response to teaching. Chapters 7 through 11 offer examples of the wide range of needs, interventions, and outcomes that can be documented. Sources of evidence of individual patient and family learning include: organizational policies and procedures, patient progress notes, flow sheets, referral and consultation notes, interviews with staff, written information provided to the patient and family, and interviews with staff and patients.

JCAHO Standards PF.1 Through PF.4

Four standards comprise the directives for patient-focused teaching. The reader is encouraged to review the standards as they are published by JCAHO to appreciate the many examples of practical application.

Standard PF.1

The patient and family are provided with education to increase their knowledge of their diagnosis, needs for treatment, and skills needed to participate in their recovery and rehabilitation.

Teaching Targets. The patient and family should understand the current health problem or the reason for admission. This sounds obvious and simple, but many patients do not know why they are hospitalized or cannot express it in their own words. Understanding the purpose of the hospitalization and acknowledging the episode or symptoms that precipitated it are important lessons in managing chronic illness. The patient and family should also be taught about the proposed treatment plan and the role they will play. Even before a final drug, diet, or exercise regimen may be prescribed, teaching should include the expectation that, for example, cardiac patients will participate actively in their recovery in these three areas. Finally, in addressing standard PF.1, patients should receive an overview of the survival skills needed for discharge and explore their individual learning needs.

Evidence. All patients receive instruction. In addition, priorities for teaching are noted based on the reason for admission, length of stay, and individual safety needs. Many nurses have described to us the interaction initiated by a JCAHO surveyor with patients. Patients are asked why they are in the hospital, what staff are doing to help them prepare for discharge, and what things the patients expect they will need to do to participate in their own care.

Standard PF.2

The patient and family receive individualized education specific to their assessed needs, abilities, readiness, and length of stay.

Teaching Targets. Priorities for teaching are based on survival and safety issues. Patient assessment is key. Chapters 7 and 8 discuss the process of assessing critical learning needs. The following targets indicate priority areas that must be addressed if they apply to the patient: medications, medical equipment, food-drug interactions, diets, rehabilitation skills, community resources, and ongoing health care needs. Patients must be informed about how to obtain further treatment, including possible emergency treatment as well as follow-up appointments.

Evidence. Patient assessment should include the patient's current understanding of the health problem, statements in the patient's "own words" that reflect an understanding of the health problem and willingness to participate (readiness), and prior knowledge, beliefs, or values which influence care (cultural aspects). Refer to Chapter 7 for guidance in teaching nurses these patient assessment skills.

Standard PF.3

Discharge instructions are given to the patient and the organization responsible for continuing care.

Teaching Targets. Patients receive written instructions that are understandable to them. See Chapter 9 for information on preparing one-page discharge instructions that promote patient understanding. Discharge planning clearly involves the patient and family and instructions promote safe, continuing care.

Evidence. Documentation reflects discharge and patient preparation. A copy of discharge instructions is in the patient record and has been forwarded to appropriate parties. Instructions are readable, usable, and understandable. A JCAHO surveyor might ask a patient what kinds of written information have been provided and to explain what it means.

Standard PF.4

The organization plans and supports coordinated learning activities and resources based on patient and family needs.

Teaching Targets. The organizational assessment described earlier in this chapter has resulted in the provision, coordination, and evaluation of quality learning interventions that are based on specific needs. They may include classes, community resources, videos, reading materials, presentations, and a variety of other formats. The process of patient teaching is interdisciplinary, well organized, and not overwhelming to the patient. Health care team involvement strengthens, streamlines, and individualizes care to address the

patient's functional problems. Patient teaching focuses on each patient's functional problems; it is not dictated by medical diagnosis. Nurses and other team members focus teaching on answering the question "How does this diagnosis affect this patient?"

Evidence. The patient's attendance at classes and participation in individual teaching sessions and the use of closed circuit television provide documentation. Chapter 11 provides examples of documentation. It is important that learning activities are selected based on individual priority needs and length of stay. Nursing staff and other team members should acknowledge that they may not be able to meet all the learning needs of the patient; instead the focus is to teach less and reinforce more. The organization-wide needs assessment, resulting programs including standardized approaches, and educational resources used to promote learning are also documented. It is important to remember that well-prepared staff are the most critical resource for providing patient education.

Preparing for Patient-Centered Care: Profile of a Teaching Program for Nurses and Other Staff

With new standards to address and with staff representing a diversity of interests and experiences in teaching, a formal teaching program can be effective in centralizing organizational values and approaches for patient education. We have found that full-day workshops best meet this need, with content and learning activities carefully planned to promote teamwork and critical thinking. Table 2-3 outlines a workshop developed by one of the authors and offered numerous times with interdisciplinary audiences.

Workshop participants should include staff nurses, educators, nurse managers, and interested members of other disciplines. The content includes material from Chapters 7 through 11 of this text. Participants are instructed that regardless of setting, there are always three "universal goals" of patient education: developing survival skills, recognizing problems, and making decisions. Just as we do with patients, limiting concepts to only three or four critical items promotes retention. The workshop begins with a simple set of concepts, which are reinforced throughout the day. Participants often come to the workshop feeling overwhelmed at the prospect of teaching sicker patients in less time. The workshop is intended to empower staff, giving them permission to teach smarter instead of faster and harder. The three universal goals are then tied to the chart of four JCAHO standards, demonstrating how the goals are a template for accreditation. Using small group discussions and case study analysis, participants are asked to examine how the JCAHO might survey for outcomes and to provide examples of learning outcomes that could be accomplished in a

wide variety of settings, from intensive care to long-term care. We also discuss methods to streamline documentation and at the same time provide a "snapshot" of the patient's involvement in learning. The ways patient education is currently provided by the participants is explored, often exposing issues over discipline turf battles and lack of coordination, which adversely affect patient-centered approaches.

The focus of the workshop then shifts to the process of patient education from a patient's perspective. The issue of compliance comes to light as workshop participants are asked to answer a survey about their own health behaviors (smoking, seat belt use, diet, exercise, medication use). Participants, in analyzing why they often do not practice what they preach to patients, identify the chal-

TABLE 2–3. Workshop: Patient-Centered Approaches to Patient Education

Objectives	Content (Topics)	Time Frame	Methodology
I. List three goals of patient education	I. JCAHO Standards and Scoring Guidelines	8:40–9:40 am	Lecture, discussion, handout
II. Identify four levels of patient learning outcomes	II. Four levels of evaluation	9:40–10:00 am	Lecture
III. Describe how the Health Belief Model can be used to understand and influence patient behavior	III. A. Cooperation vs. compliance B. Barriers to cooperation C. Patient motivation D. Application of model E. Patient decisions	10:15–11:00 am	Lecture, group exercise, dyads, discussion, handouts
IV. List five concerns of hospitalized patients	IV. A. Pain B. Cure C. Scarring/deformity D. Burden on others E. Dying	11:00–11:30 am	Discussion, handouts
V. List four questions a nurse can ask to determine priorities for patient teaching	V. A. Safe discharge B. Complications/readmission C. Past experience D. Equipment used at home	12:45–2:00 pm	Lecture, case studies, discussion
VI. Discuss guidelines to improve the effectiveness and safety of videotapes and written discharge instructions	VI. A. Content B. Format C. Organization D. Emergency plan E. Follow-up	2:15–3:30 pm	Lecture, discussion video preview/evaluation
Wrap-up/Evaluation	Review Objectives I–VI	3:30–4:00 pm	Q & A, discussion

lenges of motivating patients to change their behaviors. The wisdom of expecting three or four simultaneous lifelong behavior changes is questioned. The steps of the Health Belief Model are reviewed with strategies for addressing barriers and influencing patient decisions toward healthy life-styles. Patient concerns, which are addressed in Chapter 8, are discussed and recommendations offered for sequencing patient education based on the priority concerns of patients. Priority for education about pain and pain management is discussed.

Critical needs for patient teaching are identified based on the content of Chapters 7 through 10. Principles for streamlining teaching are introduced and then applied to case studies. This is often a time of lively discussion and differing opinions, based on the practice and education backgrounds of the participants. With the use of case studies, practice and feedback are provided in identifying no more than three or four critical learning objectives for each patient, finding ways to teach and observe performance as an integral part of care, and documenting based on what the patient accomplished or demonstrated.

Due to the importance placed on media for patient learning, the workshop concludes with a lecture and critique of patient education handouts and videos. These tools for teaching must reflect the same targeted, streamlined approach based on length of stay and their effectiveness must be evaluated. The content is derived from Chapter 9. Examples of short, effective instructions are provided. The importance and challenges of creating a single, one-page, interdisciplinary set of discharge instructions is emphasized. As video technology and computer-assisted instruction become more sophisticated and affordable, they will allow practical application for patient education in homes as well as hospitals. Continuing education offerings such as this one will need to prepare staff to use these technologies wisely and to evaluate their effectiveness (Redman, 1993; Wasson & Anderson, 1994).

Throughout the workshop, participants are asked to describe barriers in their work setting that may prevent them from effectively providing patient education. As staff development practitioners know so well, administrative as well as educational issues are often identified by learners. Educators must then carry the messages between staff and management and help to address the barriers.

Confronting Barriers to Patient Teaching

Four recurring themes documented in the literature (Boswell et al., 1990) are identified in our workshops as barriers that limit staff nurses' abilities to teach patients effectively. When the following barriers are addressed with ongoing training and management support, patient education and staff satisfaction can be significantly enhanced.

1. *Time restrictions interfere with teaching.* Teaching is perceived as time consuming, unrealistic, and competing with other facets of work. Nurses often perceive that patient education is an activity separate from routine care and formal in design. Due to this perception, which often arises in settings where teaching has historically been provided by a patient educator or clinical nurse specialist, staff nurses benefit from coaching and example to incorporate teaching into every patient encounter. Attempting to apply outdated protocols or teaching plans also makes teaching in today's environment virtually impossible. Staff development's role is to assess the work setting and determine how to break down barriers. Can patient education experts be used for coaching staff? Do teaching plans need to be streamlined and accompanied by new teaching materials? Finally, do demands of paperwork, staffing, and supervision legitimately prevent staff from the patient contact required for teaching?

2. *Nurses state they lack the skills needed for teaching.* Specifically, they ask for modeling and coaching from experienced teachers such as clinical nurse specialists and patient educators. Chapter 9 offers guid-

ance in designing individual and group teaching. We have heard from many nurses that they have little confidence in their teaching and would like to observe expert teachers to benefit from their technique. This request goes beyond a class in which the expert shares tips for teaching. A precepting model of observation, demonstration, and coaching can potentially create much greater productivity from the expert teachers as they develop a staff of confident teachers and become resources for difficult teaching situations.

3. *Nurses often identify patient teaching efforts as haphazard and not directed to discharge priorities.* Patient teaching materials are not readily available or are outdated; many teaching programs are outdated. For example, one postpartum nursing unit had a new flow sheet designed to streamline documentation of patient teaching with a check-off format. However, it contained more than 40 learning objectives that staff felt responsible for teaching. Because most patient stays were less than 48 hours, teaching was not feasible and left staff frustrated. When one of the authors met with the nurses to discuss how to streamline teaching, it was discovered that some items were repetitive and a few were best taught after discharge. The remaining items were divided into four topical areas with four key learning objectives related to feeding, hygiene and rest of mother, managing baby's schedule and mother's needs, and trouble signs that needed immediate attention. Staff then felt confident focusing their teaching and assessing patient outcomes on only four areas. To accompany the streamlined teaching plan, a new discharge instruction sheet was developed, following the same format.

In many situations, interdisciplinary approaches to patient education depend on leadership from staff development and an honest appraisal of "sacred cows" that exist in the institution. If teaching plans are unrealistic, new documentation forms create more work instead of streamlined work, and staff are unable to create pa-

tient-centered approaches, staff development personnel step in to strengthen the group's work with additional training.

4. *Nurses state that patient education is not noticed or rewarded.* They believe that more recognition should be given to involvement in patient education and it should be evaluated in the performance appraisal system. Patient education is creative work, requiring astute assessment and energetic involvement with the patient and family to make every moment count. If staff perceive that rewards and recognition are based on the number of patients cared for, the number of committees served on, or the ability to troubleshoot technical equipment, they are likely to place priority on these activities. Patient education is often "invisible" in the eyes of management because it is frequently undocumented, not monitored, and underappreciated for the skill and experience it demands. Patient education efforts should be described, monitored, and marketed so that nurses receive credit for their work and strive to increase the amount of teaching that is provided (Goldrick et al., 1994). Staff development's role includes improving documentation and visibility of teaching efforts, promoting accountability of all staff through performance reviews, and sponsoring special events that recognize patient education efforts. An annual "Patient Education Week" that includes displays, guest speakers, special awards to individuals and units, and recognition of patient education outcomes and commitment by top administrators can also provide a needed boost for staff.

Promoting Skill Acquisition in Patient Education: Individualized Staff Development

Despite intensive educational efforts to teach, coach, and standardize approaches for patient education, staff development professionals recognize that nurses have different developmental needs in the process of becoming expert teachers. This is explained by the work of Patricia Benner (Benner et al., 1992), which has so convincingly explained that nurses live in different clinical worlds.

The clinical judgment and intuition needed to streamline teaching, provide culturally sensitive care, and engage with patients and families requires that nurses move from a theoretical, abstract base to a concrete world. Developing judgment and intuition occurs as the nurse learns through experience and reflection. Only by passing such developmental milestones can nurses eventually arrive at the expert stage of practice. The expert nurse is able to grasp the whole situation, set priorities, and confidently individualize patient care.

Applying Benner's work, the strategies that most effectively promote development of expertise in patient education can be incorporated in staff development efforts. Staff development can be targeted to reach out to different clinical worlds and build teamwork to accomplish patient education.

Figure 2-1 is based on Benner's description of the process of skill acquisition. One cornerstone of this process is the nurse's ability to translate theoretical knowledge into nursing's art and "know-how" and to be guided by principles rather than explicit directions. The nurse also becomes able to use intuition, recognizing what is salient in an individual situation. The nurse is able to pick up on subtle cues. Clinical knowledge enables the

nurse to attend to the patient's situation and needs as a whole, with teaching the patient and family as an integral part of care. Rather than feeling overwhelmed, expert nurses feel confident and powerful in complex situations and adapt care based on individual patient priorities. Clinical judgment is embedded in practice (Benner et al., 1992).

What is required for a novice nurse to successfully progress to expert practice? Benner describes the developmental steps associated with advanced beginner (generally the first 2 years of practice), competent, proficient, and expert. By understanding each stage, the capacity of the nurse to accomplish patient education is better appreciated. This understanding also helps staff developers to design effective coaching and precepting interventions to support nurses' development of expertise in patient education. Benner's work helps educators to carefully choose preceptors who best match the needs of their learners. Although many organizations traditionally assign precepting responsibilities to their expert nurses, Benner leads us to question this wisdom and to use the expertise of nurses at all stages of development to support one another in practice.

Table 2-4 applies Benner's work to identify both the interests and educational needs of nurses at each stage of development.

The *advanced beginner* must master technical skills and learn to organize nursing care. Attuned to rules and procedures, the nurse is

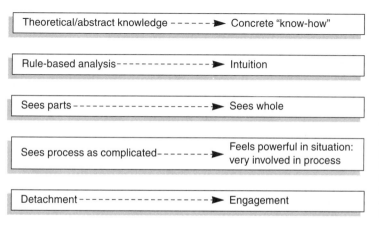

FIGURE 2-1. Patient education science and art: a process of skill acquisition. (Adapted from *From Beginner to Expert: Clinical Knowledge in Critical Care Nursing* [video], by P. Benner, C. Tanner, & C. Chesla, 1992, Athens, OH: Fuld Institute for Technololgy in Nursing Education.)

dependent on the availability of a preceptor to provide teaching and coaching in each situation. The nurse does not feel fully responsible and is often overwhelmed with the simultaneous demands of a situation. Staff development efforts for advanced beginners are often best fulfilled by unit-based preceptors and focus on the following: awareness of agency standards, resources, standardized teaching programs and critical paths; ways to integrate patient and family teaching into all aspects of care; "how-to" aspects of teaching individual patients; developing explanations of diagnoses and procedures to share with families; and documenting the outcomes of learning.

Nurses in the *competent* stage of practice begin to see patterns and recognize relationships among the various aspects of a situation. This is due to having experienced similar situations and learned from them. The nurse no longer views the patient and family as adding to the demands of providing care but begins to engage with them and personalize care. Still desiring to limit the unexpected, the nurse engages in deliberate planning and goal setting and feels the burden of all aspects of the patient's care. Staff development efforts to support the competent nurse may include classes or workshops in family assessment, group teaching skills, learning

TABLE 2-4. Promoting Skill Acquisition in Patient Education

Benner's Stages	Developmental Focus	Educational/Institutional Support
Advanced beginner	• Technical mastery and organization • Needs other staff to "delegate up" • Manages situations by rules, procedures • Learns by situation • Does not feel fully responsible	• Awareness of agency standards, resources, programs for patient education • Skills for integrating patient and family in patient's care • "How to teach" skills • Developing explanations to share with family • "How-to" of documentation
Competent	• Sees relationships among aspects of a situation; pattern analysis • Desires to limit unexpected • Deliberate planning and goal setting • Notices patient/family in new ways; personalizes care • Feels whole burden of health care team	• Family assessment • Group teaching skills • Home visits • Negotiating learning contracts • Case study analysis, exemplars • Leading/participating in health care team processes and critical path design
Proficient	• Recognizes patterns • Sees changing relevance • Increased sense of what is salient • Attuned to situation; not detached	• Documentation that supports individualized care • Clinical career ladder based on exemplars that illustrate critical thinking • Permission to "break the rules" • Support for complex patient situations
Expert	• Clinical grasp of whole situation • "At home" in rapidly changing situations • Attends to context and environment • Decisions based on qualitative distinctions/what it means for *this* patient	• Roles in case management • Teacher for competent-proficient • Facilitates patient care rounds • Designs product line models

Adapted from Benner P., Tanner C., Chesla C. (1992). *From Beginner to Expert: Clinical Knowledge in Critical Care Nursing.* Athens, OH. Fuld Institute for Technology in Nursing Education.

contracts, and case study analysis. The nurse may be interested in and benefit from making home visits as well as leading health care team conferences and serving on committees to design new critical paths. Competent nurses should be engaged in precepting beginners because they can remember how they learned and can appreciate the needs of novice and advanced beginner nurses.

Nurses in the *proficient* stage recognize patterns and see changing relevance. They confidently streamline teaching, redefine priorities, and "break the rules" in ways that benefit the patient. Proficient nurses have an increased sense of what is salient in a situation and can teach in ways that are culturally sensitive. They pick up on subtle cues and are attuned to the situation. Staff development efforts for these nurses should focus on achieving documentation that supports and reflects individualized care. Clinical career ladders based on exemplars that illustrate critical thinking help proficient nurses to demonstrate their significant contributions and development of clinical judgment. Although proficient nurses may still need support and learning resources for complex patient situations, they are skilled at coaching and precepting other nurses in most patient education situations and should be involved as teachers and mentors. Proficient nurses should define patient education successes based on the patient's learning and right to choose rather than compliance. The failure to do so may result in nurses who become disillusioned and detached, rather than engaged in their practice of nursing.

Expert nurses demonstrate an excellent clinical grasp of the whole situation and are comfortable in rapidly changing situations. They attend to context as well as environment and can make the qualitative distinctions that are crucial in complex situations. Expert nurses can provide valuable coaching for competent and proficient nurses, but they are usually a poor choice to precept beginners because they are developmentally distant from the issues beginners experience and are impatient teachers. While beginners are striving to learn and follow the rules, experts have learned the conditions under which to safely bend or break them to meet patient needs. Expert nurses are suited to roles such as case manager and clinical specialist in which they must handle complex situations. They are also valuable resources for facilitating patient care rounds and assisting in the development of multiservice product line models for patient education.

Summary

Staff development practitioners are poised to make important contributions to patient teaching efforts: providing leadership to assess needs, developing educationally sound programs, and advocating for needed resources. The work of staff development includes interpreting JCAHO standards, promoting patient-centered approaches, streamlining or replacing outdated programs, and forging alliances that are multidisciplinary and multisetting.

The role of staff development goes beyond helping the organization achieve a successful JCAHO survey. All continuing education programs must address implications for patient education. Workshops that expose staff to innovative approaches and skills for patient education should be offered and should address realistic strategies for teaching and documenting. As staff development professionals identify barriers encountered in the provision of patient teaching, they must address those issues honestly. Unit-based teaching and coaching should be provided to individual nurses to build the acquisition of skills and expertise in patient education. The strengths of nurses as coaches and teachers of others is perhaps our greatest resource for improving patient education outcomes.

Finally, staff development can increase the visibility of patient education efforts in the organization. This can be accomplished by sponsoring special events and recognitions, bringing in national experts as guest speakers, and promoting patient education activities as integral to clinical ladders and performance review systems.

Strategies for Critical Analysis and Application

1. How can the respective strengths of nurses in each of Benner's four stages contribute to the development of new or improved patient education programs?

2. Describe administrative issues that have an impact (positive and negative) on the potential for innovative patient education programs. What impact can staff development have to increase administrative support for patient education efforts?

REFERENCES

American Hospital Association. (1979). *Implementing patient education in the hospital.* Chicago: Author.

Benner, P. (1984). *From novice to expert: Excellence and power in clinical nursing practice.* Menlo Park, CA: Addison-Wesley.

Benner, P., & Tanner, C. (1987). Clinical judgment: how expert nurses use intuition. *American Journal of Nursing, 87*(1), 23-31.

Benner, P., Tanner, C., & Chesla, C. (1992). *From beginner to expert: Clinical knowledge in critical care nursing* [Video]. Athens, OH: Fuld Institute for Technology in Nursing Education.

Boswell, E., Pichert, J., Lorenz, R., & Schlundt, D. (1990). Training health care professionals to enhance their patient teaching skills. *Journal of Nursing Staff Development, 6*(5), 233–239.

Goldrick, T., Jablonski, R., & Wolf, Z. (1994). Needs assessment for a patient education program in a nursing department. *Journal of Nursing Staff Development, 10*(3), 123-130.

Joint Commission on the Accreditation of Healthcare Organizations. (1994). *Comprehensive accreditation manual for hospitals.* Chicago: Author.

Kelly, K. (1992). *Nursing staff development: Current competence and future focus.* Philadelphia: J. B. Lippincott.

Lipetz, M., Bussiget, J., & Risley, B. (1990). What is wrong with patient education programs? *Nursing Outlook, 38*(4), 184-189.

Marchiondo, K., & Kipp, C. (1987). Establishing a standardized patient education program. *Critical Care Nurse, 7*(3), 58-66.

Redman, B. (1993). Patient education at 25 years: where we have been and where we are going. *Journal of Advanced Nursing, 18,* 727-728.

Wasson, D., & Anderson, M. (1994). Hospital-patient education: Current status and future trends. *Journal of Nursing Staff Development, 10*(3), 147-151.

CHAPTER

3

Patient Education as a Tool for Normalization and Self-Regulation

Rae L. Jayne

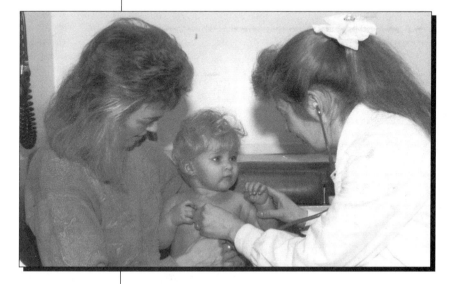

OBJECTIVES FOR CHAPTER 3

After reading this chapter, the nurse or student nurse should be able to:

1 State one rationale for using theory or frameworks in nursing practice and education.

2 List five of the six factors used in the Health Belief Model to determine a person's likelihood of complying with health care recommendations.

3 Compare the Health Promotion Model to the Health Belief Model; describe the difference in the definition of health for each model.

4 State how the Self-Regulation Model differs from the Health Belief Model and the Health Promotion Model.

5 State the interacting components of the Personal Meaning Schema.

6 Describe how nurse educators can assist patients with normalization within the constraints of chronic illness.

7 Discuss the relationship(s) between patient education and self-regulated management practices.

Patient Education: Issues, Principles, Practices, Third Edition, by Sally H. Rankin and Karen Duffy Stallings.
Lippincott–Raven Publishers , Philadelphia, © 1996.

Purpose

As chronic illness became more prevalent in our society, patient education focused on helping patients obtain knowledge and self-management skills necessary to regulate illnesses over long periods of the life span. This chapter discusses the need for nursing to provide patient education that reaches beyond the teaching of skills and strategies. In addition to knowledge about self-care, patients need assistance in learning to deal with the complexities of living with chronic illnesses.

In the past, the focus of patient education was to persuade the patient to comply with the prescribed treatment regimen. Coercing people into accepting these regimens without acknowledgement of the intrusion of such treatment plans on a person's usual daily activities resulted in frustration and dissatisfaction on the part of professionals and patients. Professionals are frustrated by their inability to motivate patients to follow treatment plans, and patients are dissatisfied with care that does not recognize their need to play roles other than that of "patient."

Role of Patient Education in Nursing Practice

Nursing has defined its roles as diagnosing and treating the human responses to illness (American Nurses Association, 1980). Leventhal and Johnson (1983) describe the nurse as the professional who acknowledges patients' perceptions of their illnesses, the impact of the illness on their lives, and the strategies they use to respond to their illness experiences. Historically, nurses have taught patients about health management. As far back as Nightingale (1859), teaching was recognized as a nursing function. Today, the nurse practice acts in many states and national guidelines from the American Nurses Association (1979) and the American Hospital Association (1972) mandate nursing's obligation to help patients learn to take care of their health and self-manage their illnesses.

In the preface of the second edition of this text, Rankin and Stallings, (1990) describe the relationship between patient education and nursing practice as follows:

> Our commitment to patient education has not changed...as we continue to view it as an essential patient empowerment tool. Feeling powerless is perhaps the most devastating aspect of illness for a patient. Patient education is the most effective means of returning control to the patient by reducing feelings of helplessness and enhancing the ability to be the chief decision maker in the management of one's health and illness problems. We view patient education as the *essence* of nursing practice. (p. viii)

As the recognition of education as an essential aspect of nursing practice grew, so has the responsibility and liability (see Chap. 5 for further discussion). As a result, practice standards for specialized nursing roles have been developed and guidelines structuring the content and goals of education now exist (American Association of Diabetes Educators, 1992; American Diabetes Association, 1993; American Nephrology Nurses Association, 1991, 1993).

Models for Explanation

As a profession, nursing has recognized the need to use theoretical frameworks to guide practice and organize nursing and patient education. Theories help structure practice by providing concepts that can be consistently applied and evaluated. Efforts at understanding motivation for health care that promotes healthier life-styles have resulted in the development of several patient education models.

A major influence on guidelines for patient education is the compliance model of treatment and education. In the seminal work by Sackett and Haynes (1976), compliance was defined as "the extent to which the patient's behavior (in terms of taking medications, following diets or executing other life-style changes) coincides with the clinical prescriptions" (p. 1). They further state that "the presentation of compliance data has clinical relevance only when it is related to the simultaneous achievement of the treatment goals" (p. 3). This definition influenced compliance research and literature in two major ways. First, it indelibly associated the control of illness with compliance to physician-directed regimens (i.e., control resulted from complying with the prescribed treatment). The physician determined the dose of medication to be given and the time it was to be taken, the specific diet to be followed, and the kind of body monitoring to be completed by the patient. Completing these actions as ordered was assumed to lead directly to control of the illness. Compliance was measured by the extent to which the patient accomplished these activities.

Second, the patient's performance of the prescribed regimen became the focus of the indices of compliance or noncompliance. Noncompliance is defined as "the failure of the patient to fulfill the clinical prescription *as it was intended by the practitioner*" (Hays & DiMatteo, 1981, p. 37). Patient noncompliance with the medical prescription suggested a lack of knowledge, rebellion, or emotional instability (Leventhal, Zimmerman, & Gutmann, 1984; Trostle, 1988).

According to this model, the educator's task involves motivating patients to accept treatment plans as valuable in attaining health or controlling illness, providing them with the skills and knowledge necessary to manage continuing care without daily professional supervision, and encouraging them to change behavior patterns to fit the requirements of the regimen. Even in the innovative nurse-managed clinics developed by Allison (1973) and Backscheider (1974), in which Orem's nursing theory of self-care was used to organize the clinic practice, the prescriptive or compliance model was the philosophical basis. The goal of nursing care was to assist the client in following the prescribed treatment plan; the individual's definition of self-care was rarely considered.

Despite prescribed regimens intended to control illness and education to inform the patient about the need to follow the medical prescription, the rate of noncompliance with treatment regimens is notoriously high. Sackett (1976) reports that compliance with short-term regimens decreases rapidly as the days of treatment increase, and the level of compliance in long-term therapy is approximately 50%.

In a classic study, Watkins and colleagues (1967) were the first researchers to observe diabetic patients in their homes. They were interested in the relationships between what people knew about diabetes, what they actually did to manage their illness, and how this manifested itself in their level of diabetes control. The results showed that 80% of the 60 patients in the study administered their insulin in an inappropriate manner, over 50% made errors in insulin dosing, 45% incorrectly or inadequately used urine test results, 73% did not match food amounts and timing to fit insulin use, and over 50% performed foot care poorly.

Health Belief Model

Studies of this kind led to an interest in trying to identify factors that influence compliance or noncompliance with a health professional's recommendations for care. One framework, the Health Belief Model was originally developed by social psychologists to predict the likelihood of a person taking recommended preventive health action and to understand a person's motivation and decision-making about seeking health services (Hochbaum, 1958). It has been adapted for use in predicting compliance with chronic illness regimens.

The model attempts to identify compliers and noncompliers by looking at six factors. The factors considered important to health care decisions are:

1. Perception of the *severity* of the illness
2. Perception of *susceptibility* to illness and its consequences
3. The value of the *benefits* of treatment
4. The consideration of the *barriers* to treat-

ment, such as degree of social support, expense, regimen complexity, length of treatment, and side effects

5. The *costs* of treatment in physical and emotional terms

6. What *cues* stimulate action taken for treatment of illness, such as illness in family or friends, television, or other media presentations—films, newspaper stories, or health pamphlets

Demographic variables such as age, gender, socioeconomic status, and ethnicity are believed to modulate a person's perceptions about the seriousness of health conditions and the need to take action for those conditions (Becker, 1974, 1979; Becker & Janz, 1985; Janz & Becker, 1984).

The Health Belief Model has been used in a number of research studies that cover a wide range of health-related decision-making situations (Eisen, Zellman, & McAlister, 1992; French, Kurczynski, Weaver, & Pituch, 1992; Galvin, 1992). However, studies using the Health Belief Model have been somewhat inconsistent in identifying the differences between those who comply with professional recommendations and those who choose not to comply. Studies show various components of the model as effective for prediction, whereas the model as a whole has not been a consistent predictor of compliance. Janz and Becker (1984) suggest that barriers and costs are the most prominent factors associated with preventive health practices or maintenance of illness regimens. Cerkoney and Hart (1980) found that subjects who perceived their diabetes as serious and responded to cues for action were more compliant with their treatment regimen. The authors state that a positive correlation of $r = 0.50$, $p < 0.01$ occurred between the subjects' total compliance scores and a composite score of their level of health motivation. This correlation only accounted for 25% of the variance in compliance levels of this sample and could not be used as reliable clinical predictors of compliance. Some of the inconsistency in results is related to the fact that the components of the model were not operationalized

in the same way or applied consistently across studies (Wallston & Wallston, 1984).

Despite the fact that the Health Belief Model acknowledges the importance of patients' beliefs in compliance, the assumption is that the variables specified regarding health beliefs are the most significant factors in decision-making about health behaviors. The model also does not offer an explanation of the relationships between the variables or how other aspects of personal experience may affect the way illness treatment is managed or ignored (Conrad, 1985).

Health Promotion Model

Another model attempting to explain how individuals arrive at decisions about behaviors directed toward health promotion was developed by Pender, a nurse (1982, 1987). Pender thought that the Health Belief Model focused on an "avoidance orientation" (1982, p. 60) related to seeking preventive care to decrease the probability of negative health and illness outcomes.

Pender believed that the Health Belief Model did not address positive actions taken to sustain or increase an individual's level of health. She maintained that the Health Belief Model had been tested on preventive actions requiring the performance of a single act of compliance and was insufficient in explaining behavior directed toward health promotion.

Pender defined health, not as the absence of disease, but as self-actualization. She felt defining health as self-actualization suggested that health was related to self-initiated behaviors directed toward attaining higher levels of health. From her perspective, defining health as adaptation or stability directed behavior toward health protection or avoiding illness and disease.

Health-promoting behaviors are operationalized as activities that are integrated on an ongoing basis into an individual's lifestyle. Actions such as exercise, optimum nutrition, stress management, and development and maintenance of social support systems are examples of health promotion behaviors. These behaviors are directed toward self-actualization and fulfillment, leading to "increased self-awareness, self-satisfaction, enjoyment, and pleasure" (Pender, 1987, p. 59).

The role of the health care professional is to assist individuals in overcoming barriers to health-promoting activities in addition to supporting preventive health practices. Assistance by health providers is accomplished by removing genuine barriers, increasing the importance of positive consequences of preferred behaviors, and by reducing the frequency of negative consequences.

The components of the Health Promotion Model were based on many of the components in the Health Belief Model and on a synthesis of health promotion and wellness literature. The Health Promotion Model, like the Health Belief Model, was organized into categories: *cognitive-perceptual factors, modifying factors*, and *participation in health promotion behavior*. Two stages, the *acquisition* stage and the *maintenance* stage, were hypothesized as possibly influencing which cognitive-perceptual factors are significant as the time frame changes from short- to long-term behaviors (Fig. 3-1).

Cognitive-perceptual factors determining health promotion activities were labeled as:

1. The importance of health
2. Perceived control on health behaviors
3. Perceived self-efficacy, the belief individuals have in their ability to perform behaviors necessary to accomplish the desired action
4. The definition of health as actualization
5. Perceived health status
6. Perceived benefits of health promoting
7. Perceived barriers to health-promoting behaviors

The *modifying factors* were defined as:

1. Demographic variables
2. Interpersonal variables such as the expectations of others and the individual's experience with health professionals
3. Situational variables such as access to health promotion alternatives

4. Biologic variables such as body weight
5. Behavioral factors or prior experiences with various health promotion choices

The likelihood of engaging in health promotion behaviors depends on *cues for action* that are defined as:

1. The desire for increased well-being
2. Interaction with others interested in health promotion
3. Advice from others, either for or against health promotion
4. Mass media sources of information about health-promoting behaviors such as television programming related to health matters or representations of health problems presented in fictionalized programs, public information on health promotion such as that found on public transportation or in public transportation depots, newspaper articles, and health promotion literature distributed within health agencies
5. An awareness of potential for growth and self-actualization

Pender (1982) reports the results of a study that was not specifically designed to test the components of the Health Promotion Model but documented the importance of health, perceived control, and perceived health status as significant predictors of health behavior. Demographic variables such as education, occupation, household size, age, and religion were also supported in this research as important in predicting health behaviors (Christiansen, 1981).

Other studies using the Health Promotion Model attempting to identify health promotion behaviors in middle-aged and elderly subjects have further confirmed the relationships between various components of the Health Promotion Model and health-promoting behaviors. Duffy (1988) reported high self-esteem, internal health locus of control, and good current health related to self-actualization, exercise, and interpersonal support health promotion activities in midlife women. Hawkins and colleagues (1988) found higher self-esteem, internal locus of control, and better health sta-

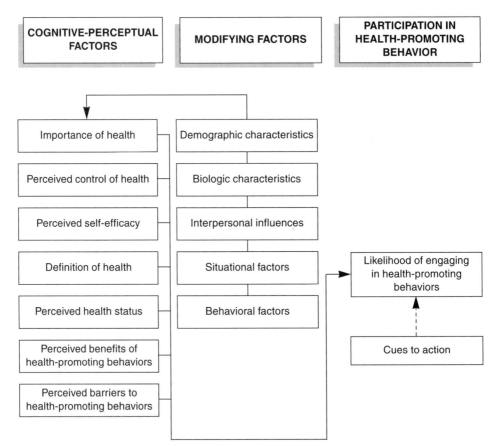

FIGURE 3-1. Health Promotion Model. (From *Health Promotion in Nursing Practice*, 2nd ed., 1987, by N. Pender, East Norwalk, CT: Appleton & Lange.)

tus related to the health promotion activities of regular exercise and sleeping 7 or 8 hours a day. Pender and colleagues (1990) reported that better health status was related to self-actualization, health responsibility, exercise, nutrition, interpersonal support, and stress management. Duffy (1993) reported that subjects who believed that their current health was good, had high self-esteem, and believed that health was under their own control more frequently practiced the health promotion activities of self-actualization, nutrition, interpersonal support, stress management, and exercise.

Even though Pender's model expands the Health Belief Model to include individual perceptions and acknowledges the importance of environmental and situational variables on health action decisions, it is not clear why the modifying factors do not have equal impact on the likelihood of taking health-promoting action; they are mediated through the cognitive-perceptual factors. The model remains a cognitive processing type in which health-promoting behavior can be enhanced by health care professionals through changing the cognitive and perceptual fields of the patient to align with the desired outcomes. One of the problems with testing the Health Promotion Model is the problem of defining health as self-actualization. This definition remains unclear and further efforts have attempted to clarify individual expressions of health (Pender, 1990).

Indications for Reframing Compliance

Some authors suggest a need to reframe compliance models to better reflect the centrality of personal rather than professional health expectations. In fact, Trostle (1988) declares that compliance is an ideology invented by medicine to maintain power and control over health decisions and is not about the efficacy of treatment at all. Hayes-Bautista (1976) suggests that patient noncompliance or treatment modification is not the result of stupidity or ignorance, but rather a means of exerting some personal control over health care. Hayes-Bautista adds that patients have their own explanations for health behaviors. They usually do not explain their behavior "in terms of age, sex, education, marital status, social class, norms, values, or other variables often used by social scientists..." (p. 233).

Common Sense or Self-Regulation Model

Another model looking at decision-making related to health care includes personal meanings and responses to illness. The Common Sense or Self-Regulation Model developed from studies looking at the effect of fear-arousing communications on preventive health care actions. Studies were conducted using the psychological framework of drive theory that suggested a drive, such as fear, would precede performance of an activity. Therefore, fear-arousing information could be used to make people comply with health-related activities (Keller, Ward, & Baumann, 1989; Leventhal & Johnson, 1983; Leventhal, Singer, & Jones, 1965).

Leventhal and colleagues (1965) realized that fear communications initiate problem-solving activities related to the subject's perception of the presence of danger. If an individual developed a plan of action to deal with the danger, the subject was more likely to take action to reduce the danger. Continuing studies led Leventhal and his colleagues to believe that people generate their own construction or representation of health threats and plan health-related action based on these representations.

Representations are constructed from accumulated experience over time and are an integration of knowledge gathered from the media, personal contacts, health professional input, symptoms and body sensations, and past experience with illness. The model views four factors as the key features of a person's construction of health threats: *identity* or identification of concrete symptoms (i.e., a headache means a brain tumor is present), *cause* such as improper food habits or stressful life events, *time line* or the perception of how long the illness will last (i.e., acute or chronic), and what the perception of the *consequences* is. Action taken will depend on: the individual's belief that he or she can *manage the health threat* and the emotional response to the challenge, the individual's *strategies* for dealing with problem situations, and the individual's evaluation of whether the *action taken is effective* or not (Keller, Ward, Baumann, 1989; Leventhal, 1982; Leventhal, Zimmerman, & Gutmann, 1985; Meyer, Leventhal & Gutmann, 1985). Interpretation and synthesis of these factors will influence how a person copes with illness (Fig. 3-2).

Research studies using the Self-Regulation Model represent an expansion of the medical model's conception of compliance as a result of fixed patient characteristics, situational barriers, and inadequate motivation or education. The concepts developed in the Self-Regulation Model suggest that a person's understanding of an illness may be the critical factor in decisions about continuing treatment or illness control.

Further, beliefs about illness will determine what symptoms people choose to monitor in evaluating health status. How symptoms are interpreted as illness threats will have an impact on actions taken to correct the problem. For example, if a diabetic patient interprets lethargy as a normal part of the label "dia-

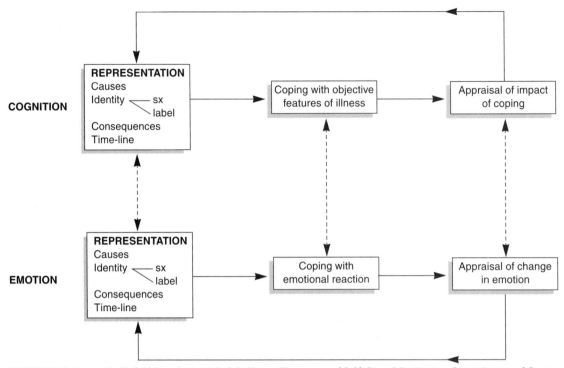

FIGURE 3-2. Leventhal's Self-Regulation Model. (From "Processes of Self-Care: Monitoring Sensations and Symptoms," by M.L. Keller, S. Ward, & L. J. Baumann, 1989, *Advances in Nursing Science, 12* (1), 54-66.)

betic," she may ignore the symptoms of hyperglycemia and fail to adjust the diet or medication. The consequences of continuous high blood sugar levels can lead to devastating disabilities over time. Assessing people's representation of illness and connecting the constructions of the illness with self-management choices provides a means of identifying at what point health information may be most helpful to the patient.

In summary, the Self-Regulation Model focuses on the patient's interpretation of illness meaning as a vehicle for explaining compliance to medical treatment. However, the model maintains a purely cognitive approach to illness management and does not pay attention to health and illness in the context of everyday life. Environmental factors such as home and work stress are only acknowledged in the research as important in the construction of beliefs about the cause of illness.

What is left unrecognized in the model is how modifications in health definitions affect emotions and social activities. It further fails to address how valued social activities affect emotional adjustment to illness, health definitions, and health practices.

Summary of Models of Explanation

The models discussed above all attempt to better discern what characteristics best describe people who would or would not comply with prescribed health promotion and treatment plans. Without consideration of the roles and obligations imposed by the environmental context of a patient, prescribed regimens may not be achievable or realistic. The following section describes an investigation about compliance with diabetes treatment regimens using a patient's perspectives to describe components of a developing model.

Negotiating Self-Regulation in Diabetes

People with diabetes are asked to lose or maintain weight by staying on a diet 365 days a year, every year, for life. Blood fats and cholesterol are scrutinized because of the high rate of heart attacks, strokes, and gangrene in the long-term diabetic patient. Constant self-monitoring of blood glucose is required by finger sticks and urine testing and is done by the patient to check sugar and ketone levels. Exercise is considered part of the treatment, but it must be planned to avoid causing elevations or severe drops in blood sugar levels; all the while, the patient must inject insulin under the skin several times per day or take oral medications. The complexity of the regimen could boggle the mind of a rocket scientist, and yet, ordinary people are asked to accomplish these tasks, and at the same time carry on a normal life of work, school, and social relationships.

One of the problems is that patients and health care professionals see the situation of managing an illness such as diabetes from different viewpoints. The professional assumes one angle, and the patient may have a totally different perspective. Anderson (1985), an educator at the University of Michigan who works with diabetes educators, stated: "While many health-care practitioners see the treatment regimen as a solution, patients may see it as another part of the problem of having diabetes....Many patients view the treatment of diabetes as more of a problem than having the disease" (p. 32). Nurses providing patient education must acknowledge this situation and find a way to evaluate and integrate the patient's perspective into workable treatment regimens.

As a diabetes educator for more than a decade, I have spent hundreds of hours talking to and observing people with diabetes. Despite standards for patient education and certification of diabetes educators and education programs, people with diabetes continue to amaze health care professionals with widely varying and individualized interpretations of prescribed medical regimens devised to control blood glucose levels. The study described here was designed to find out from people with diabetes how they developed these unique self-regulating processes for managing the treatment regimen prescribed by a health professional.

I believe that compliance with treatment regimens from the patient's perspective is related to the degree the patient's identity with diabetes is incorporated into the activities and roles of everyday life. Based on this belief, an investigation was conducted on how an individual's compliance behaviors were influenced by the interaction of personal characteristics, individual understandings of the illness, and multiple settings requiring role variations (Jayne, 1993). From this perspective, compliance is not a set of rigid or constant behaviors. Instead, compliance becomes a complex interaction between a particular setting, its role requirements, and a choice of self-care behaviors based on the priority given diabetes in that setting.

Questions used to guide the investigation were:

1. How does a person's understanding of the nature of diabetes affect the development and modification of self-regulation?
2. Under what condition and contexts does self-regulation develop? How do these conditions affect the ability to comply with treatment regimens prescribed by health professionals?
3. What strategies do persons with diabetes use to self-regulate their diabetes? How do these differ from professional suggestions? How effective are these strategies in maintaining metabolic control?
4. What implications does self-regulation have for nursing efforts to facilitate client self-management outcomes?

Subjects with insulin-dependent diabetes mellitus (IDDM) were interviewed to uncover the meanings diabetic patients give their diagnosis, discover the variety of situations they see as modifiers of their illness representations, and determine how these situations become conditions for self-regulating treatment actions.

Design

To describe and explain the process of self-regulation in people with diabetes, 30 subjects with IDDM were interviewed on two occasions, 2 to 3 months apart, using a semistructured interview guide. The first meeting with participants consisted of the interview itself, collection of demographic information, the use of a visual analogue scale (VAS) estimating the subject's perception of current diabetes control and of effort expended to attain control, and a blood sample drawn for glycosylated hemoglobin (GHb) level. The second meeting included additional interview questions, collection of the VAS data, and another blood sample for a repeat GHb level. The interview data were analyzed using a variation of grounded theory (Charmaz, 1990; Chenitz & Swanson, 1986; Glaser & Strauss, 1967) called dimensional analysis (Schatzman, 1986, 1988, 1991).

The GHb blood tests have been used over the past decade to estimate the long-term control of diabetic patients. This test replaced the older system of 24-hour urine collections in determining overall glucose control. The GHb is a blood test that measures the number of molecules of glucose that are attached to the red blood cells. Glucose attaches to proteins in a nonenzymatic, irreversible reaction. Elevation of glycosylated proteins is related to the height of the glucose concentration and the length of time the blood glucose is elevated. Because the life of the erythrocytes is approximately 2 to 3 months, the GHb indicates the average blood glucose level over the past 60 to 90 days. In this study, the GHb levels were used to compare the subjects' estimated level of control and estimated effort expended to gain control with the quantified blood sample level.

The VAS has been used to measure feelings or sensations regarding subjective phenome-

non such as severity of fatigue, intensity of pain, and sensations of dyspnea (Krupp, LaRocca, Muir-Nash, & Steinberg, 1989; Stensman, 1989; Wilson & Jones, 1989). The VAS is used in this study to measure the subjective estimate of the subject's perception of metabolic control. The scores were used to evaluate how well a person felt the self-regulating decisions, assessed in the interview, affected blood sugar control. The Estimate of Diabetes Control Visual Analogue Scale and the Estimate of Effort Expended to Attain Diabetes Control Visual Analogue Scale, developed for this study, are 100-mm solid horizontal lines anchored by words related to poor diabetes control and little effort expended at the 0 point and diabetes control as good as it can be and as much effort as can be expended at the 100 point (Fig. 3-3).

Setting

The sample population was drawn from patients who attended the diabetes training and management course at the Diabetes Center at the University of California, San Francisco. This center represents a cross section of the

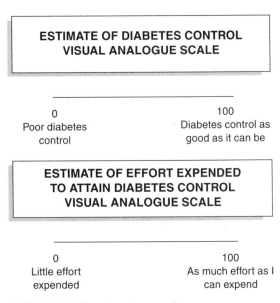

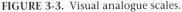

FIGURE 3-3. Visual analogue scales.

multicultural, multiethnic populations of the San Francisco Bay Area. People attending the course come from diverse socioeconomic backgrounds, receive follow-up care in both private and public settings, and represent both genders and all age groups.

Subjects

Sixteen men and 14 women representative of insulin-dependent diabetic clients who attended the course were initially chosen. Selection was based on following criteria:

1. Age between 20 and 55 years
2. Duration of illness between 5 and 20 years
3. No severe diabetes complications requiring specialized medical treatment such as renal dialysis, total blindness, or immobility due to cardiovascular or peripheral vascular disease
4. English speaking and able and willing to give consent to participate in the study

Findings

A qualitative analysis of the data using a grounded theory methodology revealed three major findings. (Numbers in parentheses represent identification code numbers for the study subjects.)

First, the data indicate that *participating in everyday life experiences is the predominant consideration in self-management decisions.* This theme occurs repeatedly and is reflected in comments such as: "I just want to live...a normal life. You know, really do whatever everybody else does."(006)

Second, the findings indicate that subjects evolved into self-regulating behaviors for managing their diabetes treatment through a series of *temporal phases* (Fig. 3-4) designated as:

Becoming diabetic: the rules are followed.
Confronting the illusion of promised normality: the rules are tested.
Pragmatic sufficiency: the rules are customized.

Getting the diagnosis happened to all of the subjects, but past experience with the illness greatly influenced self-management decisions. The spectrum is illustrated by the following:

"I knew it was diabetes because my grandmother and my uncle both had it...I knew what the symptoms were." (030)
"I had no clue. I didn't know what diabetes was, up to that point." (009)

In the phase of becoming diabetic, a person begins to "know" what the illness is. The regimen is taught and the person begins to monitor her or his status through technologic and intuitive means. Subjects described learning the regimen and how they did what the health professionals told them to do. Subjects were often told by care providers that they could live a normal life as long as prescriptions from health care providers were followed. At this point, subjects believed that normal life was possible: "This isn't going to go away...but you would be able to live a very normal life." (004)

It becomes apparent that individuals must also learn to balance life activities with the regimen. As time passes, an awareness grows that the diabetes regimen is problematic and this leads to a sense of unpredictability. Patients question how much ambiguity and unpredictability they can tolerate. The kind of

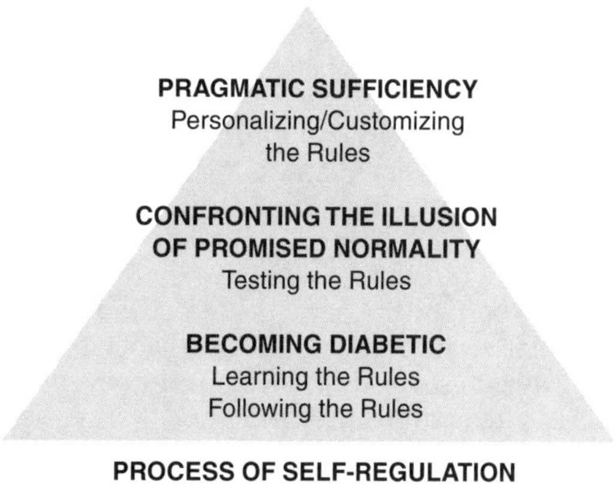

PRAGMATIC SUFFICIENCY
Personalizing/Customizing
the Rules

**CONFRONTING THE ILLUSION
OF PROMISED NORMALITY**
Testing the Rules

BECOMING DIABETIC
Learning the Rules
Following the Rules

PROCESS OF SELF-REGULATION

FIGURE 3-4. Process of self-regulation.

monitoring and the degree of adjusting an individual engages in is determined by the level of tolerance the person develops for these activities. The process of defining what diabetes means is constantly changing and evolving as time passes, and the regimen is analyzed and changed in terms of the new knowledge gained.

In the phase of confronting the illusion of promised normality, a new understanding developed as treatment progressed. Subjects realized that taking insulin is not like taking a pill for an infection. One dose does not work to control glucose levels under all conditions. Taking insulin led to fluctuations in blood glucose levels—up and down, often both in the same day. High and low blood glucose caused symptoms that interfered with normal activity and could be life-threatening. It became clear that there were no real answers to treatment problems. Medical science is not able to give perfect control because the tools are not available to do what the nondiabetic pancreas automatically does. This led to disillusionment with treatment, and the rules were tested.

> "Doctors think their patients do what they tell them, but they don't. They do for some period of time, and then they realize what doctors tell them is not realistic." (027)

> "The hardest part for me was that even when I did everything I was supposed to, I didn't get perfect control; so what was the point?" (014)

Once a person reaches the phase of pragmatic sufficiency, diabetes self-care is adapted into the rest of life. Care is defined as whatever is sufficient to keep symptoms under control so life can go on. Pragmatic sufficiency describes the situation in which the person with diabetes achieves a balance between the need to control the blood glucose levels and the need to participate in certain life activities. Decisions about the relative importance of the diabetes treatment regimen versus participation in everyday social interactions are made, and self-regulating actions are taken in response to these decisions. One subject said she could not be "a professional diabetic" because there was a constant need to pay attention to all the other things she was trying to do.

Strauss and coworkers (1984) and Zola (1981) pointed out that being a patient is only a portion of one's life from the patient's view. Health may be the primary concern of the care provider who may assume that patients share the medicalized view of the world. However, one subject expressed his thoughts in the following way: "It also struck me that it would be great if all diabetics were sort of, very pragmatic, highly organized, lived very disciplined lives, and loved schedules. Unfortunately, I think God has a sense of humor, at least in my case. He certainly married me to the wrong disease, I'm afraid." (027)

The third major finding was that a *form of natural analysis* on the part of the subjects described a process of decision-making related to self-management practices. This schema, originally developed by Schatzman (1986, 1988, 1991), suggests that the choices each person makes are based on understandings, sensitivities, tolerances, and the ability to generate options and calculate the risks and stakes involved in any problem- solving situation (Fig. 3-5).

Choices result from an individual's interpretation of events or problems in life that need decisions or solutions. Each component affects the others to influence decisions and is modified as experience with a situation changes. As the subjects in this study analyzed their changing relationships with diabetes, their self-regulation evolved. This schema helps explain the variation among individuals as each analytic procedure will be based on this private, personal analysis.

Self-regulation is, then, the coordinating or meshing of diabetes care and everyday activities to fit each person's situation. However, this does not necessarily mean better control of diabetes; this is an important point. It means that subjects moved away from getting advice from professionals and made their own decisions about care. The following quotations represent variations that natural analysis produces. Each represents self-management action, rationally analyzed, leading to different consequences:

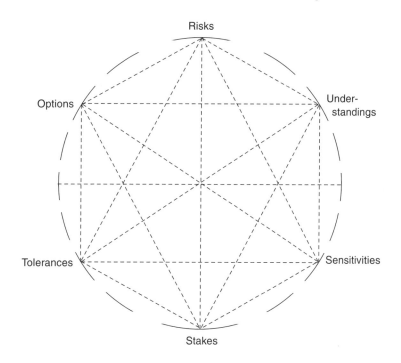

FIGURE 3-5. Personal meaning schema.

"Maybe it [the dose of Regular insulin] would go up from five to six...fish and pasta is a five; but a potato and chicken is a six." (010) In this case, the subject carefully adjusts the insulin by small unit changes based on her experience and analysis.

"Instead of eating a sandwich and an apple for lunch, I'll eat a candy bar. That's two carbohydrates and three fat [exchanges]." (011) In the second case, he is making a choice that would cause a dietitian apoplexy but is technically correct.

Implications and Conclusions of the Self-Regulation Study

Implications of this study for nursing are that the phases of development and the process of natural analysis appear to have a greater impact on treatment adherence than prescriptions imposed by health care providers. Attempts to assist patients with normalization within the constraints of diabetes may be key to developing treatment plans that are consistent with both metabolic control and the social realities of the patient.

Patient education may need to expand its role beyond telling patients what to do to take care of their diabetes. Instead, patient education needs to move toward asking what may seem to be the obvious questions of people to find out what their values and understandings are. Then problem-solving skills can be provided that will equip individuals with tools for analyzing, evaluating, and implementing self-management practices consistent with each person's definition of "living a normal life."

Patient Education for Normalization

Three issues directly related to patient education arise from the results of the study described above. If living a normal life is an important aspect of living with chronic illness, how can living a normal life be translated into treatment regimens meeting the needs of the client? The study on negotiating self-regulation suggests the possibility that as the subjects focused attention on how they managed their diabetes and analyzed their efforts at gaining metabolic control, their ability to accurately predict the actual level of blood glucose control increased. This was reflected in the increase in the correlations between the subjects' assessments of control, effort expended, and the laboratory value for glycosylated hemoglobin levels obtained at the time of the second interview (Fig. 3-6). How can this natural analysis be used in patient education by nurses to encourage better diabetes control?

It is clear that self-regulating behavior has a temporal element to it and changes over time with the disease. With this in mind, how can client education and intervention be continuously reassessed to identify the changing contexts in which decisions are made?

All three of these concerns can be addressed by nursing interventions focused on assisting clients with the analysis of their self-regulating actions and expediting problem identification and definition. Helping clients to verbally articulate their personal analysis leads to clarification of their understandings and meanings of the current diabetes state. Options for care can be explored in an atmos-phere that is consistent with clients' perceptions of how diabetes care fits into their usual life activities. With new options available, clients can set goals better reflecting their own needs, decide on expected outcomes of management practices, and develop solutions to current problems. This type of intervention allows the provider to assist the client in developing criteria for evaluating whether the new management actions are effective in meeting the goals. If the goals are not achieved, clients can be encouraged to use this information as part of further analysis to modify management strategies. The analysis can also assist both client and provider in identifying areas where further education and information may provide new choices related to care.

Applied to practice settings, the client's personal meaning schema can be translated into assessment questions that uncover the client's natural analysis. Box 3-1 provides some guidelines for probing client's feelings toward care and receptivity to change.

The findings suggest that as clients become more sensitive to consequences of the illness, such as at the onset of complications, their tolerances for uncontrolled glucose levels may narrow and more effort will go into controlling glucose levels. The reverse may also occur. With the onset of complications, tolerances for doing intense self-care may decrease if a client feels there is no point in working for controlled blood glucose levels. Each of these understandings leads to different actions and consequences. Treatment regimens should reflect current guidelines for probing changes in understanding, sensitivities, and tolerances.

Options for self-management can be explored by asking the client probing questions as suggested in Box 3-1.

The stakes may be high; an example is the pregnant diabetic woman who must make decisions that affect both her diabetes control and the health of her baby. In this case, the benefits of intensive self-management may outweigh the inconvenience and intrusion of increased testing and strict dietary adherence.

CORRELATION OF GLYCOSYLATED HEMOGLOBIN AND ESTIMATE OF CONTROL

Time 1	Neg. N.S.
Time 2	$r = -0.72$, $p < 0.001$

CORRELATION OF GLYCOSYLATED HEMOGLOBIN AND ESTIMATE OF EFFORT

Time 1	$r = -0.42$, $p < 0.05$
Time 2	$r = -0.62$, $p < 0.001$

FIGURE 3-6. Visual analogue scales and glycosylated hemoglobin correlations.

Patient education geared toward making the client a more active problem-solver changes the role of the provider from that of a controller to that of an advisor or coach. The nurse educator becomes the feedback system helping clients evaluate the viability of the options chosen. In this role, the nurse is a facilitator who functions to assist the client in analyzing progress toward stated goals. This type of nursing intervention allows greater autonomy for the client, and the nurse educator is relieved from being the only problem-solver or expert in the relationship.

Lastly, patient education using the process of self-analysis can be facilitated in cost-effec-

tive group teaching environments. If groups of clients are taught how to analyze problems using a consistent model, group problem-solving methods can increase the number of options and solutions made available to members of the group. Wallerstein and Bernstein (1988) suggest that education in groups promotes a sense of "power to act with others to effect change" (p. 380) and strengthens a person's belief in his or her ability to influence health behaviors. If these types of interventions are to proceed, nurse providers need to learn counseling techniques to help facilitate client self-assessment for informed decision-making related to diabetes care.

Anderson and coworkers (1991) discovered two common difficulties for professionals attempting to develop client-centered teaching and treatment programs. First was the problem that professionals find it difficult to encourage clients to explore and express feelings and emotions related to diabetes. Second, educators have difficulty moving away from the role of problem-solver and giver of advice about the best way to accomplish diabetes self-management goals. "The educator should facilitate and not dominate the process of helping patients come to a decision about pursuing their own diabetes goals" (Anderson et al., 1991, p. 587).

BOX 3–1. Personal Meaning Schema as Assessment Tool

Guidelines for Probing Client's Understanding, Sensitivities, and Tolerances

- What other possibilities do you see for managing this problem?
- Have other options or methods for dealing with this problem been explored?
- If other options have been thought of, the question then becomes:

    What are the costs and benefits of taking that care option?

    How much risk is there in taking such actions?

- Lastly, the concept of stake can be ascertained by asking: What value do you place on the outcome of this/these actions?

Guidelines for Probing Changes in Client's Understanding, Sensitivities, and Tolerances

- What do you think is happening right now for you to be getting these results?
- What bothers you the most about (whatever current problem is)?
- How much (of current problem) are you willing to put up with?
- What are the outer limits of your definition of acceptable control right now?
- What range of blood glucose levels do you define as your goal?

Nursing Education

As nursing moves toward increased specialization and advanced practice in the clinical specialist and nurse practitioner roles, there is a growing need to be experts in the physiologic aspects of health and illness. Increased nursing responsibility for diagnosis and treatment of health problems necessitates incorporating physiologic and pathophysiologic assessment skills into nursing education. In light of these new responsibilities, it is imperative that nursing education not lose sight of the mandate to also treat a person's responses to illness (American Nurses Association, 1980).

Nursing education for those working with diabetic clients needs to include both physiologic and psychosocial assessment skills.

The American Association of Diabetes Educators training program has attempted to set standards for expert practice. Their core curriculum (American Association of Diabetes Educators, 1993) teaches an educator the information to give clients, methods for teaching clients strategies to perform diabetes self-care activities, and strategies to test the client's knowledge of diabetes. The study reported in this chapter proposes that nurses be educated in the natural analytical process to understand how individuals with diabetes treat and use information to make decisions about diabetes self-management. Use of the natural analytical process provides a means for the nurse to overcome the problems mentioned in developing client-centered treatment—allowing clients to express feelings and emotions about diabetes and moving away from the role of sole problem-solver (Anderson et al., 1991). Nursing education needs to teach ways to integrate the products of this process into the content of teaching and treatment plans.

Patient education directed toward increasing the client's capacity to self-assess and self-generate strategies for change are an important part of the nurse educator's role. Methods for teaching professionals how to develop client-centered interventions using interactive counseling models have been developed and offer helpful suggestions that could be integrated into nursing education curricula (Anderson et al., 1991; Funnell, Anderson, et al., 1991; Funnell, Anderson, & Oh, 1994; Funnell, Donnelly, et al., 1991; Tupling, 1981).

Patient Education

Recent reports in the diabetes education literature indicate a move away from knowledge testing as a means of evaluating diabetes management skills. It is clear that giving and receiving information is not the equivalent of knowing how to respond in an independent and appropriate fashion (Funnell, Anderson, et al., 1991; Tupling, 1981). More problem-solving based education is suggested

to help clients work through situations requiring decision making skills on their part (Pichert, Snyder, Kinzer, & Boswell, 1992).

Funnell, Anderson, and associates (1991) suggest that diabetes educators attempting to help clients gain mastery over their diabetes must provide programs using an empowered client model. In this model, both client and professional are problem-solvers and caregivers. Problems, learning needs, and goals and strategies are identified by the client and supported by the professional. The goals of the empowered client model are different from those in the traditional medical model where finding ways for the client to comply with prescribed regimens is the goal of diabetes patient education. The current study supports the client-centered model as a more effective means of assisting clients in maximizing self-management practices.

Summary

This chapter has reviewed several models associated with an individual's decision-making processes as it relates to health management choices. A proposal is made for patient-centered education in which the person being educated is assisted with learning based on self-chosen goals and expectations. As noted at the beginning of the chapter, patient education encompasses all of the domains of nursing as it interacts with the patient, health, and the environment. Patient education is guided by the American Nurses' Association mandate to treat a person's responses to illness; it is the "...*essence of nursing*" (Rankin & Stallings, 1990). Nurses need to provide patient education that assists the client to define what a normal life is in the context of an illness, provide problem-solving skills related to self-management practices, and help clients reevaluate the efficacy of their self-management choices. Further, patient education assists the client and family to create a new way of life (Hagedorn, 1994) and makes the goal individually designed, self-regulated treatment plans.

Strategies for Critical Analysis and Application

1. Have students role play being a person with diabetes. Some students should be assigned the role of being a non–insulin-taking diabetic person who has to go onto a strict dietary regimen. The calories should be appropriate for the student; the idea is to follow a meal plan precisely for a week, adding no extra treats. Other students can be assigned roles with different levels of insulin therapy. For instance, a two injection per day regimen, a three injection per day regimen, and a four injection per day regimen. They all need to perform self-monitoring of the blood glucose, eat the diabetic diet, record all blood sugars and dietary intake, and inject saline in the appropriate doses per instructions. The sales representatives from the various diabetes product companies will often provide the materials necessary for this exercise. Debriefing these experiences at the end of a week can add a great deal of insight into the problems of living with a chronic illness that requires constant self-management practices.

2. Have students play the roles of educator and patient. During the conversations, have some dyads use judgmental language about why there is little or no compliance with suggestions. Use statements such as "What have you been eating to make your blood sugars so bad?" to demonstrate why patients may falsify their records or respond to the educator in a hostile manner. Have students practice using questions to assess the personal meaning of diabetes (or other chronic illnesses) to the individual. Compare the kinds of information received from the two types of communication.

3. Have students listen for references to "noncompliance" in their clinical settings. Use these reports in seminar discussions or postclinical conferences to ask students to suggest other ways to describe the problem. Practice speaking up to other professionals in these circumstances, pointing out the need to consider the context in which the patient is functioning.

4. Have students evaluate the components of the various models presented in this chapter in their clinical settings and discuss the usefulness of the models in a practice context.

REFERENCES

Allison, S. D. (1973). A framework for nursing action in a nurse-conducted diabetic management clinic. *Journal of Nursing Administration, 3*(4), 53-60.

American Association of Diabetes Educators. (1992). The scope of practice for diabetes educators and the standards of practice for diabetes educators. *Diabetes Educator, 18*(1), 52-56.

American Association of Diabetes Educators. (1993). *Diabetes education: a core curriculum for health professionals* (2nd ed.). Chicago: Author.

American Diabetes Association. (1993). Clinical practice recommendations. *Diabetes Care, 16*(Suppl. 2), 1-118.

American Hospital Association. (1972). *The patient's bill of rights.* Chicago: Author.

American Nephrology Nurses' Association. (1991). *Core curriculum for nephrology nursing* (2nd ed.). Pitman, NJ: Author.

American Nephrology Nurses' Association. (1979). *Standards of clinical practice for nephrology nursing* (3rd ed.). Pitman, NJ: Author.

American Nurses Association. (1979). *Model nurse practice act.* Kansas City, MO: Author.

American Nurses Association. (1980). *Nursing: A social policy statement.* Kansas City, MO: Author.

Anderson, R. M. (1985). Is the problem of noncompliance all in our heads? *Diabetes Educator, 11,* 31-34.

Anderson, R. M., Funnell, M. M., Barr, P. A., Dedrick, R. F., & Davis, W. K. (1991). Learning to empower patients: Results of professional education program for diabetes educators. *Diabetes Care, 14,* 584-590.

Backscheider, J. E. (1974). Self-care requirements, self-care capabilities, and nursing systems in the diabetic nurse management clinic. *American Journal of Public Health, 64*(12), 1138-1146.

Becker, M. H. (1974). The health belief model and sick role behavior. In M. H. Becker (Ed.), . Thorofare, NJ: Charles B. Slack, 82-92.

Becker, M. H. (1979). Understanding patient compliance: The contributions of attitudes and other psychosocial factors. In S. J. Cohen (Ed.), *New directions in patient compliance.* Lexington, MA: DC Heath, 1-19.

Becker, M. H., & Janz, N. K. (1985). The health belief model applied to understanding diabetes regimen compliance. *Diabetes Educator, 11*, 41-47.

Cerkoney, K. A. B., & Hart, L. K. (1980). The relationship between the health belief model and compliance of persons with diabetes mellitus. *Diabetes Care, 3*, 594-598.

Charmaz, K. (1990). "Discovering" chronic illness: Using grounded theory. *Social Science and Medicine, 30*, 1161-1172.

Chenitz, W. C., & Swanson, J. M. (1986). *From practice to grounded theory*. Menlo Park, CA: Addison-Wesley.

Christiansen, K. E. (1981). *The determinants of health promoting behavior*. Unpublished doctoral dissertation, Rush University, Chicago.

Conrad, P. (1985). The meaning of medications: Another look at compliance. *Social Science and Medicine, 20*(1), 29-37.

Duffy, M. E. (1988). Determinants of health promotion in midlife women. *Nursing Research, 37*, 358-362.

Duffy, M. E. (1993). Determinants of health-promoting lifestyles in older persons. *Image - The Journal of Nursing Scholarship, 25*, 23-28.

Eisen, M., Zellman, G. L., & McAlister, A. L. (1992). A health belief model-social learning theory approach to adolescents' fertility control: Findings from a controlled field trial. *Health Education Quarterly, 19*, 249-262.

French, B. N., Kurczynski, T. W., Weaver, M. T., & Pituch, M. J. (1992). Evaluation of the health belief model and decision making regarding amniocentesis in women of advanced maternal age. *Health Education Quarterly, 19*, 177-186.

Funnell, M. M., Anderson, R. M., Arnold, M. S., Barr, P. A., Donnelly, M., Johnson, P. D., Taylor-Moon, D., & White, N. H. (1991). Empowerment: An idea whose time has come in diabetes education. *Diabetes Educator, 17*, 37-41.

Funnell, M. M., Anderson, R. M., & Oh, M. S. (1994). Adapting a diabetes patient education program for use as a university course. *Diabetes Educator, 20*(4), 297-302.

Funnell, M., Donnelly, M., Anderson, R., & Sheets, K. (1991, June). *Noncompliance with a diabetes regimen by medical students and diabetes educators*. Poster presented at the 14th International Diabetes Federation Congress, Washington, DC.

Galvin, K. T. (1992). A critical review of the health belief model in relation to cigarette smoking behavior. *Journal of Clinical Nursing, 1*, 13-18.

Glaser, B. G., & Strauss, A. L. (1967). *The discovery of grounded theory*. Hawthorne, NY: Aldine Publishing.

Hagedorn, M. I. (1994). *A way of life: A new beginning each day—the family's lived experience of childhood chronic illness*. Paper presented at the Second International Interdisciplinary Qualitative Health Research Conference, Hershey, PA.

Hawkins, W. E., Duncan, D. F., & McDermott, R. J. (1989). A health assessment of older Americans: Some multidimensional measures. *Preventive Medicine, 17*, 344-356.

Hayes-Bautista, D. E. (1976). Modifying the treatment: Patient compliance, patient control and medical care. *Social Science and Medicine, 10*, 233-238.

Hays, R. D., & DiMatteo, M. R. (1981). Patient compliance assessment. *Journal of Compliance in Health Care, 2*, 37-53.

Hochbaum, G. M. (1958). *Public participation in medical screening programs: A sociopsychological study*. (Public Health Service Publication No. 572). Washington, DC: U.S. Government Printing Office.

Janz, N. K., & Becker, M. H. (1984). The health belief model: A decade later. *Health Education Quarterly, 11*(1), 1-47.

Jayne, R. L. (1993). Self-regulation: Negotiating regimens in insulin-dependent diabetes. *Dissertation Abstracts International, 54*(3), 1334B. Ann Arbor, MI: University Microfilms International.

Keller, M. L., Ward, S., & Baumann, L. J. (1989). Processes of self-care: Monitoring sensations and symptoms. *ANS Advances in Nursing Science, 12*(1), 54-66.

Krupp, L. B., LaRocca, N. G., Muir-Nash, J., & Steinberg, A. D. (1989). The fatigue severity scale: Application to patients with multiple sclerosis and systematic erythematosus. *Archives of Neurology, 46*(10), 1121-1123.

Leventhal, H. (1982). Wrongheaded ideas about illness. *Psychology Today, 16*, 48-55, 73.

Leventhal, H., & Johnson, J. E. (1983). Laboratory and field experimentation: Development of a theory of self-regulation. In P. J. Wooldridge, M. H. Schmitt, J. K. Skipper, & R. C. Leonard (Eds.), *Behavioral science and nursing theory*. St. Louis: CV Mosby.

Leventhal, H., Singer, R., & Jones, S. (1985). Effects of fear and specificity of recommendations upon attitudes and behavior. *Journal of Personality and Social Psychology, 2*, 20-29.

Leventhal, H., Zimmerman, R., & Gutmann, M. Compliance: A self-regulation perspective. In D. Gentry (Ed.), *Handbook of behavioral medicine*. New York: Guilford Press, 369-346.

Meyer, D., Leventhal, H., Gutmann, M. (1985). Common-sense models of illness: The example of hypertension. *Health Psychology, 4*(2), 115-135.

Nightingale, F. (1859/1992). *Notes on nursing: What it is and what it is not*. Philadelphia: J. B. Lippincott.

Pender, N. J. (1982). *Health promotion in nursing practice*. East Norwalk, CT: Appleton-Century-Crofts.

Pender, N. J. (1987). *Health promotion in nursing practice* (2nd ed.). East Norwalk, CT: Appleton & Lange.

Pender, N. J. (1990). Expressing health through lifestyle patterns. *Nursing Science Quarterly, 30*(3), 115-122.

Pender, N. J., Walker, S. N., Sechrist, K. R., & Frank-Stromberg, M. Predicting health-promoting life styles in the workplace. *Nursing Research, 39*, 326-332.

Pitchert, J. W., Snyder, G. M., Kinzer, C. K., & Boswell, E. J. (1992). Sydney meets the ketone challenge—a videodisc for teaching diabetes sick-day management through problem solving. *Diabetes Educator, 18*(6), 476-477, 479.

Rankin, S. H., & Stallings, K. D. (1990). *Patient education: Issues, principles, practices* (2nd ed.). Philadelphia: J. B. Lippincott.

Sackett, D. L. (1976). The magnitude of compliance and noncompliance. In D. L. Sackett & R. B. Haynes (Eds.), *Compliance with therapeutic regimens.* Baltimore: The Johns Hopkins University Press, 9-25.

Sackett, D. L., & Haynes, R. B. (1976). *Compliance with therapeutic regimens.* Baltimore: The Johns Hopkins University Press.

Schatzman, L. (1986). *The structure of qualitative analysis.* Paper presented at the International Sociology Conference, New Deli, India.

Schatzman, L. (1988). *Anchoring grounded theory.* Unpublished manuscript, University of California, San Francisco, Department of Social and Behavioral Sciences.

Schatzman, L. (1991). Dimensional analysis: Notes on an alternative approach to the grounding of theory in qualitative research. In D. Maines (Ed.), *Social organization and social process: Essays in honor of Anselm Strauss.* New York: Aldine de Gruyter.

Stensman, R. (1989). Body image among 22 persons with acquired and congenital severe mobility impairment. *Paraplegia, 27*(1), 27-35.

Strauss, A. L., Corbin, J., Fagerhaugh, S., Glaser, B. G., Maines, D., Suczhet, B., & Weiner, C. L. (1984). *Chronic illness and the quality of life* (2nd ed.). St. Louis: C. V. Mosby.

Trostle, J. A. (1988). Medical compliance as an ideology. *Social Science and Medicine, 27*, 1299-1308.

Tupling, H. (1981). *You've got to get through the outside layer: A handbook for health educators, using diabetes as a model.* Diabetes Education and Assessment Programme of the Royal North Shore Hospital of Sydney and the Northern Metropolitan Health Region of the Health Commission of New South Wales.

Wallerstein, N., & Bernstein, E. (1988). Empowerment education: Freire's ideas adapted to health education. *Health Education Quarterly, 15*(4), 379-394.

Wallston, B. S., Wallston, K. A. (1984). Social psychological models of health behavior: An examination and integration. In A. Baum, S. Taylor, & J. E. Singer (Eds.), *Handbook of psychology and health: Vol. IV. Social psychological aspects of psychology.* Hillsdale, NJ: L. Erlbaum Associates.

Watkins, J. P., Williams, T. F., Martin, D. A., Hogan, M. D., & Anderson, E. (1967). A study of diabetic patients at home. *American Journal of Public Health, 57*, 452-459.

Wilson, R. C., & Jones, P. W. (1989). A comparison of the visual analogue scale and modified Borg scale for the measurement of dyspnoea during exercise. *Clinical Science, 76*(3), 277-282.

Zola, I. K. (1981). Structural constraints in the doctor–patient relationship: The case of non-compliance. In L. Eisenberg & A. Kleinman (Eds.), *The relevance of social science for medicine.* Dordrecht: Reidel, 241-252.

CHAPTER

Special Populations/ Special Challenges

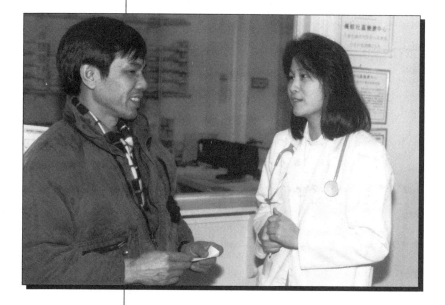

OBJECTIVES FOR CHAPTER 4

After reading this chapter, the nurse or student nurse should be able to:

1 Apply Bronfenbrenner's ecological principles of micro-, meso-, exo-, and macrosystems to patient education for children.

2 Develop a patient teaching plan for an elderly person using life-span developmental concepts.

3 Plan a teaching program for a Native American diabetic man using Kleinman's question as part of the assessment.

4 Estimate the degree of cultural embeddedness, using Tripp-Reimer's and Friedman's assessment tool, of a childbearing family living in the barrio of East Los Angeles.

5 Analyze the stressors facing a migrant family with tubercular family members forced to leave Central America for political reasons.

Patient Education: Issues, Principles, Practices, Third Edition, by Sally H. Rankin and Karen Duffy Stallings.
Lippincott–Raven Publishers, Philadelphia, © 1996.

Health Care Challenges Today

When the first edition of this book was written in the early 1980s, the United States was entering a period of optimism that technology could solve many of the health care ills and that ever- growing affluence would offer greater opportunities to establish creative and sweeping patient education programs. In the mid-1990s, this optimism has been replaced by a realization that technology has complicated rather than solved many health care dilemmas and that although health care reform is touted as an important issue for Americans, the problems related to health care are not easily resolved. The financial depression of the early 1990s and growing social problems related to alienation from "mainstream" society as well as the growing prevalence of diseases such as human immunodeficiency virus infection and acquired immunodeficiency disease that strike young adults has produced challenges for patient education previously unconsidered. Therefore, this chapter addresses patient education as it applies to special populations with theoretical and practice-oriented approaches to the special challenges confronted. Additionally, the chapter addresses in greater detail than has been done in either of the previous editions, special populations such as the elderly, children, and diverse cultural and ethnic groups. Other special populations who offer special challenges are groups who are unaware they are at risk for certain diseases, with the paradigm case of women and heart disease examined.

Developmental Frameworks as the Bases for Patient Education

Developmental frameworks, such as those of Erikson, Piaget, and Duvall, are frequently included in nursing education programs because they offer a theoretical basis to undergird nursing assessment and interventions. Nurses and other health care professionals use the concepts of Erikson's developmental theory when they prepare the young adult for surgery related to repair of a congenital heart anomaly remembering that the primary task at this developmental stage is engendering of intimacy versus despair. They teach a 6-year-old child to self-administer insulin recalling Piaget's stage referred to as preoperational development (see Chap. 14). Likewise, the nurse who prepares the family for the birth of the second child recalls that the tasks of the family with preschool children concern integration of the new family member and ways to cope with sibling jealousy. Although these developmental frameworks are useful, they are limited because they do not consider the multiple determinants that influence individual and family development. Therefore, the following two sections discuss two useful theories, Bronfenbrenner's ecological systems theory and life-span development theory, for understanding the dynamic nature of development and its influence on patient education.

Ecological Systems Theory

Publication of *Ecology of Human Development* in 1979 by Urie Bronfenbrenner, a child developmental psychologist, highlighted the importance of considering the context of individual development. Bronfenbrenner argues that it is impossible to understand the developing person without also understanding the "ecological niches" that govern favorable, or unfavorable, maturation. An "ecological niche" is formed by the intersection of a combination of personal attributes and demographic characteristics (Bronfenbrenner, 1989). Not only is the concept of ecological niche important to understanding development, but it also influences the process of patient education. Thus, an ecological niche in a situation involving a newly diagnosed diabetic adolescent might consist of an upper middle class, two parent and three children urban, Caucasian family, with both parents working and the child attending a private school. The ecological niche for this adolescent may be favorable to patient education and the learning of necessary self-care management skills. Contrast this ecological niche and its influence on patient education with a diabetic adolescent, who is a high school drop-out, living with a single, unemployed parent, and six siblings in a rural southern U.S. household.

Bronfenbrenner contends that the individual is an actor in this process of development that is influenced by the environmental context and the reciprocity of the organism. Therefore, in the example given above we cannot assume until more information is available that the second adolescent would not be capable of developing diabetes self-management skills, although at first glance his ecological niche appears less favorable.

Other important concepts key to understanding Bronfenbrenner's ecological systems theory include four levels of nested concentric structures that are a model for interactive systems that influence and are influenced by the developing person (Fig. 4-1). These interactive systems are: microsystems, mesosystems, exosystems, and macrosystems.

Microsystems are the patterns of activities, roles, interpersonal relationships, and mater-ial characteristics with which the developing individual interacts (Bronfenbrenner, 1979; Bronfenbrenner & Crouter, 1983). Important microsystems with which the child interacts are the family, peer group, and school. Microsystems are the most basic level of system influencing development. In terms of patient education and its intersection with microsystems, the health care professional who is working with a child should consider the quality of family, peer, and school life and how these in turn might influence the child's ability to be receptive to patient teaching.

Mesosystems are interrelated microsystems, such as the interrelationships that occur between a child's family and the school (Bronfenbrenner, 1979). These interrelationships have an impact on the development of the child. Implications for patient education include such examples as children who are enrolled in schools where the family and school together are able to create private environments for children to monitor their blood glucose levels if they wish to conceal their diabetes. When the family and school have limited understanding of each other or interact negatively, the child will not have

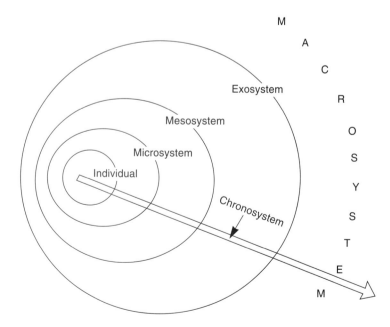

FIGURE 4-1. Bronfenbrenner's ecological framework.

the environmental supports to maintain the self-care activities taught by the health care professional.

Exosystems are environments and conditions external to the child that exert indirect effects on the child's development. Examples of exosystems are parental occupational environments and parental friendships (Bronfenbrenner, 1986). Exosystems are systems the child infrequently enters, but they are structures that can have major effects on the child's maturation. Implications for patient education include parental friendships that affect the manner in which health teaching is interpreted by parents. For example, parents who are encouraged by their friends to send their child to diabetes camp may open up new avenues of patient education for the child who has never before been exposed to other diabetic children. The hospital and health care community are also examples of important exosystems. Schmidt (1990) found that hospitalized children did not have the same levels of fears or postoperative behavior problems as had been reported in an earlier study by Visintainer and Wolfer (1975). This was interpreted as a result of greater parental involvement in the exosystem (i.e., hospital) and more knowledge on the part of children and parents about this influential exosystem. Implications for patient education include enhancing knowledge of parents and children through the schools and the media, especially television, regarding hospitalization so that hospitals as an exosystem are more amenable to children's needs when hospitalized.

Macrosystems are the broadest and most indirect system influences on the child. Macrosystems include the impact of culture, subculture, and embedded belief patterns on the developing child. Macrosystems affect the child through their relationships to the micro-, meso-, and exosystems. Macrosystems and their influence on patient education will be examined later in the chapter in the section on culture and its importance to patient education.

Chronosystems include the dimension of time and were added by Bronfenbrenner in 1986 to expand the theory so that the effects

of change, and continuities, on the developing individual could be better understood (Bronfenbrenner, 1986). Chronosystems are typically conceived as life transitions. The chronosystem is an important thrust that intersects the other systems and thus is illustrated in Figure 4-1 as an arrow. The importance of understanding chronosystems as related to patient education and children entails a constant attendance to the transitions that children and adolescents encounter during the first 20 years of life. For example, the 12-year-old youth who is diagnosed with insulin-dependent diabetes mellitus (IDDM) is most likely entering the tumultuous years associated with adolescence where peer relationships and being part of the crowd are more important than euglycemia. On the other hand, a 3-year-old child diagnosed with IDDM is still within a parentally controlled orbit where peer relationships are secondary to the family sphere. Thus, the life transitions, or chronosystem effects, encountered by the a 12 year old can be postulated as making adjustment to diabetes more difficult than for a 3-year-old child.

A poignant example of the power of the chronosystem and life transitions was seen when I facilitated a support group for parents who had diabetic children. One mother told the story of her 12-year-old son who had been relatively compliant in terms of insulin injections, diet, and self blood-glucose–monitoring (SBGM). She related that as he began spending more time after school in the company of friends she began noticing candy wrappers in his pants pockets. At first he denied he had been eating candy and then he showed her his SBGM log book that he had filled in indicating his blood glucose levels were within acceptable guidelines. Finally following an episode of an upper respiratory infection, he was hospitalized in diabetic ketoacidosis. When he began SBGM again, the nurse noted that he was incorrectly performing the process so that he "fooled" his blood glucose monitor, resulting in false low readings. When confronted with his SBGM technique, he readily admitted what he had done but told his parents it was more important to him that he be "part of the gang" than that he have acceptable blood glucose readings. The ability to normalize is discussed in Chapter 3 from the perspective of diabetic adults with IDDM. Nurses and other health care providers should realize that chronosystem influences are frequently more significant than long-term health outcomes to patients. Understanding patients from the perspective of life transitions can add greater clarity and direction to patient teaching.

In summary, Bronfenbrenner's ecological systems theory can be a means of sensitizing the health care professional working with children and adolescents to the various dimensions influencing development not commonly considered in traditional approaches. Although the theory is encumbered by the jargon used by Bronfenbrenner, the importance of considering individuals in the broadest context of development is an important contribution from Bronfenbrenner's work.

Life-Span Development Frameworks

Life-span development frameworks, also referred to as life-course perspective, evolved in the 1960s and 1970s, as a result of life-span developmental psychologists and life-course perspective sociologists and their research that looked at the interrelated effects of age, cohort experience, and nonnormative life events on development. Unlike Bronfenbrenner who added the concept of chronosystem almost as an afterthought, the life-span developmental psychologists had long been involved in longitudinal studies of various U.S. cohorts. Their work was also influenced by the "stage developmentalists" such as Erikson and Duvall, but as in Bronfenbrenner's case they realized that there was more to development than simply an orderly progression through stages. Although ecological systems theory is a useful device for considering the many influences on development and, in turn, their influence on patient education, it pertains primarily to children and adolescents. Life-span developmental frameworks,

however, are applicable to people across the life span and add a particularly salient dimension to the work of health care professionals with aged adults.

The life-span developmental framework as outlined by various social scientists (Baltes, Reese, & Lipsitt, 1980; Featherman, 1981; Schaie, 1986) is a useful conceptual approach for considering the dynamic, integrated aspects of human functioning (Fig. 4-2). A basic assumption of this model is that biologic, environmental, and behavioral determinants, in conjunction with specified developmental influences, shape the life span of individuals and families. Important developmental influences that should be considered by health care professionals appraising the effects of adult development on patient education include normative age-graded factors, that is, person-related biologic and environmental variables that exhibit a high correlation with chronological age; normative history-graded factors, for example, the historical events that influence particular birth cohorts; and nonnormative factors, that is, life events that occur asynchronously with the life course or are not experienced by the population at large.

Normative age-graded factors overlap with the psychological and cognitive stages outlined by developmental theorists such as Erikson and Piaget; they also coincide with normative physical development. Although normative age-graded factors are frequently taken for granted when planning patient education, the importance of considering the effects of age on patient education is illustrated below in the case of women with coronary heart disease (CHD).

The fact that women are usually older than men when they experience an acute myocardial infarction (MI) has implications for recovery and rehabilitation from MI and may also be related to their greater incidence of death from MI (Dittrich, Gilpin, Nicod, Cali, Henning, & Ross, 1988). Older women are likely to have preexisting comorbidities that may limit participation in cardiac rehabilitation programs and exercise regimens. For example, limited mobility as a result of

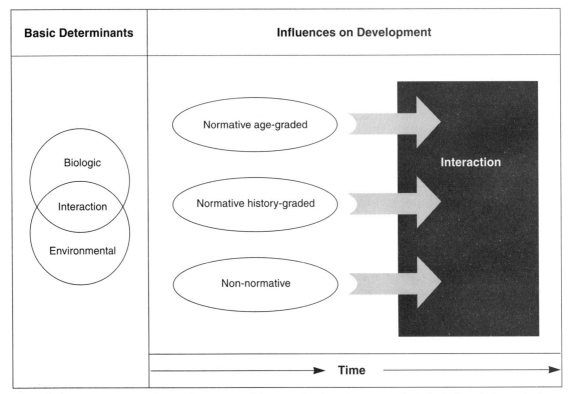

FIGURE 4-2. Determinants and influences on life-span development: a methodological and theoretical approach. (From "Life-span Developmental Psychology" by P.D. Baltes, H. W. Reese, & L. P. Lipsitt, 1980, *Annual Review of Psychology, 31,* p.65.)

osteoarthritis and rheumatoid arthritis, peripheral vascular disease, and orthopedic impairments are comorbid conditions that may impinge on the ability of older women to participate in cardiac rehabilitation programs. Thus, any attempts to effectively educate the older woman post-MI must contemplate preexisting comorbidities and plan methods of exercise that consider them.

Implications of Normative Age-Graded Factors for the Elderly

A meta-analysis of diabetes patient education research examining the effectiveness of diabetes patient teaching interventions found that across 73 studies normative age-graded factors were especially important (Brown, 1992). Brown's meta-analysis revealed that

diabetes teaching interventions were less effective for older patients and that for patients older than 55 years, glycosylated hemoglobin levels were only minimally improved by teaching interventions. She surmises that older diabetic patients may need more individualized instruction than younger patients and that rather than mixing diabetes management regimen (i.e., insulin versus oral hypoglycemic versus diet) across group participants, it might be better to segregate by diabetes type and regimen.

Continuing with the example of older women and MI, important *normative history-graded influences* can be identified as attitudes toward health promotion, health restoration, and health maintenance. Health promotion, restoration, and health maintenance activities relating to CHD include cigarette smoking and eating and exercise patterns. Cigarette smoking has been identified as the most prominent risk factor for heart disease in women (Castelli, 1988; Corrao, Becker, Ockene, & Hamilton, 1990). Smoking appears to have synergistic effects because it increases the risk for heart disease and MI if used in conjunction with oral contraceptives and if hyperlipidemia is present (Corrao et al., 1990; Murdaugh, 1990). The cohort of women who are presently experiencing CHD and MI were naive to the harmful impact of tobacco on the cardiovascular system when they began smoking and thus did not have the benefit of the information available to younger women who are currently making decisions regarding smoking. Although they now are privileged to the same information acquired by younger persons, patient education strategies need to be oriented toward improving the quality of life they have left rather than preventing the onset of coronary artery and other vascular diseases as is done with teenagers and young adults.

Other prominent health promotion and restoration activities related to CHD include dietary intake and exercise. In a similar fashion to information regarding cigarette smoking, dietary information was not available to women when they were young and establishing health promotion activities. Today's cohort of women with CHD and MI may have amended their current eating patterns, but prior behavior may have already established irreversible atherosclerosis. Exercise to establish adequate cardiovascular health has health promotive and health restorative functions. However, the cohort of women who are experiencing CHD and MI today were less likely to engage in health promotive vigorous exercise when they were younger than is found in their more youthful counterpart. Additionally, only a small percentage of women experiencing MI are likely to engage in structured cardiac rehabilitative exercise for health restoration (Wenger & Hellerstein, 1992). Therefore, health care professionals seeking to provide cardiac rehabilitation and its attendant patient education to older women must consider these history-graded factors and amend cardiac rehabilitation programs so that they appeal to older women and are based on their own life experience.

Health maintenance history-graded effects include the belief by most women that they were not at risk for CHD and MI because it was considered a male disease. Such beliefs, which have also been prominent in the health care community, have resulted in less attention given to the clinical symptoms with which women present with CHD and MI, and thus fewer diagnostic procedures and laboratory tests have been performed that may have assisted in earlier identification of CHD and better management. The patient education implications for these health maintenance history-graded effects include the fact that women across the life span need education informing them of their risk for CHD and the symptoms that may indicate the occurrence of angina or MI.

Nonnormative factors, or those events that occur unexpectedly during the life span, often offer the greatest challenge to the health care professional conducting patient education because they include the onset of acute or chronic illnesses at times seemingly asynchronous with usual occurrence. For example, most women are unprepared for the diagnosis of MI at the age of 40; indeed, 40-year-old men are equally unprepared. Unexpected and severe illnesses are generally unexpected in young children and thus challenge the health care professional who must educate the parents and help the family cope. The family that discovers it must be prepared to manage IDDM in their 18-month-old child is faced with a nonnormative event of such monumental proportions that the parents will probably require additional teaching time as well as additional support in managing the potential future losses envisioned. Therefore, nonnormative factors should be recognized by the nurse during the assessment process as conceivably requiring more time and greater resources than normative age-graded or normative history-graded factors that may influence patient education strategies.

Ramifications of the Life-Span Framework for Patient Education

All too often nurses and other health care professionals do not consider the multiple factors that influence a particular patient's receptivity to patient teaching. If we assess patients within the multiple constraints of life-span development, we can better particularize the nature of our teaching. Examples using the life-span approach were cited above for older women with CHD. Consideration of the normative age-graded influences remind us that at different ages people will approach learning from distinct vantage points. Remembering that patients are products of the historical eras in which they matured also should give us indications of what is appropriate for different birth cohorts. For example, women born during the baby boom era (1946–1964) have willingly embraced physical exercise in many different forms. Their mothers, on the other hand, were less likely to exercise to the point of maximal cardiovascular capacity. The female baby boomers who have MIs will probably be open to cardiac rehabilitation, whereas their mothers are less likely to become involved. Attitudinal differences toward sexuality, reproductive health, and raising children are major cohort effects found in these two generations of women. These are only a few disparities in these two generations; the health care provider must constantly consider history-graded factors, or cohort effects, when planning patient education. Lastly, nonnormative factors challenge the nurse to further individualize patient education efforts so that the patient's own particular experience is viewed from an appropriate perspective.

Special Challenges Involved in Teaching the Patient From a Different Ethnocultural Group

The first and second editions of this text relegated patient education with clients from different cultural backgrounds to appendices or the Roundtable chapter. This approach is representative of the inadequate attention that has generally been given to patient education with members of different cultural groups during the past two decades. The growing realization that the United States is not a "melting pot" where immigrants are assimilated into American mainstream culture but is instead a country of many cultures has led to a growing appreciation of different ethnocultural groups. This realization has resulted in various attempts to provide culturally sensitive patient education. One of the problems, however, is that it is virtually impossible for health care providers to learn the cultural dynamics of all of the various ethnocultural groups in the United States. Parenthetically, the provision of culturally appropriate patient teaching is also recognized in other countries experiencing large scale immigration. The Netherlands, for example, has attempted innovative strategies to sensitize providers to the needs of Turkish and Moroccan patients, although Dutch health education specialists readily admit the limitations of their strategies (Glastra & Kats, 1992). The problem is twofold: is there a generic assessment approach that can help providers learn to assess clients from many different cultural backgrounds, and how can providers become more sensitive to the needs of multicultural clients? We believe it is presumptuous to specify patient education approaches for different cultural, racial, and ethnic groups because so many variations exist among and between groups. Therefore, because no health care provider can become knowledgeable about all of the different ethnocultural groups, we believe it is more useful to present overall frameworks from which to assess culture and to refer readers to the many excellent texts available on different ethnocultural groups.

Before presenting a generic approach to understanding ethnocultural influences on patient education some basic definitions should be outlined. *Culture* is generally viewed as a blueprint for ways of living, thinking, and behaving (Friedman, 1986). Culture is learned within the family and guides the ways in which we solve problems and live our daily lives. *Ethnicity* is closely related to culture although it usually implies a particular cultural group or race that interacts and has common interests. There is as much diversity within ethnic groups as between them. For example, Hispanics are often stereotyped as an ethnic group; however, there are enormous differences between Cubans and Mexicans even though they share Spanish surnames.

Understanding Explanatory Models of Illness and Their Influence on Patient Education

Arthur Kleinman is a psychiatrist and anthropologist who has endeavored to help health care professionals understand the meanings that people attribute to illness (Kleinman, Eisenberg, & Good, 1978; Kleinman, 1988). In the attempt to attribute meaning to seemingly disordered events, patients and families develop means of interpreting the events, symptoms, and illnesses they experience. Kleinman has developed a concept called explanatory models of illness that is especially applicable to chronic illness. Explanatory models of health and illness are shaped by cultural factors that govern the perception, labeling, explanation, and valuation of discomforting symptoms or diseases experienced by individuals (Kleinman et al., 1978). Kleinman points out, as have others, that *illness* is the understanding patients have of what is happening to them. Illness is the uniquely personal experience of disease, whereas *disease* is the health care professional's biomedical understanding of the problem.

Kleinman was one of the first health care professionals to recognize the importance of the various domains of influence on individuals beliefs and actions related to disease and illness. These domains comprise professional, popular, and folk areas of influence (Kleinman et al., 1978; Kleinman, 1988). The *professional* domain is the one within which the health care professional operates. Within the professional domain knowledge related to diseases is learned and therapeutic strategies are used. The *popular* domain includes the family,

relatives, other kith and kin, and the community. This domain is probably the most powerful influence on patients and one with which the tactical patient educator will constantly interact. The popular domain is consulted first by patients in approximately 70% to 90% of all situations involving illness in western and nonwestern cultures (Kleinman et al., 1978). The third domain, *folk*, comprises nonprofessional healers. Examples of folk healers are the curanderas/curanderos who are important in many Hispanic groups. Other important healers who may be consulted in illness situations are Native American medicine people and Chinese herbalists. The nurse educator should constantly be aware of the other two domains and not assume that the professional domain is the only one consulted by or important to the patient.

To reconcile the patient's and health care worker's understanding of the situation, Kleinman and his colleagues (1978) suggest eight questions that are useful in understanding the meaning given to the problem by the patient (Box 4-1).

By asking the patient and the family these questions before patient education is initiated valuable information is received that assists in focusing the presentation of needed material.

BOX 4–1. Eight Questions to Reveal a Patient's Illness Perspective

- What do you think has caused your problem?
- Why do you think it started when it did?
- What do you think your illness does to you? How does it work
- How severe is your illness? Will it have a short or long course?
- What kind of treatment do you think you should receive?
- What are the most important results you hope to receive from this treatment?
- What are the chief problems your illness has caused for you?
- What do you fear most about your illness?

For example, Rankin recently completed a study of Chinese Americans with non-IDDM (R21 Institute of Diabetes, Digestive, and Kidney Diseases DK45184; Rankin, Galbraith, & Johnson, 1993). The purpose of the study was to develop an understanding of the meanings that diabetic Chinese Americans attributed to their diabetes so that patient education programs could be planned that more specifically met their learning needs. We were surprised to find in answer to question seven that 33% of the participants felt stigmatized by their families and coworkers because of their diabetes. They stated that either they or their family members believed diabetes was contagious. One young father who recognized the fear of contagion said "my wife won't let me serve my children food with my chopsticks." Acting on this information, the health care professional should realize that fears related to contagion can be alleviated although feelings of being stigmatized are more difficult to influence. Other themes that were noted included answers to question five regarding treatment. For example, it was common for participants to discuss treatment in terms of "powerful others," a term we identified as suggestive of the power health care professionals, especially physicians, had in influencing management. Implications for this explanatory model and patient teaching entail involving physicians in the patient education enterprise in some way.

Use of Kleinman's eight questions can assist the health care provider who is from a different cultural or ethnic background than the patient respond in a more creative and less judgmental manner than otherwise. Because the patient's interpretation of illness is more significant than the health care provider's representation of the disease, it behooves the health care provider to teach from a position of mutual understanding rather than a traditional western medicine stance with which the provider may feel more comfortable but is less efficacious.

Assessing Cultural Embeddedness

Dr. Marilyn Friedman (1986, 1992), building on the work of Tripp-Reimer and associates (1984), has developed a useful approach, which we have turned into questions, to determine the degree of family embeddedness in one's native culture. These questions expedite the process of assessing for acculturation so that the nurse or other health care provider has some indication of the extent to which the patient's native cultural practices may influence patient teaching.

Below are the questions that are useful in assessing acculturation:

1. How recently has immigration occurred? Was it desired or forced? Were there intermediate countries in which the patient was either detained or in which he lived before leaving for the United States? Usually, it can be assumed that the more recent the immigration the less the acculturation. If the patient was forced to leave his native culture and was detained in other countries in the process of leaving, as has happened with many southeast Asian immigrants, the process of acculturation is more likely to be delayed because of painful experiences during the process.

2. From what country did the patient immigrate? How different is the native culture from U.S. culture? If the patient immigrated from a western European country, acculturation problems are minimal. However, the patient who immigrates from a nonwestern European country, an Asian, an African, or South American nation, may take longer to become acculturated and comfortable in the U.S. medical system.

3. Are the patient's friends from the same ethnic group, or does he have friends from the predominant ethnocultural group? Because most people seek a level of comfort in their daily interactions, it is not uncommon for new immigrants to associate only with others from their native culture. It may

take more than one generation before the immigrant group feels comfortable associating with the predominant ethnocultural group and even then most friends may not be of this group. The implications for patient education are primarily that the greatest influence on responses to illness may not be those with which we are familiar.

4. Are religious, social, and recreational activities within the cultural group of origin? The answer to this question also gives the nurse an idea about the degree of cultural embeddedness. Religious beliefs may influence the openness of the patient and family to patient teaching and thus should be assessed.

5. Where does the patient live? Is it an ethnoculturally diverse neighborhood or is it ethnically homogeneous? The recency of immigration can frequently be traced through the neighborhood within which the patient lives. In the United States, it is possible for immigrants to remain within a community in which the native language is the primary language spoken; street signs are in the native language, and newspapers are also in this language. Chinatown in both New York and San Francisco is a good example of this phenomenon. Thus, a patient who is embedded in the original culture may not have as many neighborhood contacts with the predominant cultural group and may be a greater challenge in terms of patient teaching.

6. Does the patient maintain traditional dietary habits and dress? Traditional dietary habits are frequently maintained for many generations, whereas traditional dress is usually given up sooner unless it is also closely associated with religious beliefs (e.g., Muslim women). Traditional dietary habits should be acknowledged and worked into patient teaching plans. Traditional dietary habits of native peoples are almost always healthier than U.S. eating habits because there is little use of processed foods or overuse of animal fats. We have found that when immigrant diabetic pa-

tients return to their original dietary patterns their diabetes is easier to manage.

7. Is the native language spoken exclusively or only in the home? If the native language is spoken exclusively, the patient can be assumed to be more culturally embedded. In these cases an interpreter is usually necessary. Guidelines for culturally sensitive patient teaching using an interpreter are below.

8. What is the territorial complex of the patient? Does the person leave the ethnocultural neighborhood or does he frequent it exclusively? Patients whose territorial complex is comprised exclusively of the ethnocultural neighborhood are usually more culturally embedded than those who leave the neighborhood. Implications for patient education include the necessity of clear directions to the health center or hospital or, better still, the possibility of a home visit for purposes of patient education.

9. Does the patient use a folk medicine or traditional healer? Use of a folk healer or native healing practices is not an unusual occurrence and is frequently one that can be encouraged as long as the practices are safe. The American Academy of Nurses Expert Panel Report on culturally competent health care suggests that an 800 telephone number could be established for nurses who need additional information about cultural practices (Davis, Dumas, Ferketich, et al., 1992). Such a resource would allow the patient educator to tailor the teaching for the patient with whom she is working.

10. Is there discrimination against the ethnocultural group to which the family belongs? If discrimination exists, the process of acculturation will be more difficult. The history of racism, ethnocentrism, and intolerance for others who do not reflect the ethnocultural practices of the mainstream have been well documented. Nurses and other health care providers are just as guilty of such discrimination as other U.S. citizens. A recognition of discrimination toward the immigrant patient should suggest to the patient educator that acculturation will be

hindered and that attitudes of trust and respect are imperative for establishing a climate conducive to patient education.

11. Anderson, a Canadian nurse researcher, adds another question that can be helpful to the health care professional who is trying to assess the degree of acculturation (Anderson, 1987). Is the patient from a rural or urban area in the country of origin? Immigration from a rural area implies less knowledge of western medical practices and the dominant cultural group. This is especially true of rural immigrants from Asian, African, and South American countries.

Important nursing leaders who have developed models of cultural assessment and transcultural nursing theory include Tripp-Reimer and Leininger. Tripp-Reimer's work is referred to in this chapter. Leininger's theory of transcultural nursing is outlined in her book, *Transcultural Nursing: Concepts, Theories, and Practices* and in more recent publications in the journal *Nursing and Health Care*.

Tripp-Reimer and Afifi (1989) describe the above assessment as the first stage of cultural assessment. The next stage of assessment in situations comprising patient teaching involves obtaining information regarding the specific clinical domain. Knowledge about the clinical domain can be obtained using the questions suggested by Kleinman. For example, if a newly arrived immigrant man has just been diagnosed with hypertension, it is helpful to ask the eight questions suggested by Kleinman to find out how he interprets hypertension. The answers to these questions can then be understood within the broader cultural assessment developed by Tripp-Reimer and colleagues (1984), expanded by Friedman (1986, 1992), and outlined above.

Tripp-Reimer and Afifi (1989) characterize the third stage in assessment for purposes of patient education as the eliciting of detailed cultural considerations that may influence intervention strategies. For example, if the intervention strategy involves insulin injections, then data must be obtained about cultural attitudes toward injections. We found that many of the diabetic Chinese Americans did not want to use insulin and were willing to tolerate higher blood glucose levels to avoid self-injections. In some situations underlying fears are connected to intervention strategies that may not be recognized by the health care provider. For example, we found that some diabetic Chinese Americans feared taking insulin because they knew others who began insulin and became blind. Although health care providers know the causal agent was not insulin, it is difficult to convince persons whose belief systems, and limited experience, embrace such a view. The Kleinman questions that deal with the interpretation and meaning of illness are again useful in terms of gathering data related to this type of detailed assessment. Cultural considerations related to such topics as death, sexuality, childbirth, and women's health are frequently topics poorly understood in terms of their cultural implications by the health care provider and should be probed with care and respect.

Bringing About Effective Patient Education With Different Ethnocultural Groups

Once the cultural assessment has been completed tactics to achieve effective patient teaching with culturally diverse populations must be considered. Tripp-Reimer and Afifi (1989) suggest that the process must include "cultural negotiation" or "cultural brokerage." These processes use as a basis the patient's interpretations and meanings as discussed above in light of Kleinman's work. For example, once the health care provider obtains an answer to question five, cultural negotiation can take place in terms of bargaining for a treatment regimen that is acceptable to patient and provider. An illustration of such a situation was found when Rankin conducted her study with diabetic Chinese Americans. Because the practice of Chinese medicine often includes the use of herbal teas and special broths, Chinese patients were encouraged to use these non-western treatments once it was ascertained they were not harmful. On the other hand, these same individuals were encouraged to use the prescribed western medicines such as oral hypoglycemics and insulin. Another example of effectively joining western and Chinese traditional medical approaches was seen in dietary teaching. A Chinese dietitian cleverly used the beliefs about cold (yin) and hot (yang) foods and the importance of achieving balance to plan meals that were acceptable to her diabetic patients.

An example of conflict that can occur between the health care professional attempting patient education and the patient involved an elderly Chinese immigrant who consistently had blood glucose readings of 400 mg/dL or higher for which he refused to take insulin. In answer to the question about what he feared most about his illness he stated that he feared dying in the United States without having anyone from his family, from whom he was alienated, willing to take responsibility for proper burial according to traditional beliefs. He had no particular fears about his diabetes and was totally unwilling to conform to western medical practices. We acknowledged the lack of agreement between our two positions but did not prevent him from returning to the comprehensive health center for additional information regarding diabetes nor did we affirm his position. This type of situation tends to be trying for the health care professional who wants the patient to do what she or he believes is correct. However, the autonomy of the adult patient must be recognized and respected; at best we can only hope that the patient will change his mind.

Frequently the use of health care providers from the patient's own culture is recommended as a means of achieving more effective patient education and better responses to desired outcomes. Although this approach may be successful, we have found that if there is a tremendous chasm between the beliefs of providers and patients, and if providers have become westernized, the disdain with which

they view the traditional beliefs may cause them to be nontherapeutic with members of their own cultural group. Thus, we cannot always assume that a match between language and culture will ensure effective patient education.

Using Interpreters for Patient Education Purposes

Once the assessment process has been completed including the components outlined in Chapter 7 as well as the approaches outlined above, the implementation of patient teaching begins. However, if the nurse or other health care professional is not fluent in the patient's language then it is necessary to obtain interpreter services. The use of interpreters is preferred over the use of translators. *Interpreters* are usually professionally trained persons who interpret the meaning of words and phrases from the health care provider's language to the patient's language. A *translator* does not typically have the same fluency in both languages and may lose the cultural nuances and meanings that an interpreter is skilled at conveying. Frequently, family members are asked to act as translators if there is no one else who can act as an interpreter. Family members are probably the least desirable source of translators because they may filter what the health care provider is trying to tell the patient and, conversely, what the patient is trying to tell the health care provider. Using family members as translators also puts undue stress on both the patient and the family member. The family member may attempt to protect the patient by not revealing what the health care provider has said or, on the other hand, may believe that the health care provider would not be interested in the patient's information.

When the nurse or other health care provider is using the services of an interpreter, it is important to remember that rather than speaking to the interpreter it is best to speak directly to the patient. Patient educators should also be cognizant of their own body language and make certain that it is culturally sensitive. Many large institutions use their own employees to serve as volunteer translators. Although this method is usually successful, the health care provider should be sympathetic to such issues as gender when the information that must be taught involves sexuality or female or male reproductive health. It is also undesirable to let employees who know the patient serve as translators if the material to be taught is especially sensitive. Whether translators or interpreters are used, the health care provider should speak slowly, avoid undue of medical terminology, and arrange for the patient to ask questions. If possible, the patient should be given the opportunity to return demonstrate the material that was taught.

Migration as a Special Stressor in Situations Involving Patient Education

Migration, whether desired or forced, is becoming an important factor in the delivery of health care in the United States. Nurses and other health care providers should be attuned to the implications of migration when they are providing patient education.

In 1979, Sluzki described a pattern that is still useful in understanding the stresses that accompany migration (Fig. 4-3). The first stage is the *preparatory stage* during which the migrating individual and family experience a period of excitement that is similar to euphoria.

Although this period may be accompanied by some doubts, it is frequently a time when the migration is seen as an answer to all of the family's problems. The second stage, *migration*, is a transition period, but unlike many other important transitions it has no accompanying rituals. This lack of rituals means the family must accommodate the experience without the help of prescribed behaviors.

Following the migration or physical act of leaving is a *period of overcompensation* that lasts for approximately 6 months. During this period the family makes extreme efforts to adapt to the new environment. Although the family may cling to hope of returning to the country of origin, maximal efforts are being made to adjust to the new setting. Children are enrolled in schools, attempts are made to find work and suitable housing, and adults may enroll in English as a second language classes. Eventually, disillusionment sets in and a *period of decompensation or crisis* occurs. During this fourth period the family is attempting to shape a new reality for itself. Sometimes a crisis occurs because the children may adapt more quickly than the parents and make more demands on the parents than had been made in their native countries. Finally, the family adjusts at some level to the migration; citizenship may be applied for and gained, and adaptation occurs to a greater or lesser extent. Sluzki states that a *transgenerational impact of migration* occurs that must be faced by later generations. For example, whatever issues have been avoided

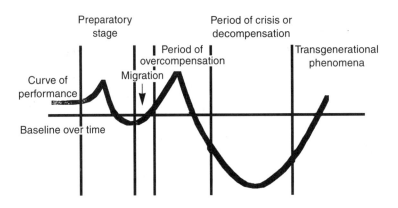

FIGURE 4-3. Migration and stress. (Adapted from "Migration and Family Conflict" by C. E. Sluzki, 1979, *Family Process, 18,* p. 381.)

by the first generation will cause clashes between the first and second generations.

For the health care provider faced with issues of patient teaching, a knowledge of the stage of migration in which the individual and family are situated is important. If the family is in the period of overcompensation and presents to the nurse, opportunities for patient teaching may be better than during the period of decompensation. An example of this involved adolescent immigrants at a high school for new immigrants on the West Coast of the United States. Many of the adolescents were from southeast Asia where rates of tuberculosis are high. Parents and children typically were fairly compliant in terms of taking isoniazid during this period of overcompensation because of a desire for the children to obtain an education. Indeed, during this period parents and children were amenable to patient education involving issues of basic health and safety. As time went on and the harsh realities of daily life led to decompensation, some of these adolescents began consuming large quantities of alcohol and cigarettes. The initial healthy diets from their homelands were discarded and American junk foods were consumed. Thus, the window of opportunity may be narrow in terms of instituting new health practices for migrant adolescents.

The transgenerational impact of migration is illustrated beautifully in such popular literature as Amy Tan's books, *The Joy Luck Club* and *The Kitchen God's Wife*. In terms of patient teaching, we have found situations involving diabetic Chinese migrants who maintain traditional Asian treatment strategies, whereas their acculturated children want them to avail themselves of western medicine. The challenge for the health care provider is not to become involved in the transgenerational struggles but to respect the two positions and allow opportunities for teaching that recognize the importance of both generations.

Undesired migration, or *forced relocation*, is another special stressor that should be considered in situations of patient education. If migration is not desired, then patient teach-ing may be more difficult. The characteristics of undesired migration are different from those of desired migration and are outlined below as originally developed by Tyhurst (1951) and elaborated more recently by others (Scudder & Colson, 1982). The *motivation to emigrate* may be based on desire to escape an overwhelmingly negative situation. For example, many migrants from Haiti, El Salvador, and Yugoslavia experienced physical and psychological terrorism in their own countries before migration.

A second characteristic is that *vertical mobility* is limited in the country of origin and may be limited in the United States. Many Haitians migrating to the United States have experienced overwhelming poverty in Haiti and have not had the opportunity to obtain an education or job skills, thus limiting their access to economic opportunity in the United States. A third characteristic of undesired migration is that there may have been *repeated moves or frequent changes* before and after the migration. These frequent changes can lead to *physical and psychological rootlessness* that can result in physical manifestations of stress. Morbidity and mortality increase in such situations above the rates experienced in desired migration.

Chaotic circumstances of the move such as having to leave the country of origin in haste and with few belongings add to the sense of rootlessness once relocation has occurred. Lastly, *prolonged exposure to extreme stressors* exacerbates undesired migration. For example, Vietnamese families who left Vietnam in the late 1970s and early 1980s frequently were moved from one refugee camp to another before arriving in the United States. Family members were separated and reunited only after many years apart.

Therefore, the patient educator must be attuned not only to the stages of migration but to the process by which migration occurred. If migration was undesired, the process of patient education will be fraught with more difficulties than if it had been desired. The Hmong people, a group of southeast Asians from Laos, are a good illustration of the adversities inherent in forced migration. The

Hmong, originally a group of subsistence farmers, suffered terrible persecution in Laos following the Vietnam War. Following the war and subsequent flight, thousands of men, women, and children died in attacks by Pathet Lao Communist soldiers, exposure to biologic warfare, or hazards encountered in the jungles. Once they escaped from Laos to Thailand they were frequently shifted from one immigrant camp to another before arriving in the United States. Of all recent immigrants they had the least education, and minimal exposure to modern technology and western health care (Sherman, 1988).

Acculturation in the United States has been made more difficult by their unfamiliarity with western conveniences, the lack of a written language, minimal education and work skills except for farming, and religious belief systems that are different than those of most health care providers. The Hmong have experienced a high incidence of NIDDM after immigration, a phenomenon that is common to migrating peoples who make vast life-style changes in terms of exercise, diet, and exposure to stressors. Health care providers attempting patient education with diabetic Hmong adults are confronted with multiple problems related to ethnocultural assessment and also with the overlay of forced migration. The challenges that the Hmong present to health care providers are not atypical in the United States or Canada today.

Summary

This chapter presents frameworks for understanding the special populations and special challenges with which the nurse and other health care professionals are constantly confronted in today's changing health care environment. Using Bronfenbrenner's ecological systems framework helps the nurse consider influences on children that may impede attempts to successfully perform patient education. Similarly, viewing older adults within a life-span perspective that considers multiple developmental influences offers an opportunity to tailor patient education to match the age and cohort effects that may influence patient education outcomes.

A generic approach to understanding the power of culture and its influence on patient education is presented because we believe that it is presumptuous to specify patient education approaches for different cultural, racial, and ethnic groups. The questions that Kleinman developed are suggested as methods of learning more about the ethnocultural group of interest and their beliefs about illness. Additionally, questions developed by Tripp-Reimer as a means of assessing cultural embeddedness are presented so that the patient educator can develop a rudimentary understanding of the possible influence of culture on any teaching efforts. The unique stressors associated with forced immigration are discussed with the Hmong from southeastern Asia used as an example.

Although the special challenges engendered by other than the prototypical patient teaching situations can be anxiety provoking, they can also offer some of the greatest rewards in terms of patient education. Nurses and other health care providers are encouraged to use the frameworks suggested in this chapter to enrich their practices.

Strategies for Critical Analysis and Application

1. You are the nurse caring for Randy, a 7-year-old Caucasian boy with multiple episodes of acute asthma, two of which have required hospitalization in the last 6 months. At home with Randy are his 5-year-old sister who also has asthma, although hers is better controlled, two favorite cats, and his single-parent mother. Randy has been playing soccer as part of the YMCA's program and is doing age-appropriate second grade school work. Randy's father lives in an adjacent community and has a girlfriend who thinks Randy is "wimpy" because he cannot keep up with her 7-year-old daughter when he has an exacerbation of his asthma.

   Using Bronfenbrenner's ecological systems theory, identify the different systems impacting Randy and their influence on your attempt to derive a patient education plan.

2. Frank Wilson is 72-year-old World War II veteran who has had a triple coronary artery bypass graft at the local Veterans Administration hospital. You are the health care provider who sees him in the outpatient clinic for his first postoperative check-up 5 weeks after surgery. During your assessment you find out that he has not walked or exercised at all since his surgery, he and his wife have not resumed sex, he has major sleep disturbances and vivid nightmares, and he is certain that the surgery has made him worse and he will die.

   Using the life-span developmental framework, derive a patient teaching plan for Mr. Wilson.

3. Jane Leander is a 54-year-old Pima Native American woman living on a reservation in the southwestern part of the United States. Ms. Leander was diagnosed with NIDDM at the age of 44. Her blood glucose levels have been consistently high, she has gained 14.5 kg (32 lb) since she was diagnosed, and she has been reluctant to begin using insulin since her diabetic brother became blind after he was put on insulin.

   How might Kleinman's eight questions help you, the nurse, understand Ms. Leander better?

   Role play Ms. Leander and her non-Native American nurse who asks her Kleinman's questions to try and understand Ms. Leander's explanatory model. Based on the data gathered from the role play, plan a teaching session for Ms. Leander.

4. The Hernandez family, consisting of two parents and four children, arrived 2 weeks ago in East Los Angeles from El Salvador, which they fled because of Mr. Hernandez' political activities. Mr. Hernandez was a teacher and his wife finished the eighth grade but had never worked. Mrs. Hernandez is 7 months pregnant and has arrived at your clinic for her first prenatal visit.

Only the two oldest children have had any immunizations and the infectious disease status of the family (e.g., tuberculosis, hepatitis, intestinal parasites) is unknown.

Using the questions to determine cultural embeddedness and the pattern described for understanding forced migration, describe how you would assess the famil's cultural embeddedness and how you would plan for patient education to accompany childbirth and integration of the children into the local community's health care system.

REFERENCES

Anderson, J. M. (1987). The cultural context of caring. *Canadian Critical Care Nursing Journal, December,* 7-13.

Baltes, P. B., Reese, H. W., & Lipsitt, L. P. (1980). Life-span developmental psychology. *Annual Review of Psychology, 31,* 65-110.

Bronfenbrenner, U. (1979). *The ecology of human development.* Cambridge, MA: Harvard University Press.

Bronfenbrenner, U. (1986). Ecology of the family as a context for human development: Research perspectives. *Developmental Psychology, 22,* 723-742.

Bronfenbrenner, U. (1989). Ecological systems theory. *Annals of Child Development, 6,* 187-249.

Bronfenbrenner, U., & Crouter, A. C. (1983). The evolution of environmental models in developmental research. In W. Kessen (Ed.), *History, theory, and methods.* Vol. 1 of P. H. Mussen (Ed.), *Handbook of child psychology* (4th ed., pp. 357-414). New York: John Wiley & Sons.

Brown, S. A. (1992). Meta-analysis of diabetes patient education research: Variations in intervention effects across studies. *Research in Nursing and Health, 15,* 409-419.

Castelli, W. P. (1988). Cardiovascular disease in women. *American Journal of Obstetrics and Gynecology, 158,* 1553-1560.

Corrao, J. M., Becker, R. C., Ockene, I. S, & Hamilton, G. A. (1990). Coronary heart disease risk factors in women. *Cardiology, 77*(Suppl.), 8-24.

Davis, L. H., Dumas, R., Ferketich, S., Flaherty, M. J., Isenberg, M., Koerner, J. E., et al. (1992). Culturally competent health care: The AAN expert panel of culturally competent nursing care. *Nursing Outlook, 40,* 277-283.

Dittrich, H., Gilpin, E., Nicod, P., Cali, G., Henning, H., & Ross J. (1988). Acute myocardial infarction in women: Influence of gender on mortality and prognostic variables. *American Journal of Cardiology, 62*(1), 1-7.

Featherman, D. L. (1981). *The life-span perspective in social science research.* Paper commissioned by the Social Science Research Council for the National Science Foundation. New York: Social Science Research Council.

Friedman, M. M. (1986, 1992). *Family nursing: Theory and assessment.* East Norwalk, CT: Appleton-Century-Crofts.

Glastra, F. J., & Kats, E. (1992). Culturalizing the ethnic patient: Educational films and images of interethnic relations in health care. *Health Education Research, 7,* 487-496.

Kleinman, A. (1988). *The illness narratives: Suffering, healing and the human condition.* New York: Basic Books.

Kleinman, A., Eisenberg, L., & Good B. (1978).Culture, illness, and care: Clinical lessons from anthropologic and cross-cultural research. *Annals of Internal Medicine, 88,* 251-258.

Murdaugh, C. Coronary heart disease in women. *Journal of Cardiovascular Nursing, 4,* 35-50.

Rankin, S. H., Galbraith, M. E., & Johnson, S. (1993). Reliability and validity data for a Chinese translation of the Center for Epidemiologic Studies-Depression (CES-D). *Psycholological Reports, 73,* 1291-1298.

Schaie, K. W. (1986). Beyond calendar definitions of age, time, and cohort: The general developmental model revisited. *Developmental Review, 6,* 252-277.

Schmidt, C. K. (1990). Pre-operative preparation: Effects on immediate pre-operative behavior, post-operative behavior and recovery in children having same-day surgery. *Maternal-Child Nursing Journal, 19,* 321-330.

Scudder, T., & Colson, E. (1982). From welfare to development: A conceptual framework for the analysis of dislocated people. In A. Hansen & A. Oliver-Smith A (Eds.), *Involuntary migration and resettlement: The problems and responses of dislocated people.* Boulder, CO: Westview Press.

Sherman, S. (1988). The Hmong in America: Laotian refugees in the land of the giants. *National Geographic, 174*(4), 596-610.

Sluzki, C. E. Migration and family conflict. (1979). *Family Process, 18,* 379-390.

Tripp-Reimer, T., Brink, P., & Saunders, J. M. (1984). Cultural assessment: Content and process. *Nursing Outlook, 32*(2), 78-82.

Tripp-Reimer, T., & Afifi L. A. (1989). Cross-cultural perspectives on patient teaching. *Nursing Clinics of North America, 24,* 613-619.

Tyhurst, L. Displacement and migration: A study in social psychiatry. *American Journal of Psychiatry, 107,* 561–568.

Visintainer, M.A., & Wolfer, J.A. (1975). Psychological preparation for surgical pediatric patients: The effects on children's and parents stress responses and adjustment. *Pediatrics, 56,* 561–568.

Wenger, N. K., & Hellerstein, H. K. (1992). *Rehabilitation of the coronary patient.* New York: Churchill Livingstone.

5

Informed Consent: An Important Concept in Patient Education

Ellen M. Robinson

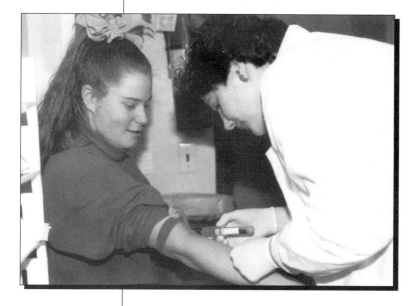

OBJECTIVES FOR CHAPTER 5

After reading this chapter, the nurse or student nurse should be able to:

1 Describe the importance of informed consent to the professional nurse's role as patient educator.

2 Discuss the legal and ethical basis of informed consent.

3 Identify the elements of informed consent as they relate to nursing.

4 Discuss exceptions to informed consent as these exceptions relate to the professional nurse's role.

5 Discuss a philosophical position on informed consent relative to the independent and collaborative practice roles of professional nurses.

The Relationship Between Patient Education and Informed Consent

Educating patients and their families is closely linked to the concept of informed consent in nursing practice. In their role as educators, professional nurses are continuously assessing the understanding these clients have of a disease state or proposed medical or nursing intervention. Patient education often involves disclosure of information to patients and families that will assist them in making decisions about their health care. Therefore, a thorough understanding of the concept of informed consent is important for nurses as patient educators.

The doctrine of informed consent is important to nurses for reasons related to both their collaborative and independent practice and research. The *collaborative* role of nurses involves an active partnership with physicians in the assessment and management of patients' medical problems. The *independent* practice of nurses is concerned with patients' responses to actual or potential health problems (American Nurses Association, 1980).

In collaborative practice with physicians, nurses are frequently in a position to carry out medical therapies or to assist with procedures that require informed consent. Examples might include ventilator management or assistance in the insertion of invasive monitoring devices, such as Swan-Ganz catheters. Nurses are often in the best position to assess a patient's understanding regarding medical treatments or to ascertain if the patient has chosen freely in accepting treatment.

In the independent domain of practice, nurses are increasingly prescribing and implementing nursing interventions that may warrant consent from patients. Some examples would be therapeutic touch, guided imagery, and interventions to restore skin integrity (Bulecheck & McCloskey, 1992). In addition to being important in clinical practice, the collaborative and independent research roles of nurses require that we be experts in informed consent. Many nursing authors have addressed this topic in detail (Cassidy & MacFarlane, 1991; Cassidy & Oddi, 1986; Davis, 1989a; Fry, 1989; Lynch, 1988; Rempusheski, 1991; Wintz, 1992; Woods, 1988).

This chapter provides information to assist practicing nurses in meeting the challenge of incorporating the principles of informed consent into their roles as patient educators. It presents an overview of the legal and ethical foundations of informed consent, presents legal cases pertinent to nursing, defines informed consent by its five elements, presents nursing research on informed consent using the five elements as an organizing framework, and outlines the exceptions to eliciting informed consent. The chapter concludes with an argument for a philosophical position for nursing on informed consent that embraces existential advocacy and the subjective standard of disclosure as the major concepts for the position.

A common conceptualization of informed consent is an active, shared decision-making between a health care provider and the recipient of care. This process of decision-making is based on mutual respect and participation (Silva & Zeccolo, 1986). The members of the President's Commission for the Study of Ethical Problems in Biomedical and Behavioral Research thought the issue so important that three volumes were dedicated to the topic (President's Commission, 1982). The Commission decided early on to address informed consent from a context of relations and communications between patients and health care providers. The goal was to see whether a means could be found to promote a fuller understanding by patients and professionals of their common enterprise so that patients could participate on an informed basis and, to the extent they could do so, make decisions regarding their health care.

Foundations in Legal Theory

According to Faden and Beauchamp, (1986) two areas of law are relevant to the concept of informed consent. These are *tort law* and *constitutional law*, with the former being most prevalent. A *tort* is a civil injury to one's person or property that is intentionally or negligently inflicted by another and that is measured in terms of and compensated by money damages. *Constitutional laws* are those laws that have been established in the United States Constitution, such as a personal right to freedom and equality.

Battery and negligence are the theories of liability that have been applied to court cases on informed consent. *Battery* is defined as the act of offensive touching that is done without the consent of the person being touched, however benign the motive or effects of touching (Prosser, 1971). The source of liability in *negligence* theory is unintended harmful action or omission (Faden & Beauchamp, 1986). Battery theory was applied frequently in the past and negligence theory is more commonly applied today.

A landmark case often cited that demonstrated application of battery theory and clear recognition of the legal principle of self-determination is *Schloendorff v. Society of New York Hospitals* (1914). This case involved a physician surgically removing a fibroid tumor from a woman who had consented to a laparotomy, but not to the removal of the fibroid tumor. Justice Cardoza's opinion is widely quoted and stands as a classic statement regarding a patient's right to self-determination: "Every human being of adult years and sound mind has a right to determine what shall be done with his own body; and a surgeon who performs an operation without his patient's consent commits an assault, for which he is liable in damages" (Schloendorff, 1914, p. 127). This notion of self-determination has proved important in future cases. Of note, however, is that "consent" is expressed through this right of self-determination; the notion of "informed" was not yet included.

Salgo v. Leland Stanford University Board of Trustees (1957) was an important case because it added the notion of "informed" to informed consent. In this case, Martin Salgo had undergone a translumbar aortography and sustained permanent paralysis. He suc-

cessfully sued his physicians for negligence in that they failed to disclose this risk, which he argued would have entered into his decision whether or not to have the procedure. This case emphasized the components of informed consent: the nature, consequences, harms, benefits, risks, and alternative treatments as information required by patients to make meaningful decisions regarding treatment (Faden & Beauchamp, 1986).

Application of negligence theory was pioneered in the case of *Natanson v. Kline* (1960). Although she consented, Mrs. Natanson sued her physician for administering cobalt radiation treatment to her after a mastectomy, claiming that he had not disclosed to her the risks inherent in the therapy. After suffering radiation burns, she sued Dr. Kline for negligence, claiming that he did not obtain her "informed consent" for a new treatment because he did not warn her of the risks. The decision for Natanson offered additional support for disclosure as an obligation, as well as continued recognition of self-determination.

Self-determination as the sole justification and goal of informed consent was further affirmed in *Canterbury v. Spence* (1972). This case was also significant in that it shifted focus from the professional practice standard of disclosure to a reasonable person standard. In this case, a patient had undergone a laminectomy for severe back pain and after falling from bed became paralyzed. The patient sued the physician, claiming that he had not been warned of the possibility of paralysis.

Regarding constitutional law, the right to privacy is relevant to informed consent. This right is based on the first, ninth, and fourteenth amendments of the Constitution. The theme is prevention of governmental interference with personal health care issues from abortion to treatment refusal (Purtilo, 1984). Currently, many states have enacted legislation for informed consent, thus reflecting the importance of the concept. According to informed consent legal experts Meisel and Kabnick (1980), the doctrine has been largely unchanged in statutory reform as compared to common law.

Recent Legal Cases Involving Nurses

The role of the professional nurse has been questioned in several recent legal cases involving informed consent (Tammelleo, 1985, 1990, 1993a, 1993b, 1993c). Although not directly related to patient education, these cases demonstrate the salience of the nurse's role around issues that involve informed consent. The first three cases to be described point to the nurse's role in collaboration with the physician; the last two cases presented are more specific to the nurse as an independent practitioner.

A controversial responsibility that is often assigned to the nurse in an acute care hospital is to obtain the patient's signature on a consent form for a procedure that is clearly to be carried out by a physician. The case of *Foflygen v. R. Zemel, MD* (1992; Tammelleo, 1993a) demonstrates the difficulty of this for nurses. A patient named Janice Foflygen went to a physician seeking a type of surgery described as a gastric diversion that she had read about in a newspaper as an effective treatment to alleviate obesity. The physician involved in the case had instructed a nurse to obtain the patient's signature on a standard hospital consent form, which was entitled "Consent for Operation, Anesthetics, and Special Procedures." The nurse did as asked by the physician. The patient underwent the surgery, sustaining several complications including pulmonary embolism, acute respiratory distress, phlebitis of the arm, acute bronchitis, stroke, and a right carotid artery occlusion. Ms. Foflygen brought suit against all health care providers, including the nurse, claiming that she had never been apprised of the risks of the surgery, or of any alternatives to surgery that would treat the obesity. The court, regarding the case as a battery to the patient, removed the action against the nurse because she did not perform the operation. Although the nurse was not convicted, Tammelleo (1993a) urges nurses not to lead or mislead a patient into signing a consent form unless they are satisfied that the patient has

been properly informed. He further adds that the physician who is to perform the procedure on the patient has a duty to obtain the patient's informed consent (p. 4).

In the case of *Brown v. Delaware Valley Transplant Program* (1992; Tammelleo, 1993b), a patient named Lawrence Brown was brought to the emergency room of a hospital suffering from a gunshot wound. Within 24 hours of his arrival, Mr. Brown was declared to be brain dead and noted to be a candidate for organ donation. His next of kin, sister Virginia Brown, was not notified until after Mr. Brown's organs were removed. She sued the hospital, arguing that a good faith effort to notify her was not made. Although the hospital was granted immunity based on the Uniform Anatomical Gift Act (1987), legal expert Tammelleo (1993b) warns nurses that their participation in procedures such as harvesting organs from a patient when informed consent has not been obtained or attempted to be obtained is "reprehensible and should be condemned" (p. 1).

A similar case in keeping with the idea of the nurse's collaborative role appears in the case of *Miller v. Rhode Island Hospital* (1993; Tammelleo, 1993c). Mr. Craig Miller was in an automobile accident and was brought to Rhode Island Hospital for treatment. He was documented to be intoxicated by blood alcohol level, and therefore thought to be incompetent to give informed consent for exploratory surgery to rule out internal bleeding as deemed necessary by the attending surgeon. Mr. Miller protested the intervention verbally; however, his protests were disregarded and the surgery performed. The morning after surgery, Mr. Miller left the hospital against medical advice and filed a suit against the hospital. A superior court ruling was in favor of the plaintiff; however, at appeal, the hospital was found innocent. This follow-up decision was based on expert testimony that this was an emergency situation and that because Mr. Miller was intoxicated, he was incapable of giving informed consent.

The two preceding cases alert practicing nurses to tread carefully in situations where patients are judged not able to give informed consent for their care. Although not named specifically in these cases, nurses must take responsibility for their own professional actions (American Nurses Association, 1985), being certain that the exception to informed consent is in fact a valid exception.

The following two cases summarized by Tammelleo (1985, 1990) specifically emphasize the nurse's independent role in patient care. In the first case, *Juneau v. Board of Elementary Secondary Education* (1984—1985), a nurse named Jane Juneau who was practicing in a special education center was responsible for the care of a 12-year-old orthopedically handicapped child. The child's behavior became disruptive, and rather than implement the policy supported by the institution to place the child in a quiet, secluded area for observation, Ms. Juneau took it on herself to subject the child to a cold shower. This is a type of aversive therapy whose goal is to discourage disruptive behavior. Ms. Juneau was dismissed from her nursing position. She appealed her case to the Court of Appeals of Louisiana, which upheld the decision, stating that the nurse had used aversive stimuli, which can only be used if approved by the institution's human rights committee and if consented to by the patient's parent or legal guardian (Tammelleo, 1985, p. 4). Neither of these two conditions had been fulfilled. This case emphasizes that nursing interventions, particularly controversial ones, should not be instituted in the absence of clear institutional guidelines and informed consent.

In the case of *Roberson v. Provident House* (1990), a quadriplegic patient named James Roberson, while in a nursing home, tried to tell a nurse not to insert a Foley catheter because in the past such catheters had caused him to have bleeding and infection. Rather than heed the patient's objections, the nurse instructed the patient to "shut up." The patient did in fact develop infection and bleeding and was hospitalized for several days. Roberson brought suit against the nursing home. The court voted in favor of the nursing home and explained its decision by the lack of expert testimony to an applicable standard of care. A dissenting opinion by a Louisiana justice, however, clearly pointed to the fact that this patient's right to informed consent was violated, drawing on Justice Cardoza's statement (1914) that "every adult human being of sound mind has a right to determine what shall be done to his own body." Clearly, the nurse violated this legal precedent in this patient's care. Both the Juneau and the Roberson cases (Tammelleo, 1985, 1990) emphasize that any intervention without baseline assessment and informed consent is ludicrous and can be harmful to patients. These cases demonstrate that nurses, as independent practitioners, will have to answer for their actions.

In 1988, a group of patients and some of their legal guardians from the state psychiatric hospitals in North Carolina filed a class action suit against the Secretary for Human Resources in the state of North Carolina in the case entitled *Thomas S. v. Flaherty* (1988). Among the multitude of complaints involving substandard care was one related to lack of education and inappropriate administration of antipsychotic drugs to patients in these state psychiatric facilities. Professional and institutional nursing and medical standards clearly delineated a gap, thus pointing to the abhorrent practices around this medication issue. Physical examination of several patients in these state institutions by a physician expert in pharmacology revealed the presence of adverse drug effects due to the antipsychotic drugs. Chart review further confirmed that patients or guardians were not informed in any way about the risks, side effects, or benefits of the psychotropic medications. In addition, many of the patients receiving these medications were not documented to have diagnoses where antipsychotic drugs would even be indicated. The court found that professional and institutional standards, which provide that patients or legal guardians be informed about the risks, side effects, and benefits of specific medications including psychotropics, and that evidence of this instruction as well as the patient's response to it be documented in the patient's medical record, was not upheld. In fact, the care of these patients around the administration of and education regarding these medications was a gross violation of institutional and national professional standards. This case represents both medical and nursing malpractice. Clearly the nurse's role to educate patients and families was not upheld as evidenced by both the care delivered and the lack of documentation regarding patient education and patient response to these medications.

The nurse's legal responsibility to educate and inform patients is contained within the nurse practice acts, which have been developed by all 50 states. Not only do these acts protect the lay public from incompetent practitioners by establishing procedures for licensure, but most also define the practice of nursing. There are six basic functions covered by most nurse practice acts; the one pertaining to the provision of health guidance and participation in health education establishes the foundation for the professional nurse's involvement in patient education.

Ethical Foundation of Informed Consent

According to Faden and Beauchamp (1986), acknowledged experts on the topic of informed consent, the ethical concerns related to informed consent focus on the patient, whereas the legal concerns focus on the practitioner, as demonstrated in the preceding section. Although both autonomy and beneficence are noted to be the two principles forming the ethical foundation of informed consent, *autonomy*, or the right to self-determination, clearly is the major ethical foundation of informed consent. Each human being has a right to make an autonomous choice in the true sense of being informed (Powers, 1993). In relationships between patients and health care providers, a duty exists based on the individual's right to make autonomous choices. For nurses, this means that patients have a right to be educated about their choices. Therefore, the principle of respect for autonomy is the primary ethical principle driving the theory and process of informed consent.

Autonomy is associated with terminology such as privacy, voluntariness, self-mastery, choosing freely, and accepting responsibility for one's choices (Faden & Beauchamp, 1986; Beauchamp & Childress, 1994). The idea that informed consent has its roots in the principle of respect for patient autonomy is a commonly understood tenet in the 1990s. The definition of an autonomous person, however, poses a challenge because there are no specific defining characteristics that can be observed in every alleged autonomous person. Perhaps there is some general agreement that such persons demonstrate self-directness, a sense of purpose, and the ability to act without the control of others. It would seem logical, then, that an autonomous person would make autonomous decisions; however, this is not always the case. A person with the assumed supposed capacity to act autonomously may or may not choose to make herself or himself aware of critical information or may be the victim of some temporary mental or physical disorder that is preventing the execution of an autonomous act. Therefore, Faden and Beauchamp (1986), make a distinction between autonomous persons and autonomous actions. Because informed consent and informed refusal represent actions, the focus with informed consent is on autonomous action rather than autonomous persons.

Autonomous action is further analyzed by Faden and Beauchamp (1986) and Beauchamp and Childress (1994) according to the concepts of intentionality, understanding, and control. *Intentionality* is defined in two parts. The first is the idea of a thought or an intention. This can be explained as a desire by a person to carry out a particular action. Take note, however, that the desire alone does not constitute entirely the definition of intentionality. Persons may intend to do many things, and never do so. This leads to the second component of the definition, which is the action. Faden and Beauchamp (1986) say that only if an action occurs, coupled with an intention to perform the action, is the action an intentional action (p. 242). An *intentional action* is a deliberate action, one that is performed after being consciously planned by the executioner of the action.

Autonomous actions are also analyzed in terms of understanding. This concept suggests that persons who carry out autonomous actions, in fact have a reasonable grasp of all that the particular actions will entail for them. This condition can be considered on a continuum from perfect understanding to no understanding. One may argue that most patients can never achieve total understanding. Even patients who are health care professionals cannot be versed in the theoretical and technical knowledge in all medical specialties. One can even make the point that a health care professional offering treatment only understands to the degree that knowledge has been discovered and made available in that field. For patients, there does, however, need to be a "substantial satisfaction" of this condition, meaning that enough information is understood by the patient to make a reasonably informed choice (Beauchamp & Childress, 1994). The amount of information to satisfy the substantial satisfaction standard is probably context dependent.

The third criterion by which autonomous actions are analyzed relates to the external control to which the person making the decision is subject. The health care provider needs to be comfortable that the patient making the decision is doing so of his or her own volition. As participants in society, persons are influenced by the institutions to which they belong, such as religious groups, family, ethnic groups, government, and so on. Like understanding, there are degrees of control, and what needs to be achieved is an acceptable level of "lack of control." As human beings we are social and have a desire to be independent as well as a part of institutions or groups. Therefore, there may always be some degree of external influence present in informed consent decisions. This, too, is a context- dependent variable, and what is required to meet the condition of autonomous action is a reasonable affirmation of the absence of control by the individual making the decision (Beauchamp & Childress, 1994).

Unlike understanding and control, which can be analyzed in terms of reasonable degree on a continuum, intentionality must decisively be a yes or no. Intentionality is not a matter of degree; it is either present or it is not (Faden & Beauchamp, 1986). Fulfillment of all three criteria constitute what Faden and Beauchamp (1986) regard as informed consent in the sense of the moral definition. As defined, this is informed consent as the autonomous authorization of an intervention by a patient that occurs when the patient with "substantial understanding and in substantial absence of control by others intentionally authorizes a professional to do something" (p. 278). Effective consent, on the other hand, is defined as fulfilling the policy requirements of institutions that have rules and regulations governing informed consent (Fader & Beauchamp, 1986, p. 280). Obviously, the moral sense of the definition of informed consent is the optimum and that which health care providers should strive to achieve.

The second ethical principle that constitutes moral grounding for informed consent is that of beneficence, which is the idea that health care providers ought to do good for patients. This ethical principle has been a mainstay in the health professions. As professional nurses, we assume an obligation to do good. Before the patient rights movement, the actions of all health care providers were primarily governed by the principle of beneficence. Beauchamp and Childress (1994) outline four elements of this principle as one ought not to inflict evil or harm, one ought to prevent evil or harm, one ought to remove evil or harm, and one ought to do or promote good.

Reliance on the beneficence principle alone in regard to informed consent encourages paternalism to run amok. *Paternalism* is defined as the health care provider deciding what is best for the patient, as a parent would decide what is best for a child. In years past, the delivery of health care based on the principle of beneficence was considered to be acceptable and well-intentioned care. However, in the age of patient rights (American Hospital Association, 1972), the principle of beneficence cannot stand as the sole principle by which members of the health professions guide their practice.

Although beneficence is clearly a foundational value, in most cases autonomy is considered the primary principle particularly when dealing with the conscious competent patient or the incompetent patient who has left evidence of his or her intentions regarding health care decisions via an advance directive or health care proxy (Omnibus Budget Reconciliation Act, 1990). In addition, there are exceptions to the informed consent doctrine, which will be outlined later in the chapter, wherein it can be seen that beneficence plays a prima facie role.

The American Nurses Association Code of Ethics (1985) reflects evidence of development based on the principles of autonomy and beneficence. Patient education is a cornerstone nursing intervention that provides an avenue for the professional nurse to fulfill the tenets of the Code for Nurses (Box 5-1). In the role of patient educator, the nurse is able to assess the level of knowledge of the patient and family concerning a particular health care issue and then provide the information that will fill the gaps for them. Patients can make autonomous decisions only if given the information they need to do so. Whether it be in the role of facilitator in respect to medical interventions or as primary practitioner for independent nursing interventions, the nurse plays a key role in assisting patients and families to arrive at informed decisions.

Definition and Nursing Research on Informed Consent

Beauchamp and Childress (1994) define informed consent, as described in the President's Commission Report on Making Health Care Decisions (1982), as consisting of five elements. These elements are competence, disclosure, understanding, voluntariness, and consent. Each element will be defined, followed directly by current nursing research related to that element. Figure 5-1 depicts the

---

BOX 5–1. The American Nurses Association Code For Nurses

1. The nurse provides services with respect for human dignity and the uniqueness of the client, unrestricted by considerations of social or economic status, personal attributes, or the nature of the health problems.

2. The nurse safegaurds the client's right to privacy by judiciously protecting information of a confidential nature.

3. The nurse acts to safeguard the client and the public when health care and safety are affected by the incompetent, unethical, or illegal practice of any person.

4. The nurse assumes responsibility and accountability for individual nursing judgements and actions.

5. The nurse maintains competence in nursing.

6. The nurse exercises informed judgement and uses individual competence and qualifications as criteria in seeking consultation, accepting responsibilities, and delegating nurses activities to others.

7. The nurse participates in activities that contribute to the ongoing development of the profession's body of knowledge.

8. The nurse participates in the profession's efforts to implement and improve standards of nursing.

9. The nurse participates in the profession's efforts to establish and maintain conditions of employment conducive to high quality nursing care.

10. The nurse participates in the profession's effort to protect the public from misinformation and misrepresentation and to maintain the integrity of nursing,

11. The nurse collaborates with members of the health professions and other citizens in promoting community and national efforts to meet the health needs of the public.

---

interrelationship between the process of informed consent in terms of its five elements to the process of patient education.

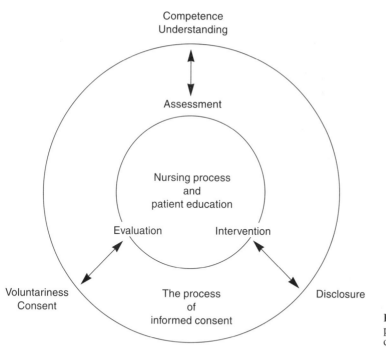

FIGURE 5-1. The relationship of patient education to informed consent.

Competence and Its Relationship to Informed Consent

The concept of competence has generated a great deal of discussion as it relates to informed consent. Jurchak (1990) summarizes four general categories into which competency falls as described by Applebaum and Grisso (1988). These are the ability to communicate choices, ability to understand relevant information, ability to appreciate the situation and its consequences, and ability to manipulate information rationally. Nurses as patient educators are familiar with these conceptual areas. Baseline assessment of the patient's mental status and ability to understand and manage new information is an essential first step for the nurse who is planning to educate and inform patients.

The landmark work of Roth and coworkers (1977) on competency identified five categories of competency tests commonly used in practice: making a choice, reasonable outcome of choice, choice based on rational reasons, ability to understand, and actual understanding. In addition, their work has demonstrated that the same subject may be found competent or incompetent depending on the measure used.

With respect to the discussion of competence and how it relates to informed consent, Davis and Underwood (1989) present a timely discussion of the nurse's role as related to assessment of competency and consent. They distinguish between informed consent for medical-surgical procedures and informed consent for nursing care. Competence as a concern of nurses is not merely an issue related to whether a patient can agree to participate in a medical or surgical intervention. The nurse's role should not be debated in terms of obtaining or witnessing consent for physician procedures; in fact, these authors advise nurses not to play such a role. Rather, nurses need to explore the meaning of informed consent for independent nursing practice. Although this conceptualization needs further delineation, it seems clear that the concept of informed consent as applied to nursing care has potential for growth.

Turnquist (1983) reports on the difficulties faced by psychiatric nurses in administering neuroleptic medications to psychotic patients in an acute stage of mental illness. One ethical justification here is exercise of therapeutic privilege, described by Faden and Beauchamp (1986) as the right of a health care provider to withhold information because of the harmful effects of the disclosure on the patient. Another justification is the fact that the patient is incompetent to make a rational decision. The health care provider must make a risk-benefit analysis for the administration of neuroleptic medications. Tardive dyskinesia, a side effect of these drugs, which manifests as involuntary motor movements especially of the face, lips, and tongue, can be permanent. Rachlin (1974), on the other hand, speaks to the fact that the liberty of the psychotic is no freedom at all. This notion suggests that to intervene with paternalistic action is to preserve a wider range of freedom from psychosis. The problem of autonomy conflicting with beneficence is not readily solved even after the objective of treatment, that is, absence of the acute psychiatric episode, is achieved. Is the patient now competent to make a decision regarding continued pharmacologic treatment? Is the therapeutic privilege still justified? Difficult as these cases may be, nurses in conjunction with family members are in a position to assess best the competency of patients given their constant attendance with the patient.

Disclosure and Its Relationship to Informed Consent

Disclosure is defined as the legal obligation of professionals to share information that professionals and patients usually consider material in deciding whether to refuse or consent to an intervention. This is to include the professional's reommendation, the purpose of seeking consent and the nature of consent as au-

thorization (Beauchamp & Childress, 1994). Three standards of disclosure have been described: the professional practice standard, the reasonable person standard, and the subjective standard.

The *professional practice standard* states that adequate disclosure is determined by traditional practices of the professional community. Faden and Beauchamp (1986) articulate three problems with this standard of disclosure. One is that it may be questionable to what degree a standard exists, and the second is that a negligent standard could exist and be upheld. The last and most fundamental objection is that it can undermine a patient's autonomous choice because an individual's situation cannot be reduced to what the professional community holds as sacred. Application of this standard in court would require expert professional testimony.

The *reasonable person standard* (Beauchamp & Childress, 1994) states that the kind and amount of information to be disclosed is determined by reference to a hypothetical reasonable person. This standard shifts the focus from the health care provider to the patient. The difficulty lies in ascertaining what a "reasonable person" would want to know. Interpretation of the reasonable person standard in court leaves the practitioner at the mercy of the jury, who in a particular case would be in the position to judge the adequacy of this standard (Faden & Beauchamp, 1986).

The *subjective standard* (Beauchamp & Childress, 1994) describes information disclosure specific to the needs of the individual patient. This is a preferable moral standard of disclosure because it truly espouses the principle of respect for autonomy. The subjective standard considers individual needs that are extremely important in decision-making. Those who oppose this standard claim it places an unfair burden on the practitioner, leaving the practitioner at the mercy of the patient. I believe that it is a standard consistent with the philosophical position of nurses. Nurses are concerned with the impact of illness on the lifestyles of their patients. The holistic patient assessment framework espoused by nursing speaks precisely to the subjective standard of disclosure. That is, the nurse assesses with the patient the impact of illness on that patient's life-style and, therefore, is in a position to tailor disclosure to the individual patient and family in collaboration with medicine.

Nursing research studies that address the element of disclosure have been reported.

Farkas (1992) reported on a study of informed consent in using therapeutic paradox as an approach to therapy. Therapeutic paradox was defined by Farkas (1992) as reverse psychology in which a client is told not to change as a way to get the client to change. This author cited several instances where this approach has been successful, such as in school phobia, marital therapy, and therapy for the chronically mentally ill. The concern with this type of therapy is the absence of informed consent that is inherent in the paradoxical procedure. If the therapist informs the patient, the therapy is not as likely to be effective. Farkas designed an exploratory study that examined the responses of 34 nonpsychiatric outpatients to a request for hypothetical informed consent for therapeutic paradox. Sixty-six percent of this sample never had sought counseling, and 27% were currently in counseling. After reviewing the detailed consent form and a vignette describing a successful case in which therapeutic paradox was used, 81% agreed to consent to therapy using this technique. Their qualitative comments, however, revealed internal reservations. The results of this study raise questions regarding the reservations that patients may in fact have when they sign informed consent documents.

Davis and Jameton (1987) reported on a study of nursing and medical students' attitudes toward nurse-physician role responsibilities on disclosure to patients through use of vignettes. The 28 nursing respondents and 28 medical respondents differed significantly on 20 of 87 items on the questionnaire. Nursing students tended to favor disclosure by nurses more than did medical students. Also of note is that nursing students favored more independent thinking on treatment decisions rather than encouraging absolute trust in the physician. These authors suggest that a patient's right to know and to be informed is so significant that it should override traditional professional distinctions on who is to be responsible for disclosure (Davis & Jameton, 1987). The interest of nurses in disclosure, in these authors' view, may be emanating from nursing's concern for patient and professional autonomy.

Understanding and Its Relationship to Informed Consent

Beauchamp and Childress (1994) identify understanding as the third element defining informed consent. Powers (1993) argues that decisions made without understanding cannot be autonomous in the true sense. This component of informed consent has been addressed in nursing research.

Silva and Sorrell (1984) reviewed empirical research studies on patient comprehension of information for informed consent. Factors promoting comprehension that were provider specific included presentation in a brief and direct manner, information presented by a nurse or health care team, allowing subjects to keep information from 1 to 3 days, and provider requests for immediate patient recall of information. Subject-specific factors noted to promote comprehension included the perception that the amount of information was just right, that information was presented clearly, higher educational and vocabulary levels, not being confined to bed, and a positive opinion toward the need for informed consent forms. Provider-specific factors inhibiting comprehension included presentation of complex or threatening information and presentation by the doctor alone. Subject-specific factors inhibiting comprehension included being confined to bed due to illness, erroneous and or selective recall, no strong opinions about the need for informed consent forms, lower educational and vocabulary levels, perception that the amount of information received was too much or too little, and a perception that the explanation was unclear. In comparing results of the studies they critiqued, Silva and Sorrell (1984) noted methodologic problems to be lack of clear definitions of terms, inconsistencies in timing of recall, and the need for more reliable and valid instrumentation.

In an exploratory study, Hughes (1993) examined the relationship between information about breast cancer treatment alternatives and patients' choices of treatment. A convenience sample of 71 women with stage I or II breast cancer was drawn from a clinic affiliated with a large tertiary care medical center. The amount of information provided to each subject as well as the nature of its presentation were tracked using an observer checklist. To determine recall of information and final decision for treatment, the researcher conducted telephone interviews 6 to 8 weeks after surgery. Results indicated that treatment decision was related to the information that the women gained from sources other than health care providers, such as lay media, relatives, and educational brochures before the clinic visit. The results also indicated that patients' recall of information about treatments and related risks was poor. Results of this study strongly support the importance of assessing the patient's current level of knowledge and understanding before intervening with information.

Silva (1985) evaluated the adequacy of information needed for informed consent to participate in a research study in 75 spouses of general surgical patients. The researcher administered an informed consent questionnaire to the subjects after they had been given the written information needed to give informed consent for a research study of spouses' responses to general surgery. The results indicated that 72 of 75 spouses had adequate comprehension of the information. The authors speculated that the reasons for the positive results were the degree of care with which the informed consent statements were read, the fact that recall was immediate, the simplicity of information on the form, and length of the consent form. All of these were carefully considered in designing the information sheet for the study because these factors had been identified as influencing comprehension of information in a previous review article (Silva & Sorrell, 1984).

Meade and Howser (1992) investigated the reading level estimates of cancer clinical trial consent forms from 44 active studies of the National Cancer Institute. Readability estimates for each consent form were calculated by the Minnesota Interactive Readability Approximation computer program, a standardized program that randomly evaluates the readability of passages from a document. Regarding the consent forms analyzed, readability estimates were from grade 12 to grade 17.5, with a mean grade level of 14.3. These study results have implications for nursing in that nurses frequently assume a role in management and implementation of research protocols. Nurses must play a more active role in developing readable forms and assisting patients to understand what is being explained to them and ultimately asked of them to participate in research.

Solomon and Schwegman-Melton (1987) measured the impact of a structured teaching program on the understanding of information desired for informed consent regarding cardiac catheterization. The hypothesis was that knowledge retained by patients participating in a structured patient education program before cardiac catheterization would be different from that retained by those who did not participate in the program. The 18 men in the experimental group received an individual teaching session, whereas the 18 men in the control group received routine information from the cardiac medicine fellow. A written knowledge test, which had been previously piloted, was administered to the experimental group on completion of the program and to the control group immediately after signing the informed consent. Results were statistically significant in comparing the two groups. The mean total score for the control group was 8.9 of a possible 13; the mean score for the experimental group was 11.5. This study provides empirical support for structured patient education in educating patients for procedures requiring informed consent, a teaching technique currently used more frequently in nursing than in any other discipline.

Sorrell (1991) conducted a study looking at the effects of writing and speaking on comprehension of information for informed consent. A posttest-only control group design was used. Eighty participants were randomly assigned to one of three groups: a writing group, a speaking group, and a comparison group. Those in the writing and speaking groups were asked respectively to write or speak regarding their impressions, questions, and concerns after reading an informed consent document requesting them to participate in a breast self-examination treatment program. After completing their assigned task (or in the case of the control group 45 minutes after reading the consent form), subjects were asked to complete a 20-item posttest. Results were statistically significant with the writing group scoring the highest (range 11–20) compared with speaking group scores (range 8–20) and comparison group scores (range 7–19). Results of this study indicate that the modalities of writing and speaking may be effective and practical interventions to enhance the patient's understanding of the content of informed consent.

Voluntariness and Consent and Their Relationship to Informed Consent

The remaining two elements specified by Beauchamp and Childress (1994) include voluntariness and consent, or authorization. *Voluntariness* is the patient's ability to act independently of manipulation or coercion. *Consent*, the final element in informed consent, is the patient giving the practitioner permission to perform the specific procedure or therapy. Nusbaum and Chenitz (1990) found no studies on voluntariness in their review of literature. This is consistent with my review. Some published research addressed the entire process of informed consent.

Nusbaum and Chenitz (1990) conducted a qualitative study examining the observed process of informed consent to ascertain if the process indeed fit with the five elements. Subjects in the study were 16 dyads of researcher and research subjects, consisting of 4 physicians, 7 registered nurses, and 5 research assistants. The findings revealed a poor fit between the elements of informed consent and the interactions during the formal consent interviews. Only the theoretical concept of disclosure was recognizable during an early stage in the researcher-subject interview. The results of this study raise serious questions regarding the implementation of the theoretical elements of informed consent to real life practice.

Carney (1987) reported on a study designed to identify communication problems between nurses and physicians in relationship to informed consent for bone marrow transplantation. Using a qualitative design, the researchers elicited the subjects' perceptions of informed consent and roles and responsibilities of nurses, physicians, and patients in the consent process. The sample included 16 nurses and 5 physicians who were experienced in caring for bone marrow transplant patients. Content analysis revealed that nurses focused on the process of informed consent, whereas physicians paid attention to options and outcomes. The principal nursing roles and responsibilities that emerged included patient advocacy and patient education. Patient advocacy was seen more as a nursing role by nurses than by physicians, who saw nurses primarily as educators. The principal role identified strongly for physicians was providing the patient with information, and secondly and less strongly, validating patient understanding. The major roles for patients as perceived by nurses and physicians in this study were to participate in the consent process and be receptive to information. The author of this study emphasized the value of the nurse advocacy role and recommended further development of advocacy as an integral component in the practice of nursing. She also spoke to the importance of tailoring information to the needs of the patient.

In a study reported by Davis (1989b) on nurses' ethical decision- making in situations of informed consent, 27 nurses (staff nurses, clinical nurse specialists, and head nurses) practicing in two clinical settings responded to four research and four treatment vignettes via semistructured interviews. Content analysis revealed that nurses felt constrained by the health care system, which in their perception was not patient focused. Perceptions of patients were that patients were in general extremely compliant, even when physician practice was in question. This made it difficult for nurses to fulfill what they perceived to be their ethical role in informed consent. Study participants reported acting differently to accommodate the behavioral differences among physician specialties. Results of particular interest were the nurses' philosophical approaches to ethical decision-making in situations of informed consent. Nurses favoring a practical approach considered manipulating factors in the institution in comparison to nurses with more philosophical viewpoints who advocated a patient-centered obligation for informed consent. Nurses with the latter perspective were able to give the patient priority and shift behaviors accordingly to the needs of the patient. Nurses interviewed for this study reported that peer support and institutional ethics committees were among supports to assist in conflict resolution. The findings of this study, particularly those related to nurses' philosophical approach, lend credibility to the subjective standard of disclosure as being consistent with an advocacy model of nursing ethics.

Exceptions to Informed Consent

Meisel (1979) outlined exceptions to the doctrine of informed consent. The exceptions to informed consent are important for nurses to consider in their roles as patient educators, so that they can recognize appropriate and inappropriate applications of these exceptions to patient situations. These exceptions include emergency, incompetence, waiver, and therapeutic privilege. Meisel presented each of these exceptions in terms of how specific evaluative approaches for each exception ei-

ther preserve or pose threats to self-determination, or the patient's ability to make autonomous choices. By keeping the purpose of informed consent in the forefront, that is, a process of enabling patients and families to make decisions for therapies based on clear, accurate information of risks and benefits, one can then clearly evaluate exceptions to the doctrine in the light of preserving such autonomy for patients.

Emergency as an Exception to Informed Consent

In an emergency, it is generally thought that a patient would desire the type of medical care that would return that patient to a healthy state. Meisel differentiated emergency situations from those when the patient is competent, such as if a limb were severed, to those when the patient is incompetent, such as when the patient is unconscious due to a motor vehicle accident. In addition to the difficulty in arriving at a commonly accepted definition of emergency, health care providers also must struggle with how much to disclose to a patient who is competent, yet severely injured and in need of immediate treatment with serious risks. Meisel (1979) used the term urgency to assist the health care provider in further delineating an emergency. The concept of urgency helps professionals to focus on the consequences that a person would endure if treatment were delayed. Meisel advocated a narrow definition of the emergency exception to those circumstances when the delay of treatment until informed consent could be obtained would result in serious harm to the patient. By advising a narrow conception, Meisel felt that individual patient autonomy is best preserved. In the case of *Miller v. Rhode Island Hospital* (Tammelleo, 1993c), described earlier in the chapter, the court's appeal decision in favor of the hospital was based on the emergency exception to informed consent. From an ethical standpoint, the physician and nurses in this case were operating under the principle of beneficence, which in this case was found not to be appreciated by the patient who had brought suit against the hospital.

Incompetence as an Exception to Informed Consent

Incompetence was also identified by Meisel (1979) as an exception to informed consent. First, it is necessary to clarify that incompetence in this sense would not be coupled with an emergency. Incompetence in fact often co-exists in an emergency, as in the case of *Miller v. Rhode Island Hospital* (Tammelleo, 1993c), but is analyzed separately from the sense of incompetence that does not occur in an emergency setting. The issues in assessing patient competence are outlined in a preceding section of the chapter (Roth et al., 1977). Both Meisel (1979) and Macklin (1987) spoke to the difficulty in objectively defining and measuring competence and incompetence in patients. Macklin (1987) summarized a proposed model for making assessments of patient competency that has been described by Drane (1984). This model incorporates a sliding scale with three standards to assess competency with the two goals of preventing a competent person from being disqualified to participate in treatment decisions and protecting an incompetent person from the harmful effects of a bad decision (Macklin, 1987, p. 91). The standards begin with low stringency for competency for low-risk decisions such as choice of pain reliever to high stringency for competency for high-risk decisions, such as death if treatment is not administered.

In considering the exceptions of emergency and incompetence, the role of the family cannot be underestimated as providers of information regarding what the patient might want. Since 1990, with the implementation of the Patient Self-Determination Act, some patients have stated their wishes for care in the form of an advance directive or through a designated health care proxy who is frequently, although not always, a family member. In such cases where the patient's wishes are known, it is the obligation of the

health care provider, and most often the nurse, to honor such wishes.

Waiver as an Exception to Informed Consent

Patient waiver is another exception to the informed consent doctrine identified by Meisel (1979). He reported that for at least four decades, the Supreme Court has defined *waiver* as a voluntary and temporary relinquishment of a known right. In patient education and informed consent, a waiver might apply if it were recommended by a physician that a patient have open heart surgery, and the patient agreed to the surgery but declined learning about the risks, benefits, and postoperative care. The important thing to note with waivers is that the patients be clear that they do have a right to information regarding proposed treatments, risks and benefits, and alternatives to therapy, along with the right to accept or refuse such therapy. Again, the family can provide a useful resource for nurses to communicate with in such situations. Beauchamp and Childress (1994) presented the potential solution of setting up rules against waivers for the purposes of protecting patients, with committees to determine the appropriateness of allowing a waiver in a specific patient context. Again, the intent would be to preserve patient autonomy by keeping limits around the waiver exception.

Therapeutic Privilege as an Exception to Informed Consent

Therapeutic privilege is the last of the exceptions to informed consent as identified by Meisel (1979). *Therapeutic privilege* is invoked when a health care provider, most frequently a physician, decides that disclosure of information to a patient would be more harmful than helpful to the patient in coming to an informed decision, and performs or withholds an intervention without the patient's consent. The problem with this paternalistic practice is obvious in that such an approach totally violates the patient's autonomy. Acceptance of such a practice constitutes an abuse of the patient's rights (American Hospital Association, 1972), as well as having tremendous potential for abuse, because it shifts the power of decision-making from the patient to the provider. With increased recognition of patient involvement in decision-making, and the increased recognition that the physician is no longer the "captain of the ship," practice of therapeutic privilege has diminished, and when practiced, is difficult to justify.

A Philosophical Position for Nursing Related to Informed Consent

The nursing profession is currently grappling with some important issues related to informed consent that will be significant to our theoretical and scientific growth as a profession. The dual role of nurses in collaborative and independent practice requires a unique and critical examination of current practices and future directions around informed consent. In our collaborative role with physicians, the overemphasis on the act of witnessing and in some cases obtaining the signature of patients for physician-performed treatments has blinded nursing to our real concerns. Nurses need to see beyond this narrow view and begin to conceptualize a new philosophy of informed consent (Davis & Underwood, 1989). Clearly it is not within the purview of the nurse to obtain consent from patients for a medical or surgical procedure that the physician will perform to satisfy the institution's policy for effective consent. The physician who is to perform the procedure on the patient has a duty to obtain the patient's informed consent, as was demonstrated in the case of *Foflygen v. R. Zemel, MD* (1992; Tammelleo, 1993a) and supported by others in nursing (Brooke, 1988; Murphy, 1988; Richardson, 1993; Varricchio & Jassak, 1989).

More importantly, nurses practicing in the collaborative realm play a vital role in ensuring that patients have a clear understanding of therapies with their risks and benefits to the extent that this understanding allows patients to make autonomous choices specific to their individual situations. The existential advocacy model described by Gadow (1983) is instructive in delineating a philosophical approach that may be applied to informed consent in the collaborative realm of nursing. She conceptualizes the patient as if on a continuum between consumerism and paternalism. When health care providers opt to take a consumerist view, they present the patient with a range of options with little regard as to where the patient might be in terms of values and knowledge. The paternalistic view is at the other extreme, essentially "making" the choice for the patient who is vulnerable secondary to his or her plight.

The position of advocacy is based on the freedom of individual self-determination as the highest value in the nurse-patient relationship. As a partner with the patient, the advocacy nurse meets the patient where the patient is, thus being able to help the individual learn what is needed to come to the best decision. This is essentially an operationalization of the subjective standard of disclosure. In my opinion, this philosophical position for the nurse regarding informed consent is consistent with the principle of self-determination, the legal and ethical grounding of informed consent, and patient education. Adoption of this philosophical approach in nursing will clarify collaborative practice of nurses with physicians. Nurses will then be able to contribute to the informed consent process in a meaningful way that is consistent with their philosophical underpinnings and their professional roles.

The research review in this paper confirms a precedent for application of Gadow's existential advocacy model (1983, 1989a, 1989b) to be applied to informed consent. Davis and Jameton (1987) found that nurses favor a move toward enhancing patient and professional autonomy. Hughes (1993) argued for a need to assess the patient's current level of understanding before imparting treatment alternatives. Studies on comprehension (Silva & Sorrell, 1984; Silva, 1985; Sorrell, 1991; Meade & Howser, 1992) support nursing's legitimate concern for patient understanding. Carney (1987), and a study not mentioned previously by Davis (1988), spoke to nurses seeing their role as advocates. Davis' study is particularly relevant because the sample were all master's-prepared nurses, who are thought of as leaders in clinical practice. The results of Nusbaum and Chenitz's (1990) qualitative study pointed to the gap between the espoused elements of "good informed consent" and the realities in practice. This research suggested that the addition of qualitative methods to the study of informed consent is appropriate and needed.

The idea that informed consent is important for treatment is gaining increasing recognition in professions other than traditional medicine (Clawson, 1994; Davis & Underwood, 1989; Rule & Veatch, 1993; Scofield, 1993). Nursing is one of those professions. There are three reasons for this in nursing. One is that patients in the current age are much more aware of their active role in health care decision- making. This more active role has been delineated in the President's Commission (1982) as well as through the Patient Self-Determination Act (Omnibus Budget Reconciliation Act, 1990). Secondly, nursing interventions are becoming increasingly sophisticated with the goal of achieving specific outcomes for patients. Lastly, economic forces in health care will make patients more conscious of services they are obtaining from all health care providers. Although less clear at this point, nurses are beginning to explore the ramifications of informed consent in their independent domain of practice. Davis and Underwood (1989) argued that attention to this issue will have positive outcomes for nursing that will enhance the autonomous nursing role in practice.

From a theoretical standpoint, the existential advocacy model (Gadow, 1983, 1989a, 1989b) fits well with informed consent in nursing practice in both the collaborative and independent domains. Clarification of this philosophical approach to informed consent will enhance the added value of nurses in collaboration with physicians. Attention to the implications of informed consent in our independent practice as nurses will contribute to a clearer definition of nursing practice for both patients and nurses. Continued research using quantitative and qualitative methods to examine the elements of informed consent as they relate to the subjective standard of disclosure and the connection of informed consent to the existential advocacy model are recommended for the advancement of nursing science and ultimately nursing practice based on that science.

Summary

This chapter provided a theoretical and practical guide for the practicing nurse on the concept of informed consent. Nurses as patient and family educators will continue to be in the best position to evaluate the knowledge and comprehension that patients and families have regarding their health status and proposed interventions and therefore inform and educate these clients accordingly.

Strategies for Critical Analysis and Application

1. Discuss the principles of autonomy and beneficence as the ethical foundations of informed consent. Give an example of when one principle might override the other.

2. A surgeon asks you to obtain a patient's signature on an informed consent form. Mr. B. is a 63-year-old man with early signs of dementia, who is scheduled to have a malignant tumor removed from his colon the following day. You know that Mr. B. and his wife have several questions regarding the surgery, such as whether the tumor is malignant and whether he will need a colostomy. You try to tell the surgeon that Mr. and Mrs. B.

have these questions, but he tells you to "get the signature, and I'll be back later to talk with the patient." You know that he is rushing off to start a complex, late afternoon case, and your patient is scheduled for surgery at 7:00 the following morning. Discuss your actions, both short and long term.

3. Name two exceptions to informed consent. Describe the professional nurse's role from an ethical and legal standpoint for each exception.

4. Discuss the importance of documentation as it relates to patient education and informed consent.

REFERENCES

American Hospital Association. (1972). *A patient's bill of rights.* Chicago: Author.

American Nurses Association. (1980). *Nursing: A social policy statement.* Kansas City, MO: Author.

American Nurses Association. (1985). *Code for nurses with interpretive statements.* Kansas City, MO: Author.

Applebaum, P. S., & Grisso, T. (1988). Assessing patients' capacities to consent to treatment. *New England Journal of Medicine, 319,* 1635-1638.

Beauchamp, T. L., & Childress, J. (1994). *Principles of biomedical ethics* (4th ed.). New York: Oxford.

Brooke, P. S. (1988). Informed consent: An ethical dilemma having life/death and legal implications. *Clinical Nurse Specialist, 2*(3), 157-161.

Bulecheck, G. M., & McCloskey, J. C. (1992). *Nursing interventions: Essential nursing treatments* (2nd ed.). Philadelphia: W. B. Saunders.

Canterbury v. Spence, 464 F.2d 772, 775 (DC Cir. 1972).

Carney, B. (1987). Bone marrow transplantation: Nurses' and physicians' perceptions of informed consent. *Cancer Nursing, 10*(5), 252-259.

Cassidy, J., & MacFarlane, D. K. (1991). The role of the nurse in clinical cancer research. *Cancer Nursing, 14(3)* 124-131.

Cassidy, V. R., & Oddi, L. F. (1986). Legal and ethical aspects of informed consent: A nursing research perspective. *Journal of Professional Nursing, 2*(6), 343-349.

Clawson, A. L. (1994). The relationship between clinical decision making and ethical decision making. *Physiotherapy, 80*(1), 10-14.

Davis, A. J. (1989a). Informed consent process in research protocols: Dilemmas for clinical nurses. *Western Journal of Nursing Research, 11*(4), 448-457.

Davis, A. J. (1989b). Clinical nurses' ethical decision making in situations of informed consent. *Advances in Nursing Science, 11*(3), 63-69.

Davis, A. J. (1988). The clinical nurse's role in informed consent. *Journal of Professional Nursing, 4*(2), 88-91.

Davis A. J., & Jameton, A. (1987). Nursing and medical student attitudes towards nursing disclosure of information to patients: A pilot study. *Journal of Advanced Nursing, 12,* 691-698.

Davis, A. J., & Underwood, P. R. (1989). The competency quagmire: Clarification of the nursing perspective concerning the issues of competence and informed consent. *International Journal of Nursing Studies, 26*(3), 271-279.

Drane, J. F. (1984). Competency to give an informed consent. *Journal of the American Medical Association, 252,* 925-927.

Faden, R. R., & Beauchamp, T. L. (1986). *A history and theory of informed consent.* New York: Oxford, 1986.

Farkas, M. M. (1992). Use of informed consent with therapeutic paradox. *Issues in Mental Health Nursing, 13,* 161-176.

Fry, S. T. (1989). Ethical issues in clinical research: Informed consent and risks versus benefits in the treatment of primary hypertension. *Nursing Clinics of North America, 24,* 1033-1039.

Gadow, S. (1983). Existential advocacy: Philosophical foundation of nursing. In C. P. Murphy & H. Hunter H (Eds.), *Ethical problems in the nurse-patient relationship* (pp. 40-60). Newton, MA: Allyn & Bacon.

Gadow, S. (1989a). Clinical subjectivity: Advocacy with silent patients. *Nursing Clinics of North America, 24*(2), 535-541.

Gadow, S. (1989b). An ethical case for patient self-determination. *Seminars in Oncology Nursing, 5*(2), 99-101.

Hughes, K. K. (1993). Decision making by patients with breast cancer: The role of information in treatment selection. *Oncology Nursing Forum, 20* (4), 623-628.

Jurchak, M. (1990). Competence and the nurse-patient relationship. *Critical Care Nursing Clinics of North America, 2*(3), 453-459.

Lynch, M. T. (1988). The nurse's role in the biotherapy of cancer: Clinical trials and informed consent. *Oncology Nursing Forum, 15*(Suppl. 6), 23-27.

Macklin, R. (1987). *Mortal choices: Bioethics in today's world.* New York: Pantheon.

Meade, C. D., & Howser, D. M. (1992). Consent forms: How to determine and improve their readability. *Oncology Nursing Forum, 19*(10), 1523-1528.

Meisel, A. (1979). The "exceptions" to the informed consent doctrine: Striking a balance between competing values in medical decision making. *Wisconsin Law Review, 1979(2),* 413–488.

Meisel, A., & Kabnick, L. (1980). Informed consent to medical treatment: An analysis of recent legislation. *University of Pittsburgh Law Review, 41,* 407.

Murphy, E. K. (1988). OR nursing law informed consent: Part II. *AORN Journal, 47,* 1294-1298.

Natanson v. Kline, 350 P.2d 1093 (1960).

Nusbaum, J. G., & Chenitz, W. C. (1990). A grounded theory study of the informed consent process for pharmacologic research. *Western Journal of Nursing Research, 12*(2), 215-228.

Omnibus Budget Reconciliation Act of 1990. Public Law No. 101-508.

Powers, M. (1993, June). Lecture on autonomy. Kennedy Institute of Ethics, Intensive Bioethics XIX. Georgetown University, Washington, DC.

Prosser, W. L. (1971). *Handbook of law and torts* (4th ed.). St. Paul, MN: West Publishing.

President's Commission for the Study of Ethical Problems in Biomedical and Behavioral Research. (1982). *Making health care decisions. 1, 2, & 3.* Washington DC: U.S. Government Printing Office.

Purtilo, R. B. (1984). Applying the principles of informed consent to patient care: Legal and ethical considerations for physical therapy. *Physical Therapy, 64*(6), 934-937.

Rachlin, S. (1974). With liberty and psychosis for all. *Psychiatric Quarterly, 60,* 410-420.

Rempusheski, V. (1991). Elements, perceptions and issues of informed consent. *Applied Nursing Research, 4*(4), 201-204.

Richardson, J. I. (1993). Informed consent: Whose responsibility? *Texas Nurse, 67*(2), 3, 15.

Roth, L., Meisel, A., & Lidz, C. (1977). Tests of competency to consent to treatment. *American Journal of Psychiatry, 134*(3), 279-284.

Rule, J. T., & Veatch, R. M. (1993). *Ethical questions in dentistry.* Chicago: Quintessence Publishing.

Salgo v. Leland Stanford University Board of Trustees, 154, Cal. App. 2d 560, 317 P.2d 170 (1957).

Schloendorff v. Society of New York Hospitals, 211 N.Y. 125, 128, 105 N.E. 92, 93 (1914).

Scofield, G. R. (1993). Ethical considerations in rehabilitation medicine. *Archives of Physical Medicine Rehabilitation, 74,* 341-346.

Silva, M.C. (1985). Comprehension of information for informed consent by spouses of surgical patients. *Research in Nursing and Health, 8,* 117–124.

Silva, M. C., & Sorrell, J. M. (1984). Factors influencing comprehension of informed consent: Ethical implications for nursing research. *International Journal of Nursing Studies, 21*(4), 233-240.

Silva, M. C., & Zeccolo, P. L. (1986). Informed consent: The right to know and the right to choose. *Nursing Management, 17*(8), 18-19.

Solomon, J., & Schwegman-Melton, K. (1987). Structured teaching and patient understanding of informed consent. *Critical Care Nurse, 7*(3), 74-79.

Sorrell, J. M. (1991). Effects of writing/speaking on comprehension of information for informed consent. *Western Journal of Nursing Research, 13*(1), 110-122.

Tammelleo, A. D. (1985). Nurse uses aversive therapy: Dismissal. Case in point: Juneau v Bd. of Elem. secondary Ed, 506 So.2d 756-LA. *Regan Report on Nursing Law, 28*(2), 4.

Tammelleo, A. D. (1990). Nurse orders objecting patient to "shut up." Case in point: Roberson v Provident House, 559 So.2d 838-LA (1990). *Regan Report on Nursing Law, 31*(3), 4.

Tammelleo, A. D. (1993a). Patient sues nurse for failure to obtain informed consent. Case in point: Foflygen v R. Zemel, MD, 615A, 2d 1345-PA (1992). *Regan Report on Nursing Law, 33*(10), 4.

Tammelleo, A. D. (1993b). Caveat to nurses in "John Doe" organ harvests: Brown v Delaware Valley Transplant Program, 615A, 2d 1379-PA (1992). *Regan Report on Nursing Law, 33*(10), 1.

Tammelleo, A. D. (1993c). "Informed consent" by intoxicated E. R. patient not required: Miller v Rhode Island Hospital, 625A, 2d 778 (1993). *Regan Report on Hospital Law, 34*(3), 2.

Thomas S. v. Flaherty, 699 F. Supp. 1178 (1988).

Turnquist, A. C. (1983). The issue of informed consent and use of neuroleptic medications. *International Journal of Nursing Studies, 20*(3), 181-186.

Uniform Anatomical Gift Act of 1987. 1–17, 8A U.L.A. (1989).

Varricchio, C. G., & Jassak, P. F. (1989). Informed consent: An overview. *Seminars in Oncology Nursing, 5*(2), 95-98.

Wintz, C. J. B. (1992). A nurse's research dilemma. In G. B. White (Ed.), *Ethical dilemmas in contemporary nursing practice* (pp. 129-145). Washington, DC: American Nurses Publishers.

Woods, S. L. (1988). Informed consent in research and the critically ill adult. *Progress in Cardiovascular Nursing, 3,* 89-92.

6

Educational Theories for Teaching and Motivating Patients

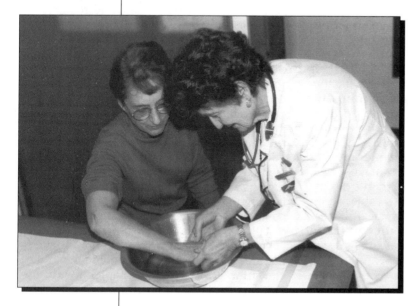

OBJECTIVES FOR CHAPTER 6

After reading this chapter, the nurse or student nurse should be able to:

1 Distinguish between compliance and cooperation as desirable outcomes for patient education.

2 Define three components of empowerment and apply them to a patient education situation involving mammography.

3 Compare and contrast the Health Belief Model, self-efficacy theory, and stress and coping as useful bases of patient education.

4 Describe the sequence of events in learning and recount examples of the events as applied to patient education.

Patient Education: Issues, Principles, Practices, Third Edition, by Sally H. Rankin and Karen Duffy Stallings.
Lippincott–Raven Publishers, Philadelphia, © 1996.

The Essence of Patient Education

In the preceding chapters, we examined issues that pertain to the provision of patient education by health care providers. We focused on issues that arise based on system constraints to effective patient teaching as well as contextual and environmental influences that condition the learning situation. This chapter considers the issues the patient faces as a result of a complex variety of factors, including attitudes and beliefs and their influence on motivation. Additional factors influencing these issues include teaching and learning theories and their impact on individual patient learning.

These issues cause each patient to affect the health care system in a unique way and influence the person's decision-making as a consumer of health care services. We discuss situations in which the patient's values are in conflict with those of the health care provider and in which patient education does not result in the behavioral changes suggested by the provider. In our examination of teaching and learning we consider the sequence of steps involved in learning. Finally, we present major schools of contemporary learning theory so that the nurse and other health professionals have sufficient understanding of the theoretical underpinnings of patient education. Empowerment has been an important underlying component of our approach to patient education; in this third edition of the book, it is further developed using the work of Paulo Freire.

Patient Education: A Process of Influencing Behavior

One of the definitions of patient education is that of Scott Simonds (National Task Force, 1979):

> Patient education is the process of influencing behavior, producing changes in knowledge, attitudes, and skills required to maintain and improve health. The process may begin with the imparting of information, but it also includes interpretation and integration of information in such a manner as to bring about attitudinal or behavioral changes that benefit a person's health status.

This definition seems particularly applicable to the focus of this chapter.

Because patient education is a process, it occurs over a period of time and requires an ongoing assessment of the patient's knowledge, attitudes, and skills. The patient's readiness or motivation to change and the obstacles to change are important factors to be considered during the process of assessment. Chapter 7 offers an in-depth discussion of assessment for patient education. Most practitioners involved in teaching patients realize the impact of the family on the patient's behavior. A close, supportive family unit may facilitate the integration of new health behaviors although the family facing conflict or lacking understanding often poses barriers to behavioral change. Strong religious, ethnic, or cultural beliefs may also prevent or influence desired change. The potency of sociocultural belief systems in influencing patient education is discussed in Chapter 4 with suggestions made to enhance the transfer of information, knowledge, and skills to persons of different cultural and ethnic groups. A Patient and Family Education Assessment Guide, introduced in Chapter 7, provides guidance in examining factors that may promote or impede the process of patient education. The practitioner can then offer the patient and the family assistance in overcoming obstacles to behavioral change.

Compliance Orientation

We asked physicians and nurses to share with us what they considered to be obstacles in their experiences with patient education. All of them identified problems with either motivating patients or achieving patient compliance. When they were asked to elaborate, they saw the two problems as closely related. The implication was that a sufficiently motivated patient would comply with the doctor's or nurse's instructions.

Many of us have justified our involvement in patient education by asserting that it would increase patient compliance, in other words, convince patients to follow our suggestions. As research in health education expands, it becomes apparent that, despite teaching, patients frequently do not make the choices recommended to them by nurses, physicians, and other health professionals. This is often termed *noncompliance.*

We are uneasy with the term *compliance.* It implies that we dictate to the patient what is to be done or changed and that the patient is to follow instructions—to obey us. Further soul-searching makes us realize that our discomfort stems from the patient's right to choose *not* to follow our advice, even though we know what is best for him.

In sharing our thoughts and ideas on the compliance orientation with Godfrey Hochbaum, PhD (Professor, School of Public Health, University of North Carolina at Chapel Hill, conference, June 1981), we have developed a broader appreciation of the patient's position in patient education. It is natural for health professionals to want patients to choose the recommended course of action; however, what we really should strive to enlist is their partnership or cooperation rather than compliance. We want them to *choose* what we suggest.

An orientation toward cooperation rather than toward compliance causes us to think about our own effectiveness in patient education in a different light. Perhaps patient education successes have more to do with patients' preparation to make informed choices than with their compliance. If, in fact, patient education acknowledges the patient's free will to make choices, it must afford understanding of the importance of his values and wishes and his ability to participate in decision-making.

As student nurses, acute care and ambulatory nurses, clinical nurse specialists, and nurse practitioners, we have all had experiences with noncooperative patients. These experiences teach us that effective patient education requires an understanding of those factors that influence the patient in decision-making: values, beliefs, attitudes, current life stresses, religion, previous experiences with the health care system, and life goals. They also illustrate that patient education involves teaching and learning that must be accompanied by behavioral changes. Patient education providers may begin with giving information and demonstrating skills, but if the patient is not included in deciding how learning will be applied, and the goals of patient education are not mutually agreed on between the teacher and the learner, behavioral changes usually will not occur.

We must understand that although the health professional tends to view cooperation with the medical regimen as a single choice, the patient's cooperation with the regimen involves many choices every day. The choice to follow the diabetic diet, for example, means not one choice but constant (often inconvenient and anguishing) choices throughout each day. We expect him to do this every day for the rest of his life even though we cannot guarantee that he will be free of neuropathies, retinopathies, nephropathies, or other complications. We offer him our guidance and support. We must also be willing to respect the patient's right to choose although we may not agree with his choice.

We reserve the right to keep trying. Despite poor cooperation in the past, we remain hopeful that a patient may be more open to patient education messages during future encounters. We must also respect the patient's right to change his mind. He may choose to take the course of action we suggest or to turn away from it if he judges that the cost or hardship to him outweighs the benefit, as in the case of a terminally ill patient receiving chemotherapy. He initially decided to take the treatment, but later decided to discontinue the chemotherapeutic drugs because he weighed the costly and uncomfortable side effects against the benefits.

The Agenda of Education

As health care providers we bring to the educational setting our own agenda, or purpose, for the health education endeavor. Health care provider attitudes related to the purpose of education vary similarly to attitudes about compliance. Although Chandler's (1992) characterization of the purpose of education was related to students in primary and secondary schools, it is also pertinent to the agenda of various health care professionals who provide patient education. Four purposes are outlined:

1. Prepare students for assumption of adult roles
2. Provide students with an orientation to improve society
3. Maintain appreciation of the dominant culture and the status quo
4. Provide knowledge that liberates people

These purposes are illustrated in Table 6-1 with the educational theorist from whom the perspective is derived and also with a patient education corollary.

The first purpose has been a motivating force behind patient education as it also has been a force in public and private school education in the United States. The second and third purposes also reflect dominant school and patient education purposes. Providing liberating knowledge so that patients can control their own care is part of the empowerment movement, which has generated a great deal of interest but one that is difficult to institute and perpetuate, particularly at the community level (Israel, Checkoway, Schulz, & Zimmerman, 1994).

Empowerment in Patient Education

The term *empowerment*, now a "buzz" word throughout American life, was introduced in the 1970s with the work of Brazilian educator, Paulo Freire. Freire advocates a participatory educational process in which people are able to name their own problems and solutions, and through this process, transform themselves and their communities (Freire, 1970; Wallerstein & Bernstein, 1994). Freire purports that education is never neutral; it is always enmeshed in the values of educators. Additionally, people will act on the issues about which they have strong feelings; their identification of issues may not be congruent with those of the teacher or health care provider.

The participatory educational process is in opposition to some of the purposes of student and patient education outlined in Table 6-1. When the term is applied to an aggregate, such as community empowerment, expectations are that people will listen to each other, compare and contrast central issues in their lives, and together construct new strategies for change (Wallerstein & Bernstein, 1994). Community empowerment has been undertaken in such attempts as the San Francisco Homeless Prenatal Program (Ovrebo, Ryan, Jackson, & Hutchinson, 1994), the Boston Healthy Start Initiative (Plough & Olafson, 1994), the Adolescent Social Action

---

TABLE 6–1. The Purpose of Education

Purpose of Student Education	Educational Proponent	Patient Education Corollary
Prepare students for adult role positions	Bobbitt (1924), Finney (1928)	Prepare patients for compliant orderly, obedient positions
Provide students with an orientation to improve society	Kandal (1941), Kliebard (1987)	Improve patient/health care provider relationships
Maintain the status quo and reproduce the culture	Broudy (1982)	Maintain the status quo with health care providers dominant
Provide knowledge that liberates people	Anyon (1980), Freire (1970)	Provide liberating knowledge so that patients control their own care

Adapted from Chandler, S. (1992). Learning for what purpose? Questions when viewing classroom learning from a sociocultural curriculum perspective. In H.H. Marshall (Ed.), *Redefining student learning: Roots of educational change* (p. 33). Norwood, NJ: Ablex Publishing.

Program in New Mexico to decrease alcohol and substance abuse (Wallerstein & Sanchez-Merki, 1994), and in rural China with peasant women (Wang & Burris, 1994). Although community empowerment is a worthy ideal, its exploration is beyond the scope of this chapter. However, individual empowerment as a strategy to achieve better patient education outcomes is introduced below.

Individual or psychological empowerment concerns the ability of the patient to have control over his own life. Israel and colleagues (1994) view individual empowerment being similar to such theoretical constructs as self-efficacy (discussed below) and self-esteem in its emphasis on the development of a sense of mastery, control, and competence. Additionally, empowerment includes the establishment of critical thinking and analytical skills that allows the patient to better understand the resources and competencies needed to achieve the desired ends. When applied to patient education, the health care professional must provide a framework for creative thinking; assist the patient in raising such questions as why, how, and who; and establish an environment where genuine dialogue can occur. Lastly, the health care professional encourages the chosen actions and evaluates their results with the patient. A model for individual empowerment in patient education situations involving hypertension is illustrated in Table 6-2. Although the strategies involved may not be considered as desirable by many health care professionals, we would like to point out that a great percentage of hypertensive patients never comply with their medication regime because of the pharmacologic consequences. Therefore, an empowerment approach is at least as likely to achieve a reduction in blood pressure as the more traditional patient education approach.

Malcolm Knowles, the proponent of "andragogy" or adult learning, attempts to em-

---

TABLE 6–2. Components of Empowerment as Applied to Patient Education With a Hypertensive Patient

Component of Empowerment	Application to Patient Education
Sufficient knowledge to make rational, informed decisions	Nurse ascertains patient's explanatory model about hypertension (see Chap. 4). Nurse gives patient all information necessary to make informed decision about management of hypertension including nonpharmacologic (diet, exercise, herbs) and pharmacologic (side effects of medications). Patient is informed of possible complications if high blood pressure is not controlled. Nurse encourages patient to read widely on hypertension, to talk with friends and relatives.
Sufficient control and resources to implement decisions	Nurse gives patient access to clinic materials on management of hypertension as well as suggestions for other nonmedical reading. Nurse informs patient of costs of various treatment options. Nurse meets with patient when patient is ready to discuss treatment options and asks patient for decision regarding treatment.
Sufficient experience to evaluate the effectiveness of their decisions	Nurse supports patient in desire to use nonpharmacologic approach. Nurse teaches patient how to monitor his own blood pressure at home and asks him to call her with weekly readings for 6 wks. When blood pressure does not respond to nonpharmacologic approach, nurse suggests other nonpharmacologic therapies such as biofeedback. Nurse continues to monitor patient's blood pressure by telephone and continues to support patient in attempt to achieve blood pressure control without drugs.

Adapted from Funnell, M. M., Anderson, R. M., Arnold, M. S., Barr, P. A., Donnelly, M., Johnson, P. D., Moon, D., & White, N. H. (1991). Empowerment: An idea whose time has come in diabetes education. *Diabetes Educator, 17*, 37–41.

power adults through the principles he imparts. His important work is covered in Chapter 8.

Patient Decision-Making

Patient Issues: A Review of the Literature

A review of patient education literature reveals many of the variables that influence patients' choices not to follow the suggestions of health professionals. Lack of cooperation is common among patients of all economic and educational backgrounds, not just among low-income populations. Rationalization and denial are recurrent problems encountered in patient education and are often seen in the management of chronic illness. Indeed, the nature of chronic illness with its remissions and exacerbations influences patient attitudes toward adherence and patient teaching with nonadherence estimated at 30% to 60% (Cameron & Gregor, 1987). Others report even higher rates of noncompliance with prescribed drug regimens, estimating that up to 50% of all patients fail to achieve full compliance and as many as a third never take their prescribed medications at all (Schroeder & McPhee, 1993).

Additional patient issues affect the patient's participation in preventive health care, with attitudes toward automobile seat belt usage and modification of diet to prevent cardiovascular disease illustrative of American attitudes toward prevention of injury and disease (Simons-Morton, Mullen, Mains, Tabak, & Green, 1992; Mullen, Mains & Velez, 1992; Sleet, 1984). The Health Belief Model (see section below) demonstrates that the patient's perceptions about the presence of disease, the likelihood of contracting disease, or experiencing an injury are predictors of his consumption of health services (Hochbaum, 1958; Janz & Becker, 1984).

Feelings such as anxiety, depression, and anger influence the patient's understanding and, eventually, his choices (Berg, Alt, Himmel, & Judd, 1985; Devine, 1992). In addi-

tion, religion, ethnicity, family problems, and family experiences influence the patient's course of action (Tripp-Reimer & Afifi, 1989). Such variables as knowledge about disease and prior contact with the disease are identified as modifying factors in the patient's consumption of health care services.

Lindeman (1988), a noted nurse-researcher in patient education, characterizes the variables influencing human learning in patient education situations as: patient characteristics, nurse characteristics, nurse-patient interaction in teaching situations, health- and disease-specific characteristics, and health care setting characteristics. These variables are examined in more detail from the perspective of research in Chapter 15.

Other patient issues affecting patient education include the patient's coping style and locus of control. Lazarus, a cognitive psychologist working in the area of stress and coping, has recognized coping as being primarily emotion focused or problem focused (Lazarus, 1991; Lazarus & Folkman, 1984). Emotion-focused coping in situations of patient education usually includes attempts to appraise the threat involved in an illness. Generally, the efforts involved at appraising and controlling the threat preclude effective patient teaching. For example, if a patient has recently experienced a myocardial infarction (MI) and is using defense mechanisms such as denial as a form of emotion-focused coping, it is unlikely that effective patient teaching can be accomplished. On the other hand, if the situation has evolved to the point that rational, action-oriented coping, commonly referred to as problem-focused coping, is being used, then the patient will be more open to suggestions related to disease management and necessary life-style changes. For a more in-depth discussion of stress and coping theories see a later section in this chapter.

Patient education requires an openness on the part of the health professional, as well as a desire to discover the variables that influence a patient's choices. Working through, rather than around, patient issues helps us to intervene most effectively and to address the barriers that prevent patients from cooperating.

Patient education requires us to take a skilled approach in assessing patient issues and problems and in setting goals with patients. Chapters 7 and 8 help strengthen this approach through use of the nursing process.

Models and Theories as the Research and Practice Foundation of Patient Education

Various theories and models have been used as the conceptual basis of patient education practice and research. While Lindeman (1988) and Smith (1989) have argued for a singular model that would unify patient education practice and research, others have noted the complexity of the topic and pragmatically contend that different models of patient and health education are needed depending on the environment, learners' needs, and a host of other factors (Glanz, Lewis, & Rimer, 1990; Oberst, 1989). We agree with the latter group and assert that the theories used in research and practice should be carefully chosen to match all situational contingencies. The fact that most patient education research in the past has been atheoretical is characteristic of research in many disciplines, especially those that are recent arrivals on the research scene. The following section presents useful theoretical approaches for patient education.

Health Belief Model

The Health Belief Model has been the most frequently used theoretical basis for research examining the efficacy of patient eduction. The traditional Health Belief Model, also discussed in Chapters 3 and 9, was constructed in the 1950s by a group of social psychologists at the U.S. Public Health Service to predict health behaviors. Built on earlier work of Kurt Lewin, an influential social psychologist, it provides a tool for understanding the patient's perception of disease and his decision-making process in the consumption of health care services. Although the Health Be-

lief Model was originally designed to predict the likelihood of patients' taking recommended preventive action, such as obtaining screening tests and annual checkups, it has been the basis for other models adapted to consider the consumption of health care services in the presence of chronic illness (Janz & Becker, 1984) or in situations where health promotion is desirable (Pender, 1987). In addition, its application as a model in research is often for compliance prediction; it is also useful for gaining a better understanding of the patient's motivation for seeking and obtaining services.

The Health Belief Model predicts that an individual is likely to consume health care services if the following situations exist and the patient experiences the following:

1. Perceives that he has a disease or condition or is likely to contract it
2. Perceives that the disease or condition is harmful and has serious consequences
3. Believes that the suggested health intervention is of value
4. Believes that the effectiveness of the treatment is worth the cost and barriers he must confront

Additionally, demographic variables, such as age, gender, ethnicity, and socioeconomic status, as well as cues to action, are considered modifiers of the individual's perception that the disease or condition is harmful (Janz & Becker, 1984). Cues to action include mass media campaigns, advice from others, newspaper or magazine articles, or illness of a family member or friend. Readers are referred to Chapter 8 for a practical approach to using the Health Belief Model in identifying patient goals and decisions.

A review of research testing this model suggests that barriers and costs a person confronts are the most salient reasons for either engaging in preventive health behavior or behavior related to the illness regimen (Rosenstock, 1990). Susceptibility to and severity of an illness were not as powerful predictors of behavior as barriers and costs, except for those persons who already have an illness, such as coronary artery disease.

The Health Belief Model has been criticized because it is difficult to test as a complete entity and is not quantifiable. Additionally, as Rosenstock (1990) points out, the Health Belief Model and social psychology have never been able to provide a direct link between beliefs and behavior. Others have noted that it fails to account for important environmental influences such as community and public policy factors. Our students have noted that the model imposes the perspective of health care professionals with the possibility of noncompliant patients being blamed for their behavior, a type of "blaming the victim" phenomenon. Nevertheless, it remains a premier theoretical model to guide practice and research.

The Health Promotion Model as developed by Pender is discussed in depth in Chapter 3. Another model pertinent to patient education, the Self-Regulation or Common Sense Model, is also discussed in Chapter 3. The foundation for both of these models is the Health Belief Model.

The following two theories, self-efficacy and stress and coping, are generally characterized as interpersonal theories of health behavior, whereas the Health Belief Model is characterized as a model of individual health behavior. Interpersonal models of health behavior offer promise for health care providers because we can become one of the sources of change in our patients' lives according to this formulation.

Self-Efficacy Theory

One of the most promising theoretical bases for patient education is social learning theory. Social learning theory, also referred to as self-efficacy theory, promises a more comprehensive theoretical base because it accounts not only for learner characteristics but also gives direction to the teacher for managing the physical and social environment in which learning occurs (Bandura, 1977).

The self-confidence to perform certain behaviors is derived from four discrete sources of information (Bandura, 1982). These include personal mastery, vicarious experiences, ver-

bal persuasion, and physiologic feedback. *Personal mastery* is the most important of the four sources of information and refers to the patient's perceived confidence that he is actually performing the desired behavior. An example of personal mastery is the newly diagnosed diabetic patient's ability to perform home blood glucose monitoring successfully. If the patient had experienced a number of unsuccessful attempts to draw blood and read the glucometer, the sense of personal mastery, or self-efficacy, would be diminished and learning would become more difficult.

The *vicarious experiences* that patients gain from observing role models, whether they are other patients, health professionals, or family members, are especially important for the new learner. For example, the new ostomate will frequently learn better and more quickly how to manage a new ostomy if taught by another person who has also had an ostomy and can role model successful management. Vicarious experiences are more predictive of effective patient education if the role model has similar characteristics to the learner, including age, gender, and ability.

Verbal persuasion as a source of information for patients reinforces verbally the patient's competence in enacting new behaviors. In a study of recovery from cardiac surgery, patients and their spouses were coached on the telephone by nurses for 8 weeks after hospital discharge regarding various aspects of risk factor reduction (Gortner et al., 1988). Additionally, patients were verbally encouraged to walk and get other forms of exercise as their condition permitted. The encouragement and verbal persuasion were reinforced by the weekly telephone calls.

Physiologic feedback, previously referred to as emotional arousal, refers to the necessary physical cues patients receive that the behavior they have undertaken is either appropriate or inappropriate, or that alternative actions should be sought. For example, a study of post-MI patients used treadmill testing as a form of physiologic feedback (Ewart, Taylor, Reese & DeBusk, 1983). In a unique attempt to ameliorate the fears of the patients' wives, and as a form of enhancing vicarious experiences, the wives were also given the opportunity to use the treadmill, thus giving them the opportunity to reinforce desired behavior through vicarious experience and their own physiologic feedback (Taylor, Bandura, Ewart, Miller, & DeBusk, 1985).

The use of social learning theory as a theoretical framework to guide patient education research and practice offers a more coherent approach to patient education than has been present in the past. Measurement of a patient's confidence, or sense of perceived self-efficacy, usually involves measures that present a singular situation such as climbing steps and then ask how confident the person is that he can climb three steps, one flight of steps, two flights of steps, and so on. The patient is then asked how confident on a scale of not at all confident (0%) to completely confident (100%) he feels in climbing steps. In a study of cardiac patients, experimental study patients who had been coached reported greater self-efficacy in terms of walk-

ing and lifting than did the control, or uncoached, group (Gortner et al., 1988).

Self-efficacy theory has contributed to the theoretical basis of patient education by specifying mechanisms that enhance learning and also increase motivation. It has been criticized for its generality and lack of methodologic refinement. In terms of deriving interventions for practice, however, the four discrete sources of information that can result in desired behavior change provide a useful heuristic for designing programs. Table 6-3 suggests different patient education interventions for the various sources of efficacy information with application to a newly diagnosed 9-year-old diabetic child who must learn how to administer insulin to himself.

The following theories are useful in understanding patient response to threatening situations involving illness. They are also considered interpersonal theories of health behavior.

TABLE 6–3. Sources of Efficacy Expectations and Related Patient Education Activity Performance for Newly Diagnosed Type I Diabetic Children Who Must Learn Insulin Injection

Sources of Efficacy Expectations	Related Patient Education Activity Performance
Performance accomplishments	1. Participant modeling: successful injection of insulin by fearful, newly diagnosed, diabetic child 2. Performance desensitization: loss of fear of self-injections 3. Performance exposure: continued successful practice of insulin injection
Vicarious experience	1. Live modeling: demonstration by another diabetic child of insulin injection procedures 2. Symbolic modeling: successful insulin demonstration by an age- and gender-matched diabetic child
Verbal persuasion	1. Suggestion: informing the child on insulin injection techniques and methods to decrease anxiety surrounding it 2. Exhortation: persuasive coaching by parents and nurse to perform successful insulin injection 3. Self-instruction: child uses doll to learn insulin injection with persuasion from nurse
Physiologic/emotional arousal	1. Attribution: modification of the threat of injection by attributing the fear to something, or someone, else 2. Relaxation, biofeedback: modifying threat by deep-breathing exercises before injection

Adapted from Bandura, A. (1977). Self-efficacy theory: Toward a unifying theory of behavior change. *Psychological Review, 84,* 191–215.

Stress, Coping, and Social Support

Stress, coping, and social support theories comprise a group of theoretical perspectives derived by various social scientists. Those that the authors have found most useful in their own practice include the cognitive appraisal approach of Lazarus and the sociologic approach of Pearlin. Both of these approaches include social support as an important modifier of stress.

Historically, stress research was given impetus by the work of two physiologists, Cannon (1939) and Selye (1936, 1952, 1982). Selye generated a tradition, still prominent today in the work of Lazarus and colleagues (1984, 1991) and others, which posits that the response of the organism is more important than the nature of the stimulus provoking the response. This approach to stress is different from that of epidemiologists and sociologists who are more concerned with the genesis, or source, of stress (i.e., the stres-

sors). We believe that both perspectives are important to understanding the patient in situations where patient education is warranted.

The cognitive appraisal approach is important because it assists the health care provider in understanding that the individual's response to a stimulus is unique and that the evaluation of the stimulus is influenced by factors within the individual and from the stimulus itself. Psychological stress is thus the relationship between the person and the environment that is appraised as exceeding the available personal resources (Lazarus & Folkman, 1984). Cognitive appraisal is an evaluation of the situation and includes primary appraisal, "Am I in difficulty?" and secondary appraisal "What can I do about it?" A simplified illustration of the stress response according to Lazarus and colleagues is depicted in Figure 6-1.

Lazarus and his colleagues posit that coping is an ongoing process and does not occur in stages; rather it is constantly being re-

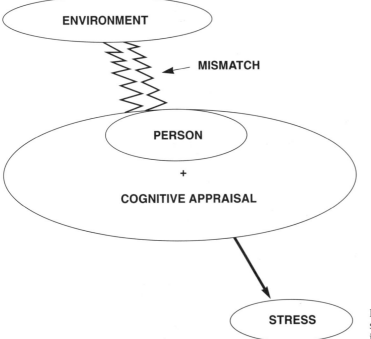

FIGURE 6-1. Depiction of the person—environment mismatch generating stress.

worked. Coping comprises cognitive and behavioral efforts to manage specific demands that are appraised by the patient as straining or exceeding personal resources. Coping resources Lazarus identifies as being available to people include health and energy, positive beliefs, problem-solving, social skills, social support, and material resources.

The health care provider will usually assist the patient in terms of developing problem-focused coping because this type of coping is most appropriate when something can be done about the situation. The nurse will offer information to enhance problem-solving and will mobilize socially supportive resources by helping the family understand how they can be most supportive during periods of stress. By referring the patient and family to a hospital social worker or case manager the nurse is mobilizing material resources. Table 6-4 illustrates, using the example of a 36-year-old woman with newly diagnosed breast cancer, how the nurse might intervene to enhance coping resources with a combination of patient education and other nursing interventions.

The sociologic view of stress is illustrated in Figure 6-2 with application to a woman who has had an acute MI. This framework postulates that the sources and mediators of stress are located within the social environment of individuals (Pearlin, Lieberman, Menaghan, & Mullan, 1981). Sources of stress are those stressors in the biologic or social environment that lead to the experience of stress. Stressors consist of life events and persistent life strains that can be physiologic or psychosocial in origin (Pearlin & Schooler, 1978). In the case of a woman with an acute MI, stressors may consist of the presence of physiologic risk factors (e.g., diabetes mellitus, hypertension) and problems of a psychosocial origin (e.g., overeating, smoking, inactivity). Mediators of stress are those social resources that assist the individual in adjusting and finally adapting to the stressors. Social support is a primary mediator of stress. Thus, for the woman with an acute MI, mediators of stress might be a supportive spouse and family.

Stress subsumes a variety of physiologic and psychosocial manifestations. Following

TABLE 6–4. Patient Education and Nursing Interventions to Enhance Coping Resources in a 36-year-old Woman With Breast Cancer

Type of Resource	Example of Resource	Nursing Action
Physical resources	Health and energy	Teach importance of diet to maintain strength and decrease cachectic effects
Psychological resources	1. Positive beliefs	1. Reinforce positive attitudes related to treatment and cure; decrease negative attitudes
	2. Problem-solving	2. Assist patient in finding solutions to problems within her purview to solve; limit scope of problem-solving to those problems in which the patient can realistically intervene.
Social resources	1. Social skills	1. Refer to American Cancer Society "I Can Cope" groups, Reach to Recovery; reinforce previously developed social skills.
	2. Social support	2. Mobilize family and friends as support. If family and friends are not supportive, refer for counseling if the patient concurs.
Material resources	Money, goods, and services	Refer to hospital social services, discharge planning, and other community agency if the patient concurs. Give information about available services.

Adapted from Lazarus, R. S., & Folkman, S. (1984). *Stress, appraisal, and coping.* New York: Springer.

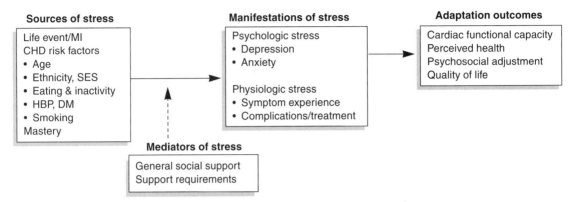

FIGURE 6-2. The stress process applied to women with acute myocardial infarctions. CHD, coronary heart disease; DM, diabetes mellitus; HBP, high blood pressure; MI, myocardial infarction; SES, socioecomonic status. Adapted from "The Stress Process," by L. I. Pearlin, M. A. Lieberman, E. G. Menaghan, and J. T. Mullan, 1981, *(Journal of health and Social Behavior, 22,* p. 337–356.)

an acute life event such as MI, stress may be manifested by depression and anxiety as well as by the experience of symptoms such as arrhythmias and pain.

Adaptation is the dynamic process of adjusting to stress. Although not part of Pearlin's original stress model, it is consistent with his work, and also a nursing perspective, to view adaptation as the logical outcome of the stress process. Adaptation includes the patient's adjustment to the MI and ongoing coronary artery disease, her perceived quality of life, her assessment of her general health, and her cardiac functional capacity. The nurse who uses a sociologic view of stress in her practice of patient education will give more attention to enhancing social resources and decreasing stressors in the social environment than will the nurse who practices using a cognitive appraisal view of stress. Both the psychological and sociologic approaches to viewing the stress process are useful and both have utility for patient education.

The next section of this chapter reviews the process of teaching and learning. The theories presented up to this point have been primarily macroanalytical theories of patient and health education, that is, they are useful in terms of understanding the broader aspects of patient education. The actual learn-ing process includes microanalytical theories that pertain to particular ideas about how information is actually learned and processed. This section of the chapter also includes a discussion of motivation.

Understanding the Process of Teaching and Learning

Definition of Learning

Learning has been defined variously as a process involving interaction with the external environment (Gagne & Driscoll, 1988) and as a change in behavior resulting from reinforced practice (Huckabay, 1980). The definition by Huckabay, a noted nurse educator, seems especially pertinent to the learning that must occur in patient teaching situations involving psychomotor skills. Chapter 8 discusses psychomotor learning in more depth, but, in brief, we define *psychomotor learning* as pertaining to learning of skills and performance. Learning that requires a change in feelings or belief, which is called *affective learning*, and learning that requires thinking, *cognitive learning*, may be more difficult forms of learning to promote and to measure.

Sequence of Events in Learning

Learning and remembering are generally thought of as an orderly sequence of events that occurs in all learners. Figure 6-3 illustrates a visual representation of the process. Bigger, 1976; Gagne, an educational psychologist, delineates the sequence of learning and remembering as one that occurs in eight phases: motivation, apprehending, acquisition, retention, recall, generalization, performance, and feedback (Bigge & Shermis, 1992; Bigge, 1976; Gagne & Driscoll, 1988; Huckabay, 1980; Lewis, Rankin, & Kellogg, 1985).

Motivation can be either internal or external. If a parent wishes to take her child home from the hospital following a fracture of the fibula and tibia, and cast care must be taught, the mother will have sufficient internal motivation to learn cast care. External motivation requires that others generate a feeling of expectancy in the learner that rewards will result from the learning.

During the *apprehending* phase, learners are exposed to the stimulus that they then take in and process in a manner that requires discriminative abilities. Patients who are mildly or moderately anxious are often good subjects for patient teaching because they attend to the stimulus with greater care than those who are not anxious. For example, most coronary artery bypass graft surgery patients and their family members are moderately anxious the day before surgery. Their discriminative abilities are heightened, and patient teaching can be extremely effective.

The *acquisition* phase includes the changes that occur in the central nervous system (CNS) and undergird and concretize the new material. Implications for the nurse in patient teaching situations are that if there is a CNS dysfunction, the new material may not be acquired. The patient with a cerebrovascular accident is an obvious example; he may be able to apprehend new information, but because of CNS damage, he may not be able to perform the desired behavior.

Retention is the fourth phase of learning, and during this phase the material that was previously apprehended is stored in the nervous system as memories. Age may be an intervening factor in terms of retention because we know that the elderly have more problems with retention of recent events and information than events or information previously retained.

Recall is retrieval; during recall the learner is able to retrieve the new capabilities for an external observer or teacher. For example, when parents are asked to demonstrate endotracheal suctioning, they recall the basics of sterile suctioning technique, then they organize the procedure systematically and are able to perform the skill safely and correctly.

Generalization, the sixth phase in the learning process, is sometimes referred to as the transfer of learning (Bigge, 1992). During generalization the patient is able to retrieve something he has learned and apply it within a different situation or context. For example, the parent who has learned the principles of

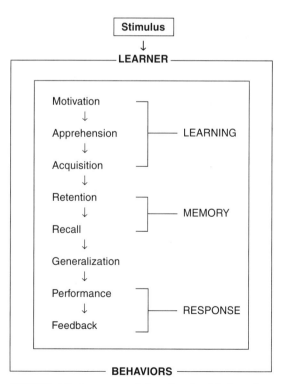

FIGURE 6-3. Sequence of steps involved in learning.

sterile technique in the context of sterile suctioning should be able to apply these techniques to other situations requiring sterile techniques.

Performance and *feedback* are the seventh and eighth phases of learning. *Performance* is the observable behavior and thus a demonstration that a change has occurred. Performance is relatively easy to observe in situations of psychomotor learning. However, in situations of affective and cognitive learning, performance is more difficult to observe and frequently must be obtained through verbal methods. *Feedback* is the last phase of learning and occurs through reinforcement. Feedback in situations of psychomotor learning is automatic because successful performance of the newly learned information serves as feedback. In situations of affective or cognitive learning, however, feedback is frequently a function of the instructor who encourages the learner by saying "good," "that's correct," and so on.

Additional Notes on Motivation

We hear constantly from staff nurses and advanced practice nurses how difficult it is to motivate patients and we have ourselves experienced this same lack of motivation with patients, family members, and friends in situations involving health and illness. Anyone who has ever tried to stop smoking, lose weight, or exercise regularly knows how difficult it is to change old behaviors. We believe that at times patients truly cannot be motivated to change their behavior. Indeed, if we espouse an empowerment viewpoint we must recognize that there are times when given all available information and after engaging in a fully participatory encounter, patients will still choose not to embrace healthy behaviors.

Gadow's work on existential advocacy that was presented in Chapter 5 further elaborates this view of motivation. She reminds us that the nurse as partner with the patient, meets him where he is and assists in whatever manner possible in coming to a decision about taking on certain behaviors (Gadow, 1983).

Gadow conceptualizes that the patient is on a continuum that stretches between consumerism and paternalism. Thus, the nurse who takes a consumerist view of the patient presents him with all of the options with little regard for the patient's personal values and beliefs. Unlike the empowerment approach, the consumerist approach does not allow for reflection and listening. At the other end of the continuum is a paternalistic position in which the nurse tells the patient what to do and makes decisions for him, a position that most nurses eschew.

Recently, however, there have been advances in attempts to understand human motivation. The following section presents an overview of the work of Prochaska and his transtheoretical model of health behavior change. One of the most appealing aspects of Prochaska's work is that his stages of change have been applied successfully to some of the most hazardous and unhealthy behaviors with moderate success.

The transtheoretical model of behavior change is an attempt to explain why some people do not modify risky behaviors despite adequate information. It has been used to study behaviors most resistant to change including addictive behaviors, diet and weight control, smoking cessation, sexual behavior related to human immunodeficiency virus (HIV) infection, and other life-endangering behaviors (Prochaska, Redding, Harlow, Rossi, & Velicer, 1994). Prochaska and colleagues propose that the stages of change are a "developmental sequence of motivational readiness" that include precontemplation, contemplation, preparation, action, and maintenance (Prochaska et al., 1994, p. 473). They point out that the stages of change are not necessarily linear and that people may go in and out of the changes as they revert to previous risk-taking behaviors. They suggest that interventions to motivate people need to be tailored for each stage. The theory is complex and includes the concept of self-efficacy, which was discussed earlier in the chapter. The interested reader is referred to the work of James Prochaska and his 15 years of publications on change and motivation. Table 6-5 lists the stage and its associated length of time and the type of intervention health care professionals can provide to increase motivation for change.

Theories of Learning

Before 1950, comprehensive theories of learning were proposed that asserted an explanation for all types of learning. However, as educational psychologists grew to understand more about the nature of learning, a realization dawned that single theories could not explain the entire realm of teaching and learning. Therefore, theories emerged that attempted to explain certain facets of teaching and learning, such as concept learning, problem-solving, skill mastery, and so on.

Tables 6-6 and 6-7 present various teaching and learning theories. The first three theories belong to the pre-1950s generation of theoretical precepts pertaining to the process of teaching and learning. They also had their earliest proponents before the twentieth century (Table 6-6).

The theories in Table 6-7 have emanated from the various schools of educational psychology that have evolved during the twentieth century. Generally most writers agree that there are individual and interpersonal

(text continues on page 116)

TABLE 6–5. Prochaska's Transtheoretical Model of Motivation and Change as Applied to Weight Loss

Stage of Change	Period of Time Associated With Stage and Characteristics of Stage	Intervention
Precontemplation	• 6 months • Very little intent to change • Resistant to change • Defensiveness regarding obesity	Consciousness raising—providing information about health risks related to obesity. Increase awareness of various approaches to weight loss.
Contemplation	• Time in this stage is variable but has been reported from 6 months to years • More serious about changing behavior • Ambivalent about the costs and benefits of changing behavior	Self-reevaluation—thoughtful attention to one's self and problems may provide an opportunity for health care professionals to influence decisions about healthy eating.
Preparation	• Variable period of time • Preliminary trying out of healthy behavior such as brief attempts to eat less	Self-liberation—belief in one's ability and commitment to change. Health care provider can reinforce belief in self through provision of support.
Action	• Usually lasts up to 6 months • Periods of weight loss interspersed with recidivism and relapse	Helping relationships—need for open, caring, honest relationships can be fulfilled by health care provider.
Maintenance	• Begins 6 months after successful behavior change in the action stage; may last for years if behavior change was successful • Relapse may occur but is less common than during the action stage	Counterconditioning—substitution of positive behaviors for negative ones. Health care provider can assist with planning meals, suggesting alternative rewards to food. Stimulus control—through restructuring of the environment access to food can be controlled.

Adapted from Prochaska, J., Redding, C.A., Harlow, L.L., Rossi, J. S., Velicer, W. F. (1994). The transtheoretical model of change and HIV prevention: A review, *Health Education Quarterly, 21,* 471.

TABLE 6–6. Important Early Teaching and Learning Theories and Their Application to Patient Education

Learning Theory and Key Persons	Attributes of the Teaching/Learning Process	Nature of Learning	Application to Patient Education
Mental Discipline Plato, Aristotle—early developers M. J. Adler, R. M. Hutchins—contemporary proponents	Teacher trains intrinsic mental power. Learner maintains strict discipline to strengthen mental faculty of attention, memory, will, and perseverance. Rote memory, repetitive drill. Teacher centered with active learners.	Discipline mind and memorization of factual material	Helpful when teaching exchange diet and basic pathophysiology. Should be used with oral drills.
Natural Unfoldment F. Froebel, J. J. Rousseau—early developers P. Goodman, J. Holt, & A. H. Maslow—contemporary proponents	Learner discovers that which nature or a creator has put within him. Teacher waits until learners expresses desire to learn before attempting to teach him. Promotes intuitive awareness of self. Learner's feelings are final authority for truth. Student centered with active learners.	Self-directed active unfolding of knowledge with intuitive awareness expressed.	Applicable to clients interested in self-care, prenatal clients, well-child care.
Apperception J. F. Herbart, E. B. Titchener—original proponents	New ideas are associated with ideas that already exist in the learner's mind. Teacher explains and learner grasps generalizations, relationships, rules, or principles. Teacher centered with passive learners.	Recognition, explanation, or use of understandings, insights, principles, relationships, concepts, theories, or laws	Applicable to clients who have previous knowledge or experience on which to build (i.e., previous surgical experiences, knowledge of medications).

Adapted from Bigge M. L. (1976, 1982). Learning theories for teachers 3rd and 4th ed. New York: Harper & Row.

TABLE 6–7. Important Twentieth Century Teaching and Learning Theories and Their Application to Patient Education

Learning Theory and Key Persons	Attributes of the Teaching/Learning Process	Nature of Learning	Application to Patient Education
Individual Learning Theories			
Conditioning—Behavioristic C. L. Hull, E. L. Thorndike—early developers E. R. Guthrie, B. F. Skinner, R. Gagne—later proponents	Involves conditioning or behavior modification. Formation of stimulus-response linkages or response-stimulus reinforcements. Teacher centered with passive learners.	Increased probability of desired response	Useful for reinforcing desired behaviors in children
Cognitive-Gestalt Information Processing (IP) M. Montessori, J. Dewey, K. Lewin, G. W. Allport, E. C. Tolman—early developers J. S. Bruner, M. L. Bigge, M. Deutsch, S. Koch, Newell and Simon, W. Kohler—later proponents	Gains or changes insights, outlooks, or thought patterns. Reorganizes perceptual or cognitive fields. Purposive involvement, problem-solving and problem-raising. Teacher-student centered with cooperative and interactive inquiry. Information processing model consists of short- & long-term memory. Long-term memory is banked and can be retrieved later for use by short-term memory.	Purposefully acquired insights, principles, relationships, concepts, generalizations, rules, theories, or laws with enhanced scientific outlook and instrumental thinking. Diagnostic reasoning	Applicable to affective learning (*i.e.*, working with parents on childrearing issues). Useful when working with groups with common problems (*i.e.*, parents of handicapped children, MI spouse groups). IP is useful for building and connecting information
Mastery-Learning B. Bloom, J. Block	Breaks down complex units of instruction into smaller learning units that build on each other. Strives for large number (90%) of learners being able to achieve or master tasks. Encourages self-development.	Increased self-esteem from learning results in changed perception of self and external world	Helpful when the information to be taught requires mastery of many skills (*i.e.*, insulin-dependent diabetics).
Interpersonal Learning Theories			
Social Learning A. Bandura, W. Mischel	Process of learning is influenced by four sources of information: personal mastery, vicarious experiences, verbal persuasion, and physiologic feedback. Learner centered. Teachers can be family members or other learners.	Increased belief that one is capable of performing desired behavior and that the performance will lead to expected outcome	Enhancement of self-confidence and self-efficacy can lead to desired health behavior changes and maintenance of desired behavior.

Adapted from Bigge, M. C., & Shermis, S. S. (1982, 1992). *Learning theories for teachers* (3rd and 5th eds.). New York: Harper Collins; Bandura, A. (1982). Self-efficacy mechanism in human agency. *American Psychologist, 37,* 122; Glanz, K., Lewis, F. M., & Rimer, B. K. (Eds.). (1990) *Health behavior and health education: Theory, research, and practice.* San Francisco: Jossey-Bass.

115

learning theories. The individual learning theories include the conditioning-behavioristic family, the cognitive-Gestalt-information processing family, and mastery learning. Interpersonal learning theory includes social learning theory. Also included in the interpersonal learning theory group, although not included on the table but discussed earlier in this chapter, are stress and coping theories.

Although the theories are helpful in explaining approaches to patient teaching and learning, we should remember that most of us make use of different theories at different times depending on the situation. Indeed, an eclectic approach probably serves our patients best. The reader should note that the attempt to apply the theories to various patient education situations is more an effort to give concrete illustrations of the theories than to imply that such situations should always be guided by these theories.

The following case study demonstrates the application of behavioristic, cognitive-Gestalt, and social learning theory principles.

❑ CASE STUDY

Claire Patterson

Brief History

Claire Patterson is a 25-year-old Caucasian woman with the onset of type I, or insulin-dependent, diabetes mellitus (IDDM), at age 16. She is 160 cm (5 ft 4 in) tall and weighs 57 kg (125 lb), placing her weight 2 kg (4.4 lb) above desired weight. She attended a comprehensive diabetes education program 5 years ago and had controlled her blood glucose levels with multidose insulin therapy since the time of her program. Her glycosylated hemoglobin level recently dropped from 13% to 7%, putting it at a desired level.

After marriage and relocation to Los Angeles, she changed physicians and insulin therapy. Her new physician prescribed 28 units of Lente (insulin zinc suspension USP) and 8 units of regular human insulin. She began having seizures in the middle of the night and was hospitalized

several times during the month of October. In December, she returned to the comprehensive diabetes teaching program for better blood glucose control.

Family Setting

Claire Patterson lived at home with her parents before her marriage. Her mother, an RN, played a primary role in managing her daughter's diabetes. Claire feels that she can openly express her feelings and concerns to her parents. Her mother hesitates between trying to "back off" and allow her daughter to be more independent in managing her diabetes and taking control of diabetes management for her daughter because, she says, it "breaks my heart" to see her having convulsions. Claire requested that her mother accompany her to another week-long session at the diabetes teaching center.

Claire's husband is in military service stationed out of state, and portions of the program were audiotaped for his benefit because he was unable to attend. Both Claire and her husband are motivated to get the diabetes under control so that they can have children.

Identified Problems

Contradicting attitudes about diabetes control resulted from Claire's insulin reactions. The family recognized intellectually that long-term complications frequently resulted from high blood glucose levels, but they believed that high blood glucose levels were safer than the threat of short-term hypoglycemic reactions. Additionally, their experiences with normal, or euglycemic, blood glucose levels led them to believe they were the antecedents of low blood glucose levels.

Goals and Recommended Interventions: Appropriate Teaching and Learning Theories

First, the patient and her family would implement an insulin regimen better suited for euglycemia. This goal presumed an understanding of multiple dose, split-mix insulin therapy. The type of learning is *cognitive-Gestalt*, in which the process of gaining or changing insights is critical. A reorganization of the family's cognitive field and problem-solving abilities was required, one of the attributes of this type of teaching and learning theory. Additionally, insights, concepts, and principles were needed to enhance the Pattersons' scientific thinking because the previous type of learning related to insulin resulted from a stimulus-response or *behavioristic-conditioning* learning process. In other words, the stimulus of hypoglycemia and convulsions resulted in a response that reinforced high blood glucose levels to diminish the undesired stimulus.

The recommended interventions were teaching Claire and her mother about her insulin requirements and the need to split the doses into four different injections so that early morning high blood glucose levels can be accommodated and finer blood glucose control could be maintained. Claire's understanding about the linkages between high blood glucose levels and diet were reinforced by having her perform her own glucose monitoring and log the results at different times during the day, and then associating these levels with her food intake. The nurse instructors used a student–teacher-centered individualized learning situation for Claire, so that she could understand the necessary relationships between diet, insulin, and exercise and then make decisions about adjusting them to maintain euglycemia.

Second, the patient would demonstrate the ability to manage her diabetes independently by telephoning the nurse instructors 2 weeks after attendance at the course to report blood glucose levels and insulin dosages. This goal presumed that Claire had learned the principles of insulin, diet, and exercise and their effects on blood glucose levels as outlined in the first goal. An appropriate type of teaching and learning theory for this type of learning situation is *social learning.*

The recommended interventions included enhancing Claire's perceived self-efficacy or self-confidence that she can manage her diabetes without her mother's intercession. The four discrete sources of information leading to perceived self-efficacy include personal mastery, vicarious experiences, verbal persuasion, and physiologic feedback (Bandura, 1982; Strecher, DeVellis, Becker, & Rosenstock, 1986). Claire gained information pertaining to personal mastery through her ability to interpret her blood glucose levels based on her intake of food over the past 48 hours. Vicarious experiences were an important aspect of teaching and learning theory as it is applied in the diabetes teaching program. Claire's observation of one of the staff nurses in the program was paramount to her learning. This nurse was diabetic and had also maintained perfect metabolic control during her pregnancy. Her sharing of her experiences contributed to Claire's self-confidence. Additionally, the sharing of experiences by other patients who had managed to artfully wrest regulation from family members was an important vicarious learning experience for Claire. An additional recommendation made to Claire by the center staff was that she attend a support group sponsored by the American Diabetes Association in Los Angeles.

Summary

It is often difficult to accept the patient's prerogative to make a decision contrary to the suggestions offered by the physician and nurse. A broader understanding of the patient's choice can be gained from the applications of the Health Belief Model, models of stress and coping, and social learning theory. Learning why these issues arise and how to deal with patient decisions helps the nurse remain committed to patient education. We recognize that the ultimate role of the health professional is to encourage patients to make informed choices about their health, rather than to guarantee compliance or obedience. Prochaska's transtheoretical model of change is presented as a vehicle for motivation and principles of empowerment theory are offered as a strategy to enable patients to advocate for their own health education needs.

Understanding the theory related to teaching and learning assists the health professional in understanding the relationship between knowledge and action. Simply knowing or understanding is not sufficient to bring about change in patients' lives; action must follow understanding. The nurse who understands the principles of teaching and learning is better able to assist the client in achieving desired health behaviors.

Strategies for Critical Analysis and Application

1. Using the concept of individual or psychological empowerment, design a program to increase use of condoms for prevention of HIV infection in sexually active teenagers.

2. Using Bandura's principles of personal mastery, vicarious experiences, verbal persuasion, and physiologic feedback, design a cardiac rehabilitation program for a 60-year-old woman who is recovering from an acute MI. Which of these principles is the most difficult to incorporate in a cardiac rehabilitation program?

3. Which stress and coping model would be most useful in understanding the teaching needs of a second generation, unemployed, Chinese American with NIDDM? Why? In what type of situation would the other stress and coping model be most useful?

REFERENCES

Anyon, J. (1980). Social class and the hidden curriculum of work. *Journal of Education, 162*(1), 67-92.

Bandura, A. (1977). *Social learning theory.* Englewood Cliffs, NJ: Prentice Hall.

Bandura, A. (1982). Self-efficacy mechanism in human agency. *American Psychologist, 37,* 122-147.

Berg, C. E., Alt, K. J., Himmel, J. K., & Judd, B. J. (1985). The effects of patient education on patient cognition and disease-related anxiety. *Patient Education and Counseling, 7,* 389-394.

Bigge, M. L. (1976). *Learning theories for teachers* (3rd ed.). New York: Harper & Row.

Bigge, M. L., & Shermis, S. S. (1992). *Learning theories for teachers* (5th ed.). New York: Harper Collins.

Bobbitt, F. (1924). *How to make a curriculum.* Boston: Houghton Mifflin.

Broudy, H. S. (1982). Challenge to the curriculum worker: Uses of knowledge. In W. H. Schubert & A. L. Schubert (Eds.), *Conceptions of curriculum knowledge: Focus on students and teachers* (pp. 3-8). University Park, PA: College of Education, Pennsylvania State University.

Cameron, K., & Gregor, F. (1987). Chronic illness and compliance. *Journal of Advanced Nursing, 12,* 671-676.

Cannon, W. B. (1939). *The wisdom of the body.* New York: Norton.

Chandler, S. (1992). Learning for what purpose? Questions when viewing classroom learning from a sociocultural curriculum perspective. In H. H. Marshall (Ed.), *Redefining student learning: Roots of educational change* (pp. 33-58). Norwood, NJ: Ablex Publishing.

Devine, E. C. (1992). Effects of psychoeducational care for adult surgical patients: A meta-analysis of 191 studies. *Patient Education and Counseling, 19,* 129-142.

Ewart, C. K., Taylor, C. B., Reese, L. B., & DeBusk, R. F. (1983). The effects of early post-infarction exercise testing on self-perception and subsequently physical activity. *American Journal of Cardiology, 51,* 1076-1080.

Finney, R. L. (1928). *A sociological philosophy of education.* New York: Macmillan.

Freire, P. (1970). *Pedagogy of the oppressed.* New York: Continuum.

Funnell, M. S., Anderson, R. M., Arnold, M. S., Barr, P. A., Donnelly, M., Johnson, P. D., Moon, D., & White, N. H. (1991). Empowerment: An idea whose time has come in diabetes education. *Diabetes Educator, 17,* 37-41.

Gadow, S. (1983). Existential advocacy: Philosophical foundation of nursing. In C. P. Murphy & H. Hunter (Eds.), *Ethical problems in the nurse-patient relationship* (pp. 40-60). Newton, MA: Allyn & Bacon.

Gagne, R. M., & Driscoll, M. P. (1988). *Essentials of learning for instruction* (2nd ed.). Englewood Cliffs, NJ: Prentice Hall.

Glanz, K., Lewis, F. M., & Rimer, B. K. (Eds.). (1990). *Health behavior and health education: Theory, research, and practice.* San Francisco: Jossey-Bass.

Gortner, S. R., Gilliss, C. L., Shinn, J. A., Sparacino, P. A., Rankin, S., Leavitt, M., Price, M., & Hudes, M. (1988). Improving recovery following cardiac surgery: a randomized clinical trial. *Journal of Advanced Nursing, 13,* 649-661.

Hochbaum, G. M. (1958). *Public participation in medical screening programs.* U.S. Public Health Service Publication No. 572. Washington, DC: U.S. Government Printing Office.

Huckabay, L. (1980). *Conditions of learning and instruction in nursing.* St. Louis: C. V. Mosby.

Israel, B. A., Checkoway, B., Schulz, A., & Zimmerman, M. (1994). Health education and community empowerment: Conceptualizing and measuring perceptions of individual, organizational, and community control. *Health Education Quarterly, 21,* 149-170.

Janz, N. K., & Becker, M. H. (1984). The health belief model: A decade later. *Health Education Quarterly, 11,* 1-47.

Kandal, I. L. (1941). The fantasia of current education. *American Scholar, 10,* 287.

Kliebard, H. (1987). *The struggle for the American curriculum.* New York: Routledge & Kegan Paul.

Lazarus, R. S. (1991). *Emotion and adaptation.* New York: Oxford University Press.

Lazarus, R. S., & Folkman, S. (1984). *Stress, appraisal, and coping.* New York: Springer.

Lewis, J., Rankin, S., & Kellogg, J. (1981). Health teaching; module 1. *Foundations of health teaching* (pp. 37-51). Long Beach, CA: Statewide Nursing Program, the Consortium of the California State University.

Lindeman, C. A. (1988). Patient education. *Annual Review of Nursing Research, 6,* 29-60.

Mullen, P. D., Mains, D. A., & Velez, R. (1992). A meta-analysis of controlled trails of cardiac patient education. *Patient Education and Counseling, 19,* 143-162.

National Task Force on Training Family Physicians in Patient Education. (1979). *Patient education: A handbook for teachers.* Kansas City, MO: The Society of Teachers of Family Medicine.

Oberst, M. T. (1989). Perspectives on research in patient teaching. *Nursing Clinics of North America, 24,* 621-628.

Ovrebo, B., Ryan, M., Jackson, K., & Hutchinson, K. (1994). The homeless prenatal program: A model for empowering homeless pregnant women. *Health Education Quarterly, 21,* 149-170.

Pearlin, L. I., Lieberman, M. A., Menaghan, E. G., & Mullan, J. T. (1981). The stress process. *Journal of Health and Social Behavior, 22,* 337-356.

Pearlin, L. I., & Schooler, C. (1978). The structure of coping. *Journal of Health and Social Behavior, 19,* 2-21.

Pender, N. J. (1987). *Health promotion in nursing practice* (2nd ed.). East Norwalk, CT: Appleton & Lange.

Plough, A., & Olafson, F. (1994). Implementing the Boston Healthy Start Initiative: A case study of community empowerment and public health. *Health Education Quarterly, 21,* 221-234.

Prochaska, J. O., Redding, C. A., Harlow, L. L., Rossi, J. S., & Velicer, W. F. (1994). The transtheoretical model of change and HIV prevention: A review. *Health Education Quarterly, 21,* 471-486.

Rosenstock, I. M. The health belief model: Explaining health behavior through expectancies. In K. Glanz, F. M. Lewis, & B. K. Rimer (Eds.), *Health behavior and health education: Theory, research, and practice* (pp. 39-62). San Francisco: Jossey-Bass.

Schroeder, S. A., & McPhee, S. J. (1993). General approach to the patient. In L. M. Tierney, S. J. McPhee, M. A. Papadakis, & S. A. Schroeder (Eds.), *Current medical diagnosis and treatment* (pp. 1-20). Norwalk, CT: Prentice-Hall.

Selye, H. A. (1936). A syndrome produced by diverse nocuous agents. *Nature, 138,* 32.

Selye, H. A. (1952). *The story of the adaptation syndrome.* Montreal: Acta.

Selye, H. A. (1982). History and present status of the stress concept. In L. Goldberger & S. Breznitz (Eds.), *Handbook of stress: Theoretical and clinical aspects.* New York: Free Press.

Simons-Morton, D. G., Mullen, P. D., Mains, D. A., Tabak, E. R., & Green, L. W. (1992). Characteristics of controlled studies of patient education and counseling for preventive health behaviors. *Patient Education and Counseling, 19,* 175-204.

Sleet, D. A. (1984). Reducing motor vehicle trauma through health promotion programming. *Health Education Quarterly, 11,* 113-125.

Smith, C. E. (1989). Overview of patient education. *Nursing Clinics of North America, 24,* 583-587.

Strecher, V. J., DeVellis, B. M., Becker, M. H., & Rosenstock, I. M. (1986). The role of self-efficacy in achieving health behavior change. *Health Education Quarterly, 13,* 73-92.

Taylor, C. B., Bandura, A., Ewart, C. K., Miller, N. H., & DeBusk, R. I. (1985). Exercise testing to enhance wives' confidence in their husbands' cardiac capability after clinically uncomplicated acute myocardial infarction. *American Journal of Cardiology, 55,* 635-638.

Tripp-Reimer, T., & Afifi, L. A. (1989). Cross-cultural perspectives on patient teaching. *Nursing Clinics of North America, 24,* 613-619..

Wallerstein, N., & Bernstein, E. (1994). Introduction to community empowerment, participatory education, and health. *Health Education Quarterly, 21,* 141-148.

Wallerstein, N, & Sanchez-Merki, V. Freirian praxis in health education: Research results from an adolescent prevention program. *Health Education Research, 9,* 105-118.

Wang, C., & Burris, A. A. (1994). Empowerment through photo novella: Portraits of participation. *Health Education Quarterly, 21,* 171-186.

7 Assessment for Patient Education: Process and Product

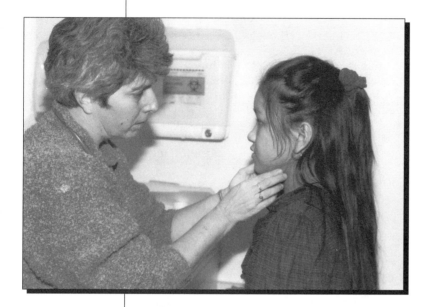

OBJECTIVES FOR CHAPTER 7

After reading this chapter, the nurse or student nurse should be able to:

1 List "red flags" used to identify patients with complex discharge planning needs as part of the assessment process.

2 Identify the four steps of the assessment process and describe how they relate to patient education.

3 Describe the limited circumstances in which you might select the following nursing diagnoses:
   a Knowledge Deficit
   b Noncompliance

4 Discuss in general terms how patient education relates to all nursing diagnoses.

5 Describe benefits of home visits for patient assessment.

Nursing Process and Patient Education

Patient education plans are part of the total plan for patient care and are patient centered. The process of patient education is an integral part of each of the four phases of the nursing process: assessment, planning, intervention, and evaluation (Fig. 7-1). It begins with early screening on admission to determine what is likely to cause trouble for this patient and to anticipate functional problems (rather than with a preset teaching plan for all patients with a common medical diagnosis, i.e., diabetes; Box 7-1).

The nurse also looks realistically at anticipated length of stay and determines how much to teach and when to teach each patient. The nursing process aids the nurse in examining her relationship to the patient. It offers a reminder that each patient is a person with individual needs and problems. Use of the nursing process encourages the application of protocols and standards that will *direct* patient care rather than dictate it in a rigid fashion. The components of the nursing process offer a framework for modifying nursing care in such a way that nurses and patients grow in a cooperative relationship. When this is accomplished, patients are cared for as individuals and can learn to participate in their own care in a meaningful and satisfying manner.

We will illustrate the use of the nursing process as a model for patient education, highlighting the important skills of assessment,

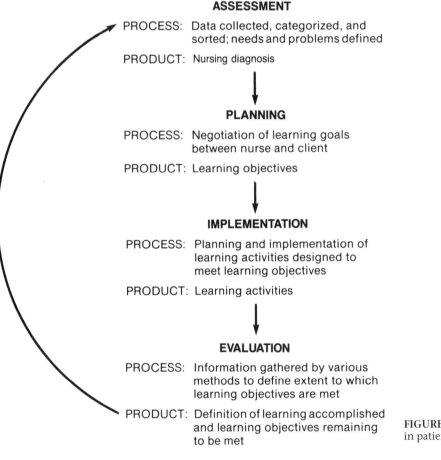

ASSESSMENT

PROCESS: Data collected, categorized, and sorted; needs and problems defined

PRODUCT: Nursing diagnosis

PLANNING

PROCESS: Negotiation of learning goals between nurse and client

PRODUCT: Learning objectives

IMPLEMENTATION

PROCESS: Planning and implementation of learning activities designed to meet learning objectives

PRODUCT: Learning activities

EVALUATION

PROCESS: Information gathered by various methods to define extent to which learning objectives are met

PRODUCT: Definition of learning accomplished and learning objectives remaining to be met

FIGURE 7-1. The nursing process in patient education.

BOX 7–1. Patient-Centered Assessment

Shift focus from medical diagnosis to
FUNCTIONAL PROBLEMS:
   How does it affect *this* patient?

planning, implementation, and evaluation, in Chapters 7 through 11. (see Fig. 7-1). Although the principles may appear simple, application of the nursing process involves a broad understanding of the patient and family and considerable clinical expertise. Case studies are offered as examples of courses of action. Because it is not realistic of us to think we can prepare the nurse by offering examples of every patient diagnosis, we offer case studies to illustrate principles of patient education rather than to be used as a "cookbook." As nurses continue to update their knowledge in their specialty areas, learning more about patient problems they encounter, this text can be used to complement the practice of patient and family education and to help nurses develop individualized teaching plans.

The Increasing Importance of Discharge Planning

As soon as patients are admitted to the hospital, assessment of the potential for discharge begins. Although nurses often think of discharge planning as occurring in inpatient acute care settings, it also occurs in emergency rooms, home health care, surgical centers, and long-term care. This is an important evaluation of actual or potential problems that must be dealt with before a safe discharge is made. Ideally all members of the health care team contribute to the discharge assessment process. For many patients, discharge planning and patient education involve similar activities. The patient and family will be taught survival skills and assume functions of health care management. But for some patients, postdischarge needs are complex. Early detection of special assistance and resources and making timely arrangements for continuing care are essential, especially in light of decreased lengths of stay.

One method of ensuring coordinated care is use of an admission data base containing questions to screen for discharge concerns. These concerns are referred to as "red flags." Interdisciplinary case conferences are common on hospital units to pick up "red flags." Nursing rounds have become increasingly popular to continue the screening and to coordinate discharge planning and patient teaching efforts. The American Hospital Association published *Guidelines for Discharge Planning* (1984) to assist hospitals in evaluating and improving their discharge planning functions, stressing that each hospital should develop a system based on its own requirements and resources and the needs of its patients. These guidelines can also provide assistance to those in settings other than hospitals. Discharge planning is a part of routine patient care and is an interdisciplinary process to help patients and their families develop and implement a feasible posthospital plan of care. Special discharge planning services are warranted when posthospital needs are expected to be complex. Hospital social workers, clinical nurse specialists, and case managers then follow complex patient situations.

Nurses often take the lead to organize the health care team in regularly scheduled meetings to review patient cases. Depending on what types of patient needs have been identified, all or some of the following disciplines are also represented: medicine, dietary, social work, pharmacy, physical therapy, occupational therapy, recreation therapy, and home health. Sometimes patients and family members are included.

Examples of "red flag" patients who are high risk and needing intensive discharge planning are given in Box 7-2. "Red flag" patients may be identified before or during admission, during routine patient care, or through the expressed concerns of significant others. The plan of care for these patients usually requires social services and a highly individualized approach.

BOX 7–2. "Red Flag" Patients

The elderly (age over 70; may include younger disabled patients)

Elderly patients suspected of being abused or neglected

Patients living alone

Children abused, neglected, or with birth anomalies

Patients transferred from other institutions

Recent admissions

Multiple readmissions

Patients who depend heavily on community resources

Patients with financial problems

Patients with terminal illnesses

Patients who live out of state or out of the country

Patients with care-intensive disease, catastrophic illness, or chronic illness

Patients with multiple chronic illnesses

Patients with newly diagnosed disease

Patients who receive few or no visitors

Substance abusers

Patients suspected of being abused, including domestic violence

Patients with family problems

Patients with psychiatric disorders

Patients with poor living conditions

Patients who speak little or no English

Patients with recent disabilities

In addition to picking up "red flag" patients, the interdisciplinary round answers other questions related to discharge planning:

1. Is the patient likely to return home?
2. Can the family or significant others handle the care that will be needed?
3. Is the home situation (or environment) adequate or appropriate for the type of care needed?

4. What kinds of assistance will be needed?
   a. Financial
   b. Equipment
   c. Manpower
   d. Community

Patient and family education is critical to successful discharge planning, which must include teaching about physical care and how it can be performed at home. Nursing assessment and counseling must prepare patients throughout hospitalization to evaluate their family resources, understand their illness and treatment, help them make changes, and manage their continuing care. In complex situations, strategies should be developed to follow up with the patient, family, and community services to determine the outcomes of discharge planning. One such situation, domestic violence or other forms of abuse, requires skilled observation and appropriate questions on the part of the nurse. The patient often hides the signs of abuse or makes excuses for injuries, which may be life-threatening. The patient may attribute recurrent episodes of injury to being "accident prone." There may be substantial delay between onset of injury and presentation for treatment. Suicidal thoughts and depression are also common. Patient groups at special risk for abuse are children, pregnant women, and the elderly (Chez, 1994).

The following questions, asked in a nonjudgmental way, can help patients "break the silence" about abuse. Acknowledge that violence is not the victim's fault (McAfee, 1993, 1994; Bash & Jones, 1994).

"At any time, has a partner or parent kicked, hit, or otherwise hurt or frightened you?"

"I noticed your bruise. How did your injury occur? Did someone hurt you?"

"Often patients presenting with these types of symptoms have a history of having been hurt by another person in the past. Has that ever happened to you?"

It is important to document the findings of suspected domestic violence with objective data and notify the patient's physician immediately. In states with a reporting law, any person who suspects abuse or neglect of a child is required by law to report this suspicion to the county Department of Social Services. This includes instances of physical abuse causing physical harm; neglect causing failure to provide for the child's basic physical, medical, educational, and emotional needs; sexual abuse such as fondling, intercourse, incest, rape, sodomy, and exhibition; and emotional maltreatment such as bizarre punishment, belittling, or psychological rejection. Be certain to assess a patient's safety in returning home. Ask if weapons are kept in the house and determine if children are in danger (Brown & Runyan, 1994). The same types of abuse can apply to all patients, including the elderly (Chez, 1994).

The Assessment Process

The first step of the nursing process is *assessment*: the collection of data to identify actual or potential health problems. Data are gathered by other members of the health care team in addition to nurses. Families play an important role in helping the nurse to assess a patient, especially when the patient is sedated, in pain, or unable to provide needed information. Families can cue a nurse about the patient's typical behavior and responses, daily patterns, and sources of comfort. A spouse may inform the nurse of a particular fear the patient is unwilling to disclose, thus helping the nurse to address it and promote the patient's readiness to learn (Tanner, Benner, Chesla, & Gordon, 1993). In the assessment process nurses continuously collect information from different sources, validate these data, sort and categorize the data, and summarize or interpret the information. The end products of the assessment are nursing diagnoses—nursing judgments based on sound data that have been systematically collected and analyzed.

The practice of nursing is founded on the ability of nurses to carry out nursing interventions based on the assessment of individual situations. Nurses respond to patients and their families when they are unable to meet their own needs. The goals of nursing care are to reinforce the client's strengths, assist the client to meet basic human needs, and help the client to regain the ability to meet these needs to the greatest degree possible. To provide appropriate nursing care we must be able to define strengths and unmet needs accurately and to state patient problems clearly.

Nursing assessment is not guesswork. It is a conscious, deliberate process, consisting of four steps. We make assessments every day in our personal and professional lives, often without realizing it. While driving to work, we quickly note that the fuel gauge reads *E* and drive into the closest gas station. We take inventory in the pantry and make a list before grocery shopping. We walk into a patient's room, notice his shortness of breath, and elevate the head of the bed. All of these actions are based on *assessment*—the ability to collect and sort information and define areas of need or problems. It is vitally important in patient education for the nurse to make an accurate assessment of strengths and problems so that learning may be tailored to the specific situation. This assessment is based on the collection of specific data from a variety of sources, a sorting of the data, and a written summary statement of problems or needs, which we call *nursing diagnosis*. Assessment should be documented to ensure accountability.

Four Steps in Assessment

In patient education, the goal of the nurse is to ensure that the patient is guaranteed his right to know and that he is given the necessary professional assistance to acquire knowledge and skills that will help him to meet his basic human needs. It is obvious, then, that taking the time to make a thorough assessment is essential for accomplishing nursing goals. There are four steps in the assessment process: (1) select area(s) to be assessed; (2) gather data; (3) sort and categorize data; and (4) write a summary statement (nursing diagnosis or diagnoses). We now look at each step in the assessment process as it is applied to patient education.

Step 1: Selecting the Area To Be Assessed

Nurses are especially aware of the need to collect data in a manner that is as organized and efficient as possible. Because data collection is time consuming, it is imperative to collect only useful information in the assessment process. Nurses must avoid the common mistake of gathering too much data because they then overlook how the information is to be used.

Learning needs are defined when a nurse assesses the patient. The assessment for patient education does not have to be separate from other patient assessment activities. Information about the learning needs of the patient and family is gathered with other data about the patient's condition. To collect information vital to an assessment of learning needs, the nurse must keep in mind the questions listed in Box 7-3.

The use of assessment instruments. Data should be gathered using a guide or a set of criteria that will direct the nurse to the areas to be assessed. Many such instruments, published in the literature, will be helpful in assessing the learning needs of patients and families. Many guides are directed toward a particular patient population such as diabetic patients, stroke patients, ostomy patients,

and so forth. Some nurses construct their own assessment tools, which may better meet individual situations. The important point to remember about assessment tools is that they should guide the nurse in a holistic view of the patient within the contexts of the family and environment. The instrument should help the nurse to focus on the total person and direct him or her in collecting data in specific areas related to what the patient needs to learn.

The health assessment instrument often begins with physiologic data: chief complaint, history of the present illness or problem, and a review of systems. It is also important to note the informant, if other than the patient. Assessment often uses many informants, including other nurses and health professionals, and, of course, the patient and family. After or during physical appraisal, the nurse also gathers psychosocial data that affect the educational process. History taking improves with practice and experience. Nurses learn to fine tune the reporting of problems and know how to look for "significant negatives," ruling out possible problems. For example, a nurse told us about her experience assessing a geriatric patient in a long-term care setting. The patient's daughter reported: "My mother can't walk." When the nurse had the patient attempt to walk, she found the patient able to balance herself but extremely short of breath and dizzy. The problems were dehydration and shortness of breath rather than a musculoskeletal weakness.

The assessment instrument may be a checklist with space included for responses, or it may be in guide form with an accompanying flow sheet for summary in the patient's chart. The tool that seems most helpful to the nurse is the one that should be used.

Depending on the setting and the amount of time the nurse has with the client, the assessment is completed in several phases. Data are gathered at different times and are used to update the plan of care. At the first encounter, the nurse "screens" for the most obvious and most acute needs. This is a starting point for beginning care. As time permits, a more comprehensive assessment can be made, and some data gathering may be dele-

---

BOX 7–3. Assessment: Vital Information

- What information does the patient need?

- What attitudes should be explored?

- What skills does the patient need to perform health care behaviors?

- What factors in the patient's environment may pose barriers to the performance of desired behaviors?

gated to other nurses working with the patient. Assessment should also look for potential problems that can be anticipated in the plan of care. Particularly in the hospital setting, nurses often ask how nursing assistants and licensed practical nurses can participate in this process. Both can contribute *observations*; however, the registered nurse should help them know what to look for and should validate their data rather than use them as the only source of information.

We constructed our own guide for assessment in patient and family teaching (Box 7-4) and demonstrate its application in this chapter. This guide is applicable to a wide variety of situations and prompts a thorough consideration of factors that will either promote learning or pose barriers to behavioral change.

The guide uses a systems theory framework for assessing the patient and the family. Systems theory encourages an assessment of the total family as the client rather than dealing with only the patient as the client. Because most patient education has ramifications for the entire family, we feel it is important to focus from the beginning on the family system.

Systems theory has gained prominence among family therapists as a method of understanding the effects of family members on one another during their ongoing interactions. The product of the interactions of the individual members, or *subsystems*, are the beliefs, goals, roles, and norms that form the *family system*. One of the corollaries of systems theory is that the system is *more* than the sum of its parts. To the patient educator, this means that the family system must be assessed and intervened with if the patient (subsystem) is to internalize and act on the information imparted. For example, if the spouse and children of a hypertensive patient are unwilling to prepare and eat low-sodium, low-fat meals, the hypertensive patient will have difficulty complying with the medical regimen.

Another aspect of systems theory that is important to the patient educator is the concept of the *suprasystem*. We have so far discussed systems and subsystems. When we consider the family as a system, the *suprasystem* is the community to which the family relates. It includes schools and churches and economic, legal, and health institutions. Assessment of the suprasystem is important in patient education because it affords the patient educator information about support systems that may be mobilized to aid in rehabilitation and financial assistance.

Patient and Family Education Assessment Guide

Philosophy. Our opinion is that patients who have the support of family members in the learning process will cooperate better with the medical regimen. We have witnessed such a correlation in our clinical experiences. As patient education clearly becomes recognized as being within the domain of the nurse, questions arise as to who will be taught.

In the past, the nursing profession centered its interest on the hospitalized patient. Any teaching that was done with a patient's family members tended to be peripheral or due to a particular necessity (e.g., if the patient was blind and unable to draw up insulin or if the patient had sensory aphasia). Most health professionals now include families in the process of patient education. We are discovering that a systems approach to patient education mandates the inclusion of family members and that teaching one isolated subsystem without dealing with the important family system can, in some instances, negate all teaching efforts.

We believe that educating the patient without including the family will frequently result in poor rehabilitation and poor cooperation with self-care measures, whether the patient is acutely ill or whether he and his family face life with a long-term chronic illness. We feel strongly that patient education should be conducted with the family present, whether in the hospital, ambulatory care setting, or at home. We developed the assessment guide to set the stage for such a teaching environment. It was first used for an adult patient and his family who were deal-

(text continues on page 130)

Box 7–4. Patient and Family Education Assessment Guide

I. Physiologic data
   A. Chief complaint
   B. History of present illness or problem
   C. Review of systems
   D. Functional, cognitive, and sensory abilities (anxiety, ability to concentrate)

II. Family profile: a word picture of the family
   A. Household composition
   B. Gender and age of members
   C. Occupations of family members
   D. Health status of family members; physical limitations
   E. Genogram: a diagram showing family relationships

III. Resources available to the family
   A. Ability to provide for physical needs
      1. Home: space, comfort, safety?
      2. Income: sufficient for basic needs and important extras?
      3. Overall ability to perform self-care
      4. Health insurance: available to the family?
   B. Neighborhood/community resources: friends, neighbors, church, and community organizations helpful and involved?
      1. What kinds of support are provided?

IV. Family education, life-style, and beliefs
   A. Educational backgrounds and attitudes toward education
      1. Do all adult family members have basic reading and writing abilities? Check ability to read aloud from patient education material.
      2. To what extent is education, formal or informal, valued? How much education does each family member have?
      3. Are there language barriers to verbal communication among the patient, family members, community, and medical personnel?
   B. Life-style and cultural background
      1. Does the family subscribe to folk medicine beliefs?
      2. Is there a conflict between cultural and life-style approach and the health professional's teaching?
      3. What are the normal diet patterns of the family?
      4. What are the family's sleep habits?
      5. What are the activities, exercises, occupations, and hobbies of family members?
   C. Learning abilities of family members
      1. Do they assimilate information easily?
      2. Are they able to apply what is taught?
   D. The family's self-concept
      1. Are family members lacking in self-esteem?
      2. Do they have feelings of powerlessness as a result of either life situation or patient's sick role?

V. Adequacy of family functioning
   A. Ability to be sensitive to the needs of the family members

(continued)

Box 7–4. *(Continued)*

      1. How is the identified patient perceived?

      2. What are the relationships of other family members to the identified patient and each other?

  B. Ability to communicate effectively with each other

  C. Ability to provide support, security, and encouragement, especially pertaining to the learning environment

  D. Ability for self-help and acceptance of help from others when needed

      1. How open is the family to the health professional's teaching?

      2. How likely are family members to request help in the future, if needed?

  E. Ability to perform roles flexibly

  F. Ability to make effective decisions

  G. Ability of the family to readjust ideas about family status, goals, and relationships

  H. Ability of the family to handle crisis situations

      1. Has the family been confronted with chronic illness in the past?

      2. How has the family reacted to situations such as accidental injury or death? Who helped them through it?

VI. Family understanding of the present event

  A. Current knowledge about the problem: ask these eight questions

      1. What do you think has caused your problem?

      2. Why do you think it happened when it did?

      3. What do you think your illness does to you? How does it work?

      4. How severe is your illness? Will it have a short course?

      5. What kind of treatment do you think you should receive?

      6. What are the most important results you hope to receive from this treatment?

      7. What are the chief problems your illness has caused for you?

      8. What do you fear most about your illness?

  B. Point in the life cycle of the family at which the problem occurred

  C. Type of onset of the illness or problem: gradual or sudden?

  D. Prognosis for survival or prognosis for restorative training

  E. Nature and degree of limitations imposed on the patient's functioning

  F. Level of the family's confidence in the health system with which they affiliate

VII. The identified patient, health problem, and educational needs

  A. The patient's educational and cultural background, especially if different from the family's

  B. The patient's self-concept and reaction to stress

  C. Physical limitations that are barriers to learning or self-care

  D. Information base of the patient

      1. Does he understand the health team management and the health team's advice?

      2. Does he know others with the same problem and have knowledge of their treatment?

      3. What are his position and his role in the family?

      4. Has he had past illnesses?

      5. What kind of physiologic feedback is he using?

  E. Are the patient and family members willing to negotiate goals with the health care team?

  F. Are the patient's perceptions and expectations congruent with those of family members?

ing with a chronic illness. With some minor changes, the guide can be adapted to a family dealing with a patient who has just suffered an acute illness or to a family trying to establish everyday health maintenance, such as one with a newborn.

Perspective. Using a systems perspective, this guide moves from the family system, its structure, function, and processes, and how the family relates to education, to the patient as a subsystem of the family, and to some of his educational needs. Integrated in the guide are factors that commonly affect the teaching of elderly patients (Deakins, 1994).

Theoretical basis. Families, like other social systems, have structures and functions. The structure of the family is important in assessment for patient education purposes. The effectiveness of a family's organization can affect the extent to which new health behavior is assumed. Problems with family organization and role definition often pose obstacles to learning.

Differentiation and specialization of roles are important in assessment. For example, the patient's roles may have to change with the onset of a chronic illness, and the provider needs to recognize this to assist the family to adapt (MacVicar & Archbold, 1976).

Family functions are closely related to family structure, as pointed out by Horton (1977). The functions that remain in the family "... are the maintenance of the household and the intimate personal relations of the family members." Family strengths relate closely to family functions and are covered in part V of the assessment guide. If the desired family strengths are absent, the wisdom of including the family in patient education must be reconsidered or planned in a careful way because the family may be more destructive than beneficial, posing barriers to the patient's learning process.

The family processes of adaptation, integration, and decision-making are important to patient and family education. A family faced with the illness of one of its members must be able to adapt and change in a healthy fashion.

The ability of the family to handle a crisis situation is a strong indication of family adaptation (Eliopolis, 1987; MacVicar & Archbold, 1976; Otto, 1963). Boundary maintenance, or the ability to meet needs by obtaining, containing, retaining, and disposing of resources, reflects important data about the ability to adapt. Assessment questions pertaining especially to obtaining and containing resources are found throughout the assessment guide. Dealing with neighborhood and community resources is of special importance. Human resources outside the family are necessary during illness or stress, and they are also indicative of the family's ability to form trusting, caring relationships with others outside of the family. As Lewis (1976) points out, this ability is one of the most significant variables in optimally functioning families.

The family process of integration is covered mainly in parts IV and VI of the guide and chiefly refers to the family norms and beliefs that help to form the bonds in well-integrated families. It should be noted that a high degree of family integration, built through cultural beliefs and life-styles, may complicate the learning process if the beliefs and values differ widely from those of the health care provider (Gragg & Rees, 1980; Leininger, 1978; Redman, 1992).

The cultural assessment in section IV.B brings to light the diversity of backgrounds among patients that most nurses recognize. Values and beliefs influence health and also the patient's care. When nurses encounter patients with beliefs and values different from their own, the cultural assessment section must be expanded to appreciate the following significant variables:

1. *Time.* In some cultures there is a "right time" to do things and the western concept of time and clocks is disregarded.
2. *Religious beliefs.* Those that may prevent the patient from seeking health care or accepting treatments must be considered.
3. *Cultural remedies and healers.* It is important to know those the patient is currently using and their meaning to the patient. Fully explore diet and dietary remedies.

4. *Language and communication.* Note what language is spoken and what nonverbal signals are used.

Cultural differences make each patient unique and, when ignored, lead nurses to treat all patients in a similar way, often resulting in a failure of patient education. Nurses who develop a broad knowledge base and become sensitive to the patient populations they serve can plan care creatively and are more likely to achieve successes in patient and family education (Orgue, Bloch, & Monroy, 1983). Chapter 4 addresses challenges and approaches to working with patients whose cultural and belief systems differ from those of the nurse. Additionally, we recommend that continuing education opportunities such as reference texts, workshops, and inservice programs be used at the work setting to prepare nurses for assessment of the diversity of cultures encountered. An excellent resource is *Transcultural Concepts in Nursing Care* (Boyle & Andrews, 1995), which sensitizes nurses to cultural differences in their practice and the needs of culturally diverse clients in a variety of practice settings.

Decision-making in the family during events of stress or illness can affect the family's future. If decision-making is not organized adequately, the family may be unable to make important choices related to health care plans or unable to assume responsibility in health care practices. When patient education is involved, it is frequently necessary for the family to decide, whether by consensus, accommodation, or de facto decision-making, who is going to learn, for example, how to irrigate a colostomy or give an insulin injection. The importance of assessing the patient as a subsystem of the family is covered in part VI of the assessment guide, drawn partially from Robinson (1974). The patient's perception of his relationship to the family, whether realistic or unrealistic, can alter the educational process and should be determined before the teaching plan is begun. The work of Kleinman (Kleinman, Eisenberg, & Good, 1978), which was introduced in Chapter 4, is integrated in the guide with eight questions listed in part VI.

Additional comments. Various guides have been drawn up for assessment of individual learner's needs, and family assessment guides are abundant in the literature as well. Our guide is based on material contained in educational, nursing, psychological, and sociologic writings. The guide considers the patient and family as a system in a potential learning environment. It also illustrates the importance of evaluating the family as a system while considering the impacts of the community, the health care system, and sociocultural influences as suprasystems. This assessment guide has worked well for us in our patient education roles. It has helped us in assessing strengths and weaknesses that influence the ability of patients and families to adapt health behaviors. Later in this chapter, we present case studies that illustrate the use of the guide. A model of patient and family education was constructed to help the reader visualize the related components that influence learning (Fig. 7-2). The model is presented and explained.

Figure 7-2 illustrates the components of assessment found in the assessment guide. This model represents a healthy educational situation, in which the family has reasonable resources and an assessment of family functioning demonstrates strengths. Two-way arrows between each component and the family system demonstrate their dual effects on each other. Finally, the entire model is encircled by a broken line to indicate the interactions among all of the components and the family.

Step 2: Gathering Data

Data should be gathered as objectively as possible. Collecting these data (using fact or measurement rather than reflecting feelings or judgments) will guide the nurse to define needs or problems accurately. Words such as seems, appears, acts, and looks should be avoided. More useful data would note direct observations or actual behaviors. Whenever possible, note what the patient said in his own words. Describe what you hear, smell, see, and feel. Share your observations with

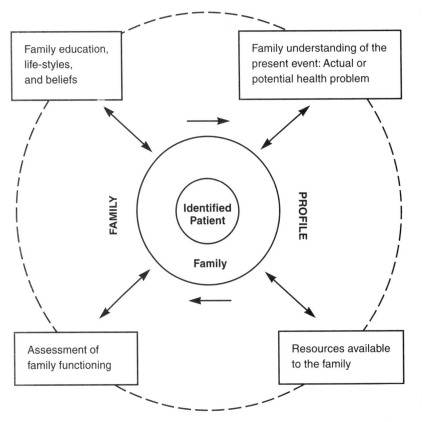

FIGURE 7-2. A model of patient—family education.

the patient to validate what you observe. Note the source of the information.

There are several methods of gathering data. The most effective follow:

1. Observation
2. Interviews with patient, family, and significant others
3. Review of patient records
4. Review of the literature: continuing education
5. Collaboration with the health care team

Observation. A significant amount of information can be collected by the use of the senses. Assessments can be made of the patient's ability to perform self-care activities, his physical appearance, and his affect. The nurse can gather valuable information in the home by observing the interactions of family members, the comfort and safety afforded by the patient's dwelling, and the facilities available to meet basic needs. Observation will also provide information about the patient's literacy level, leisure activities, and the role assumed within the family. Although the most common method of observation is through sight, nurses also rely on information from things they hear, feel, and smell. Verbal and nonverbal cues gathered by observation provide us with valuable information about what the patient thinks, feels, and believes. Questionnaires and tests are often used to assess a patient's knowledge of facts and to explore his attitudes.

Interview. Taking a patient history or performing a patient and family interview is the most reliable method of obtaining data. When patients are unable to supply information, owing to their physical or emotional condition, family members are asked to supply as much information as possible. Whether the nurse finds herself interviewing the patient or one of the family members, there are guidelines and suggestions for interviewing effectively; some of those we have used follow.

ESTABLISH A TRUSTING ENVIRONMENT. Patient must feel a sense of security and trust to confide information. They need to feel that their concerns are taken seriously and that their needs are important and respected. Communicate trust and respect to patients by concentrating attention on them, maintaining eye contact, and being an active listener. The necessity of establishing a trusting environment is illustrated by the situation that develops when a nurse deals with a patient with venereal disease. The nurse must assure the patient that all information will be held in strict confidence. After the nurse has assured the patient of confidentiality, she must then explain the importance of notifying the patient's sexual contacts so that they can be treated. Such situations are delicate, and if the client does not trust the nurse it will be impossible for the nurse to assist the client.

USE OPEN-ENDED QUESTIONS. Help the patient to provide more complete information by using the principles of active listening. Use phrases such as "Go on," or ask, "Can you tell me more about that?" and repeat the last words of what the patient has just said. This communicates an interest in what the person has to say and a desire to understand how he feels. Open-ended questions that ask for descriptions rather than a "yes" or "no" answer help the patient to give information about how he perceives his needs. If we continue with our example of the client with venereal disease (gonorrhea), the nurse can use open-ended questions such as, "Can you tell me a little more about what you know about gonorrhea?" If the nurse states to the client, "You know how you got this, don't you?" the client will probably simply respond, "Yes," because he is embarrassed, he does not want to admit his ignorance, and he feels generally uncomfortable in the presence

of the nurse. It is important in such situations, and in many other patient education settings, to avoid judgmental behaviors. The use of open-ended questions allows the client to present what he knows so that the nurse can assess what else needs to be taught.

The nurse can also use open-ended questions to determine what is most important to the patient or what troubles him most by asking, "Please tell me what is troubling you the most," or "If you could change one thing, what would it be?"

CHOOSE THE RIGHT SETTING AND TIMING. Effective interviewing occurs in a setting where the patient and interviewer can be free of distractions and where information can be shared privately. Obstacles to effective interviewing arise when the patient is too tired or too ill to share his thoughts comfortably or when the interviewer is distracted. Extremely lengthy interviews are difficult for both the patient and interviewer. Plan the interview so that critical information is obtained first; perhaps it will be necessary to have several short interviews. For example, counseling related to venereal disease must be accomplished discreetly and without family members or anyone else present. In the outpatient setting, the client should be alone with the nurse in a private room where there will be no interruptions. For other patients, the input of family members is needed.

The family can be included in assessment when they visit the patient, or if this is not practical, by telephone. The nurse might say: "Staff members are devising a plan of care for your mother, and we would like your input. Can you answer a few questions to help us?"

LET THE PATIENT "TELL HIS STORY." Allow the patient to tell you how he perceives his needs and problems. Maintain objectivity about what he says and try not to make judgments about his perceptions of his pain or his needs. Speak to the patient using language he can understand, rather than medical terminology and abbreviations. Speak slowly and clearly, allowing him time to think about your questions before he answers. If he wanders off the track, gently lead him back by repeating your question. Explain the purpose of the interview to the patient. Let him know that you want to get to know him better to care for him in the best manner possible. For example, let the chronic obstructive pulmonary disease (COPD) patient with asthma explain his perception of the problem. He may believe that his recent onset of severe symptoms is related to a specific activity, such as walking or sexual intercourse, when, in fact, the blood level for his medication is not in the therapeutic range. Once we find out what the patient believes, we may be able to correct some important misconceptions.

MAKE SHORT, DISCRETE NOTES. Notes from the interview will make documentation more accurate and more efficient. It is important, however, that you avoid writing too many notes during the interview because this may disturb the patient. Facts, symptoms, times, names, and short quotes from the patient may be recorded quickly and can be used when you are ready to document the results of the interview. Before beginning to record data during an interview, it is imperative to say to the patient, "I am going to write down a few things you say so that I don't forget anything important." Taking notes during an interview frequently makes clients uncomfortable; an explanation can alleviate such discomfort and prevent misunderstandings. With the growing use of computers at the patient's bedside, it is important to keep in mind that eye contact with the patient is essential. The focus is the patient, not the computer.

Review of patient records. The patient's medical records are often the nurse's first source of information. Although information can be gathered quickly from the patient's chart, it should be supplemented by information from other sources. Medical records supply data about the patient's health history, previous hospitalizations, past experience with the health care system, and observations others have made about him. They can give us clues to finding additional sources of information, such as a public health nurse or community agencies that have worked with the patient. Information gathered from the patient record should be validated by observation and the patient interview.

Review of the literature: continuing education. In the nursing field, which is becoming increasingly specialized and advanced, reading texts and journals to update knowledge and skills is a professional responsibility. Basic nursing education is a foundation for practice, but the ability to anticipate and intervene in areas of need depends on willingness to increase that original knowledge base through continuing education.

To intervene responsibly with patients and their families, be prepared with an understanding of the disease or health problem, its medical management, and its impact on life-styles. Nursing fundamentals textbooks are valuable resources. Many journal articles describe new approaches to teaching patients and their families or increase our awareness of self-help groups and other resources that assist in preventing, resolving, or coping with health problems. Workshops and other continuing education programs offer good opportunities for learning from experienced colleagues about patients' problems and the causes and management of these problems.

Collaboration with the health care team. Data gathered by other nurses, physicians, dietitians, pharmacists, physical therapists, and a variety of other health care professionals can validate and supplement information gathered from the sources previously mentioned. Whenever possible, team members should contribute to planning the care of the patient and family. Patient education is a concern of the team. Coordination of learning goals and activities is important for ensuring that the time of the professional and the patient and family is used productively.

Collaboration is facilitated by good verbal and written communication, team conferences, updated nursing care plans, and effective use of such opportunities as physician and nurse rounds to discuss the patient teaching plan. For example, the hospital social worker who interviews the family is frequently given lists of medications that the patient has received from various physicians. The social worker will then give this list of medications and prescribing physicians to the nurse, whose responsibility it is to share the list with the patient's admitting physician.

Step 3: Sorting and Categorizing Data Into Problem Areas

Data gathered from a variety of sources must be carefully considered, validated, and grouped into problem areas. Under optimal circumstances, the health care team agrees on assessment of patient problems and learning needs and factors affecting behavioral change for health promotion.

Step 4: Writing the Summary Statements—Nursing Diagnoses

The summary statements that describe problem areas in which the nurse can intervene are called *nursing diagnoses*. A nursing diagnosis is different from a medical diagnosis because it focuses on a patient's response to a health problem that can be prevented or altered by nursing intervention. A medical diagnosis, by contrast, describes the illness, focuses on its pathology, and guides medical orders or protocols (Eggland & Heinemann, 1994). Nursing diagnoses, statements of actual or potential health problems, are derived from the data collected in assessment. These diagnoses should be validated by the patient and family, who, while doing so, become prepared to negotiate goals with the nurse.

A standardized list of nursing diagnoses is provided by the North American Nursing Diagnosis Association (NANDA). This taxonomy has been developed by nurses in all specialties, working together since 1973, to develop the scientific basis of nursing practice. Each diagnostic category contains descriptions of etiology, contributing factors, and definitive characteristics that aid the nurse in selecting the correct nursing diagnosis. Many health care organizations have established policies and procedures supporting the use of nursing diagnoses and incorporating them in documentation systems. In 1992, NANDA updated the taxonomy of nursing diagnosis by including high-risk diagnoses (supported by risk factors

that make a person vulnerable for the condition) and wellness nursing diagnoses, such as Family Coping, Potential for Growth (Eggland & Heinemann, 1994; NANDA, 1992). We suggest that nurses who are unfamiliar with the taxonomy of nursing diagnosis learn about it through workshops and texts, such as *Nursing Diagnosis: Application to Clinical Practice* by Lynda Juall Carpenito (1992). Nursing diagnosis has gained strong acceptance throughout the nursing profession, by all specialty areas and in all areas of practice. In this text, we will use the list of nursing diagnoses approved by NANDA in 1994 (see Appendix D).

Nurses will find that all nursing diagnoses have implications for patient and family education. The diagnosis Knowledge Deficit is frequently selected to incorporate all patient learning needs related to knowledge or skills needed for self-care. We believe, however, that patient education is better integrated in the total plan of care by referring to educational needs as they relate to each nursing diagnosis. Knowledge Deficit may be best used for preoperative teaching, prenatal education, parenting skills, and so forth.

The diagnosis Noncompliance should be used carefully and specifically following a thorough assessment to describe the patient who wishes to follow a recommended plan but who is unable to because of physiologic or situational reasons. This diagnosis should not be used if the patient has made an informed decision not to comply (Carpenito, 1992).

Other nursing diagnoses related to discharge planning may be best resolved by calling in the expertise of case managers, social workers, and community agencies. These include Risk for Violence, Social Isolation, Altered Family Process and Self Care Deficit.

Management of the Assessment Process

Prioritizing Needs and Problems

It is often difficult to set priorities when faced with problems in several areas. A consideration of a hierarchy of human needs will help the nurse rank the priority of problem areas and offer guidance in how and where to begin patient teaching.

As human beings all of us have common needs that must be satisfied. The ability of patients and their families to survive depends on their effectiveness in meeting these basic human needs. When they are unable to meet basic needs, problems arise that they often cannot resolve alone. At that point, health professionals are called on to intervene. Our goal is to help clients regain the ability to meet their own needs and to foster their maximum development, both as individuals and in their relationships with others.

Maslow suggests that needs exist in various levels and that these groups of needs can be visualized as a hierarchy in which lower-level needs must be at least partially met before a person can meet higher-level needs (Maslow, 1970). A consideration of these needs helps us to prioritize needs in nursing care and in patient teaching. Many of us have discovered that learning is hampered when the family faces problems with housing, finances, or threatened self-esteem. Patients who are in pain or are fearful of pain place high priority on managing it; they will learn little else until this need is met. Because the assessment process involves not only a listing of needs but also a consideration of priorities, it is helpful to use Maslow's hierarchy of needs as a guide in doing so. The five levels are briefly presented here and are discussed in more detail in Chapter 8. Figure 7-3 illustrates examples of nursing assessment for individuals, families, and communities based on Maslow's work.

Learning During the Assessment Process

When the patient and his family have an active role in defining their problems, family learning occurs. Self-care activities depend on the ability of the patient and family to solve problems by gathering information and categorizing signs and symptoms into problem areas. We can help them build these skills by verbally sharing our thoughts during the assessment process. Let the patient and the family witness and contribute to a systematic collection of data and definition of problems. Inform them about the rationales for collecting certain kinds of data and the best ways for discovering and documenting them. The promotion of learning during assessment builds problem-solving skills, encourages validation of data with the patient and family, and serves as a motivator for future learning. Adults are more motivated to learn when they have been able to identify their own needs and to contribute toward planning a program that is tailored to their particular circumstances. The questions asked by the nurse provide families with a sense of what is important and what they will need to do to prepare for discharge.

Managing Assessment Time

Time management issues are often mentioned as impediments to the assessment process. It seldom seems feasible to dedicate an hour to collecting information in an interview or to making a detailed assessment. We would like to emphasize a few points related to time issues.

1. Assessment requires spending time in astute observation and active listening. Much time is lost when the care plan is constructed without input from the patient and family; interventions in such cases are often ineffective, and we spend additional time going back to the assessment process to discover barriers to change that were preventing our progress all along.

2. The patient and family have a need to tell their story. They must be given time to offer their perceptions of their own problems. We must take time to help them understand what is expected of them if they are later to take charge of self-care activities.

3. Assessment can be made anytime we interact with patients and their families. Gathering information need not be restricted to a 60-minute interview. Bathtime, mealtime, rounds, visiting hours,

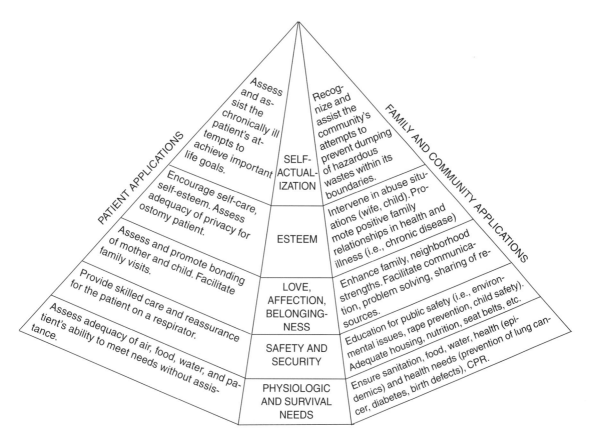

FIGURE 7-3. Applying Maslow's hierarchy in assessment of the patient and of the family and community.

and medication times are all potential opportunities for assessment.

4. Patients are sensitive to the time pressures of health professionals. They often do not know what is expected of them, whether (or for how long) they will have your attention, or how to contribute important information. We can teach them to help us with time restraints by offering statements like the following: "Mrs. Wise, I have set aside 15 minutes this morning at about 10:00. I will be asking you and your husband to answer some specific questions for me about your health problems so I can better plan your care with Dr. Mason and the nursing staff." This gives the patient an idea of what is expected of her and informs her that she will be asked specific questions instead of being put in the position of not knowing what information is important. In some instances, a questionnaire can be given ahead of time to collect initial data, which will be discussed during the interview. Whatever we can do to minimize interruptions and distractions during the interview will help to maximize productivity. Fifteen minutes of well-planned, well-used time accomplishes more toward assessment than does an hour with interruptions and lack of direction.

5. Assessment varies based on the setting and the patient. Even in the most brief encounter, the nurse can ask "What brought you here at this time?" and gain a wealth of information that is outlined in the assessment guide.

The assessment guide is a comprehensive tool for identifying barriers to learning and clues for individualizing the teaching plan. Clearly, even with such a tool, it is seldom possible to gather all this information at one time, and we are often unable to cover every aspect. The more information to which we have access, the better able we are to understand and influence patient behaviors. The guide offers direction for discovering such information during the initial assessment and throughout ongoing assessment as part of the relationship between the provider and the patient and family.

In our experience teaching undergraduate nursing students, we recommend home visits as a helpful way to learn assessment skills. Our students identified a patient in the family medicine clinic and then conducted a follow-up visit at home. A pair of students made each visit, and then wrote a summary based on the assessment guide. The following case study, adapted from Deakins (1994) is offered as an example.

❑ CASE STUDY

Mrs. Dawe

We met Mrs. Dawe when she came to the outpatient clinic for her regular appointment. She told us she had come to the clinic "to keep check on my sugar and have my blood pressure checked." She offered the information that she was a diabetic and needed help with her "weight problem." Her physician shared with us some of his frustration in caring for Mrs. Dawe. He referred to her as a "delightful lady" who was just "not compliant" despite numerous patient education efforts. We suggested making a home visit as a means of identifying factors that might be influencing Mrs. Dawe's cooperation with her self-care management in the areas of her diet, exercise, medication, and blood glucose monitoring. The physician agreed that this was a good idea and together we suggested to the patient that we make a home visit.

The following information was collected using the assessment guide.

Family Profile

Mrs. Dawe was a 73-year-old, Caucasian, obese woman. At 157.5 cm (5 ft 3 in), she weighed 77 kg (169 lb), 30% more than her ideal weight of 52.3 kg (115 lb). Her manner in the outpatient clinic was matter of fact. We had known that the patient was a retired RN. She was not going to lose any time making certain we recognized her status and competence.

An appointment for the first home visit was made during the visit to the outpatient clinic. The following information was obtained during the home visit.

Mrs. Dawe met us at the door when we arrived for the home visit. She was much more casually dressed, in a housedress with sandals and no hose, than she was at the clinic. Her white hair was neatly combed. Mr. Dawe was ready for the first visit. He was dressed in denim overalls. He was smaller in stature than his wife and was considerably outweighed by her. He was slightly deaf, but made every effort to keep up with the conversation, although he was neither as verbal nor as articulate as his wife. Mr. and Mrs. Dawe were both born in the South and had lived there all their lives.

Mr. and Mrs. Dawe were both retired. Their last jobs were at a medical center where Mrs. Dawe worked as an RN floater, and Mr. Dawe was a maintenance worker. Mr. Dawe's occupational history included various skilled and semi-skilled jobs; he had worked for railroads, textile mills, and during World War II, for the Army at a military camp.

The household had once included the Dawes' four children. The oldest child (and only daughter) was presently employed at a local governmental agency. She had been educated at a local private university and then was married and widowed within 4 years. A daughter from this first marriage, now 20 years old, was presently a freshman in a local state university. The Dawes' daughter had remarried, and this second marriage was an unhappy one involving physical abuse and separations. The Dawes' second child had married, had three children, and lived and worked in the same county as his parents. He was employed in the electronics industry. The third child seemed to be the "fair-haired boy." This son graduated from a local state university and then went to work for a large insurance company, which had steadily promoted him and transferred him around the country. This son, his wife, and three of their four children were living in Arizona and were greatly missed by Mrs. Dawe. Living nearby, with his wife and son, was the Dawes' youngest child. He worked as a painter and had recently painted the exterior of his parents' house.

The health status of the Dawes is important to consider at this point in assessment because it influences other areas in the analysis. Both of the Dawes were in robust good health well into their fifties. At that point, however, Mrs. Dawe's genetic heritage and the effects of Mr. Dawe's physically demanding work caught up with them.

At age 56, Mr. Dawe had a power-tool accident that resulted in permanent loss of function of his left hand. Ten years following surgery, Mr. Dawe suffered a myocardial infarction, from which he fully recovered. Two years later, emphysema developed and persisted, limiting Mr. Dawe's ability to engage in yard work or gardening. Mr. Dawe had smoked about a pack and a half of cigarettes per day but was able to quit. Glaucoma had been a problem but was arrested by medications. Mr. Dawe was amazingly spry, considering his ailments.

Mrs. Dawe's health history was not as long and complicated, but its implications for the future were probably more negative. Mrs. Dawe's diabetes was first diagnosed at age 56, and she was placed on insulin at the time of diagnosis. Her insulin requirements had steadily increased. She currently required a dose of 44 units/day, 29 units in the morning and 15 units in the evening (premixed 70% intermediate and 30% long-acting insulin). Her weight had steadily increased from 65.9 kg (145 lb) to 74 kg (163 lb), and her attempts at weight reduction using an American Diabetes Association (ADA) diet were fruitless. Retinopathies and a cataract, needing removal, had developed since the onset of diabetes. Mrs. Dawe's written records of home blood glucose monitoring showed very few periods of diabetic control. Hypertension had been diagnosed about 8 years earlier. As a result of coronary artery disease, Mrs. Dawe had bypass surgery 4 years ago. She currently takes 240 mg slow-release verapamil, 50 mg metoprolol, and 325 mg enteric-coated aspirin daily. She had exercised progressively less as she grew older, and the combination of obesity, diabetes, and coronary artery disease left her in poor physical health. The slightest amount of exertion made her short of breath, and she stated that she could not participate in any guided exercise program.

Resources Available to the Family

The Dawes' seven-room, completely owned home was situated in a small rural community and had aged comfortably over its 30 years. The interior of their home had been well kept, with additions such as carpeting and a new furnace added since they had first built the house themselves "piece by piece." The interior was clean, the furniture was comfortable and in good repair, and there was a homey feeling, accentuated by a pleasant clutter of family photographs, trophies, and knickknacks. Prominently displayed on a table was a photo of their second oldest son and his family, who were now located in Arizona. Photos of other children and grandchildren were in less prominent places. Mrs. Dawe gave us a tour of the home, pointing out the large size of the rooms and explaining that the candy in the dining room was not for her but for the visiting children. We also noted with interest three boxes of cake mix in Mrs. Dawe's kitchen cupboards and a cake plate sitting out in the dining room. The home was larger than necessary for their present needs because separate bedrooms had been promised to each child when the house was built. The Dawes' past lack of financial resources seemed to have been surmounted.

Income for the family was derived mainly from Social Security benefits and two pensions from the medical center. Although the Dawes'. income was limited, it did allow for travel; the previous summer they had driven to Arizona to visit their son and his family. Limited financial help was received from their children in the form of home improvements and money for traveling. Recognizing the limitations of Medicare, Mr. and Mrs. Dawe paid for additional medical insurance; the premiums were a rather large expenditure for them.

Neighborhood and community resources were informal but supportive. Neighbors watched the homes of one another, and they all kept keys to one another's homes. In the summer and fall the Dawes enjoyed their neighbors' garden produce. The family faithfully attended a local Methodist church, because it was convenient and they liked the parishioners, but both hastened to add that they were not members of the church. When questioned about involvement in community organizations, Mrs. Dawe spoke with pride of her work in the local school system when they were both employed. She told us about her initiation of an immunization program at a local elementary school. She remarked that she still had a feeling of accomplishment every time she saw the school. This was a family with informal and unstructured interface with community agencies and resources. In times of personal need, however, they had obtained services from the church, which had also helped their daughter through some difficult times.

Family Education, Life-styles, and Beliefs

Education was highly valued by the family, especially by Mrs. Dawe. She graduated from a nurses' training program. Mr. Dawe graduated from high school. All four of the Dawe children had graduated from high school and two had completed college. Books, magazines, and newspapers were evident in the household.

Mrs. Dawe denied that she held folk medicine beliefs. If Mr. Dawe subscribed to any folk medicine beliefs, it seemed certain his wife did not share them. She prided herself on keeping current with medical matters, gaining most of her knowledge from *Family Health* magazine, to which she subscribed.

The learning abilities of Mr. and Mrs. Dawe were adequate although Mrs. Dawe was unable to follow her American Diabetes Association (ADA) diet. The self-concept of this couple appeared healthy. Together they expressed the view that they had worked hard in life "but had come through in good shape." As a couple, they both seemed to have achieved psychologist Erikson's various stages and were in the eighth developmental stage, completing the tasks of ego integrity (Erikson, 1963).

Adequacy of Family Functioning

The adequacy of family functioning had to be assessed on the basis of the self-report. Mrs. Dawe appeared to be viewed by her husband with a fondness and warmth that had developed over 47 years of a marriage marked by economic and personal tribulations. Mrs. Dawe was quick to say that the marriage had been good and that they were very happy together now. Mr. Dawe laughed in a somewhat embarrassed fashion, but nonverbal clues such as nods of agreement and appropriate smiles indicated that he agreed with her assessment. Relationships with their children seemed healthy and supportive on the basis of Mr. and Mrs. Dawe's reports. Three of the four children lived in the same county and, although there was no constant interchange ("We don't get involved in their business"), there was a feeling of closeness.

Communication between husband and wife was adequate. Mr. Dawe was not as verbal as his wife and he tended to let her finish his sentences for him. These communication patterns had probably developed in the past and had tended to be reinforced by his deafness and her manner of taking charge of situations. Support and encouragement for one another were communicated in important nonverbal ways, such as Mr. Dawe's willingness to take his wife to the outpatient clinic to talk with us and his willingness to be available when we arrived. Another sign of mutual support and security was the fact that they still slept in the same double bed together. Mr. and Mrs. Dawe maintained their emotional and financial resources carefully, sharing them mainly with their children.

The family's ability to accept help, especially in areas of health care, was limited. This was mainly because of Mrs. Dawe's background as a nurse; she had a need to feel competent and self-sufficient in all medical areas. Other family members placed proscriptions and expectations on her that made it difficult for her to follow her health care plan. This was the area that caused the greatest difficulty in patient and family education. Because Mrs. Dawe was not following her ADA diet, she was placed in a constant state of jeopardy—she knew what she should do but could not, or would not, comply. As a result, her weight continued to increase, and she was left in the rather untenable position of having to justify her situation by claiming she had "a strange case of diabetes." Unfortunately, her choices would have negative outcomes for the family system in the future.

Role flexibility was not of imminent importance to this family in its life cycle. During the time of our contact with the family there was a fairly traditional delineation of work: Mrs. Dawe did the household chores, and Mr. Dawe supervised a neighborhood teenager who did the yard work.

Decision-making in this family tended to fall primarily to Mrs. Dawe as had discipline of the children in the past. Although some of the decisions were made in a de facto manner by Mrs. Dawe, there were also instances when decisions were made by the process of accommodation (i.e., a process of begrudging compromise and a questionable commitment to the decisions).

In the Dawes' viewpoint, family status, goals, and relationships were not seriously impaired by chronic illness. Adjustments to Mrs. Dawe's diabetes and to Mr. Dawe's emphysema had been smooth. The concurrent onset of chronic illness and onset of aging had, perhaps, made acceptance of the illnesses easier. Relationships had been changed as children grew up and moved out, but overall this family seemed to have adjusted well.

Crisis situations, especially serious injury or death, had been responded to by the Dawes with an immediate mobilization of energies. Because of Mrs. Dawe's background as a nurse, she immediately was called on in times of illness or injury. Besides caring for the ill or injured family member, she also carried messages from the rest of the family. Mr. and Mrs. Dawe both indicated that although they became distressed in such situations, they felt they were able to respond appropriately.

Family Understanding and the Present Event: Chronic Illness

This family had a long association with diabetes through relatives on both sides of the family. The Dawe family genogram (Fig. 7-4) shows the remarkably high incidence of diabetes and diabetes-related deaths on both sides of the family. Both partners seemed to accept the presence of diabetes philosophically—even fatalistically. When asked how he had felt 17 years before about the diagnosis of his wife's diabetes, Mr. Dawe stated, "It's just something that happens." He felt that the only way her diabetes had affected him had been in her cooking: "It's not as good as it used to be."

The fact that this chronic illness was not diagnosed until late middle age and the relatively few restrictions imposed on the family's ability to function at a preillness level had probably accounted for the relative ease with which they had handled it. Although Mrs. Dawe had to contend with a limited menu, insulin injection, blood glucose monitoring, and other medically prescribed guidelines, her role within the family was initially undisturbed. The complications of diabetes (retinopathies and hypertension) that were found in Mrs. Dawe were of more concern to the family and did interfere with daily activities. Mrs. Dawe was no longer able to drive, and this made her more dependent on her husband. Based on this information, we asked her to show us how she performed her blood glucose testing and insulin injection preparation. She was happy to do so because she saw herself "teaching us." She was able to draw up her insulin accurately with the assistance of a specially marked syringe. Her blood glucose testing was done with a digital read-out designed for patients with impaired vision. Her reading was

250 mg/dL, 2 hours after eating. This reading validated Mrs. Dawe's poor diabetic control. We took her blood pressure, which was 170/94 mm Hg, indicating problematic hypertension. As her activity level declined and her weight increased, she was unable to move around easily. This limited the mobility the couple had enjoyed during the past few years. Mrs. Dawe's role as provider of nursing care and child care for grandchildren and other family members also was restricted and would become more so.

The children of Mr. and Mrs. Dawe recognized the hereditary nature of diabetes and had their blood checked occasionally for glucose, Mrs. Dawe reported. As far as the parents knew, however, their children had no pervasive fear of diabetes.

The Identified Patient, the Health Problem, and Educational Needs

Mrs. Dawe's educational background as an RN occasionally became a problem. Her self-concept involved an image of herself as one who should be able to cope with diabetes management problems and at times she hesitated to ask for support or advice: "I just don't feel I can ask these young guys about things the way I used to when I knew them from working with them." Superimposed on the problem of daily diabetes management was her hypertension. The physiologic feedback she received (headache, occasional nausea) was symptomatic for both and, therefore, confusing.

The principles of diabetic self-care (diet, exercise, medication, response to hypoglycemic and hyperglycemic reactions, prevention of complications) were outlined for us by Mrs. Dawe. She was proud of her medical knowledge and skills. It became clear, however, that in this case (as with many other health professionals under medical care themselves), knowledge and skills were often not enough to promote healing behaviors. To assess Mrs. Dawe's learning needs accurately, we encouraged Mrs. Dawe to talk about problems with her treatment plan and her life-style. A helpful resource in this assessment was an article in which Betty Richardson (1982) offers a tool designed to confront problems with the diabetic patient's self-care regimen. Mrs. Dawe's responses to questions defined the following areas that Mrs. Dawe saw as problems:

1. Weight gain—diet is too restrictive; cannot eat "normally"; always hungry

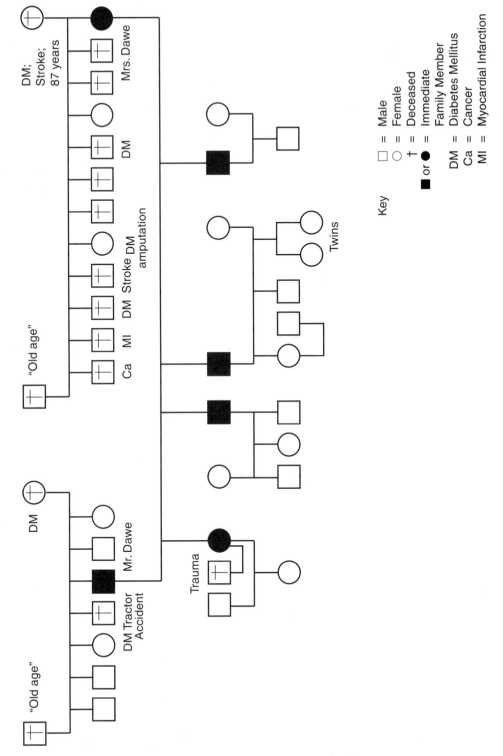

FIGURE 7-4. Genogram for the Dawe family.

2. Unable to follow exercise program due to fatigue, shortness of breath
3. Poor control of blood pressure because unable to follow low-sodium, low-fat diet; salt substitute "tastes awful"; husband likes salt used in cooking
4. Poor control of diabetes resulting in hyperglycemia, retinopathies

Mr. Dawe displayed a lack of knowledge about diabetes and its management when he was questioned. He left it "up to her" to know what to do because she was a nurse. Mrs. Dawe did not talk about her diet with him, but he noticed that her "cooking had changed some."

We concluded the assessment for patient education by discussing and validating the problem areas with Mrs. Dawe.

Nursing Diagnosis and Educational Needs

1. Altered Nutrition: More than body requirements related to nonadherence to diabetic low-salt, low-fat diet
   Educational Needs: Negotiate and coach behavior modification related to ADA diet

   Positive factors affecting behavioral change
   Patient is knowledgeable about health problems
   Patient cooks
   Patient makes decisions

   Negative factors affecting behavioral change
   Self-concept is decreased
   Environment includes availability of restricted foods
   Patient feels hungry
   Patient feels diet is too restrictive
   Husband is not impressed with seriousness of health problem
2. Activity Intolerance related to decreased mobility and obesity
   Educational Needs: Negotiate and instruct to increase activity with consistent exercise program

   Positive factors affecting behavioral change
   Interferes with role of caring for others, including grandchildren
   Patient wants to be independent and more mobile
   Symptoms bother patient

Negative factors affecting behavioral change
Patient is obese
Patient's dependence on husband has increased
Patient unable to follow diet

Nurses who work on hospital inpatient units are not afforded the time and opportunity for such extensive patient and family education assessments. Patients are often so ill in an acute episode that assessment must be conducted at various times throughout the hospitalization. This information is helpful not just in planning during the inpatient phase. With good documentation and continuity of care, the information benefits other providers such as home health nurses who can build on the assessment data during home visits. The following case study is an example.

❑ CASE STUDY

Mr. Stanley

Physiologic Data

As she began the admission data base for 60-year-old Mr. Stanley, the primary nurse gathered assessment information critical to his care. Mr. Stanley was admitted to the hospital with a medical diagnosis of asthma. His wife and daughter supplied much of the information because Mr. Stanley was "puffing" and coughing. In a relatively short time, the initial assessment was conducted.

Because asthma is a chronic disease and the patient had been diagnosed with it 15 years ago, his primary nurse knew she should gear her questioning around the cornerstones of self-care management: preventing acute episodes, using controlled breathing techniques, avoiding bronchial irritants, and using medications correctly. The prevalence of asthma and COPD were among the top diagnosis-related groups at the hospital, and a special patient education effort was aimed at improving the correct use of inhalers. It was estimated that greater than 50%

of patients using inhalers experience therapeutic failure due to incorrect technique.

Family Profile

The nurse learned that Mr. and Mrs. Stanley lived in a ranch-style house within 2 miles of their only child, a 38-year-old daughter. Mr. Stanley was a retired grounds keeper for the city and spent much of his time planning his home garden now. He also liked to fish and was active in the Baptist church. Mrs. Stanley reported that she is in good health except for discomfort from arthritis.

Understanding of the Current Event

Mr. Stanley has had progressively worse attacks of dyspnea for the last month, with occasional tachycardia. Today's episode followed working in his garden, "overdoing it," as Mrs. Stanley described. Mr. Stanley reported a decrease in appetite and difficulty sleeping. The nurse noticed that the Stanley's daughter filled out admission papers. All three family members appeared anxious. Mrs. Stanley reported that her husband worried her with his frequent use of his inhaler and increasing episodes of breathlessness. When asked to demonstrate controlled breathing techniques, Mrs. Stanley said that he had forgotten how to do them and that he just relied on his "trusty friend" (his inhaler). Mrs. Stanley told the nurse, "I've been trying to get him to go to the doctor for over a week. It finally came to this!" Mr. Stanley's prescribed medications included: Azmacort (triamcinolone acetonide) inhaler, 3 puffs, three times a day; Serevent (salmeterol-xinafoate), a long-acting bronchodilator, 2 puffs twice a day; and Ventolin (albuterol) as needed, but no more frequently than 2 puffs every 4 to 6 hours. Mr. Stanley admitted to using Ventolin on a daily basis against the orders of his physician. He had resumed smoking "a few cigarettes" lately. He had quit for 10 months after his last hospitalization.

Because Mr. Stanley became quickly fatigued, the nurse completed an initial screening of systems and flagged the assessment data base form so that additional information could be gathered in the following areas:

Observation of patient's inhaler technique
Potential environmental irritants
Income and health insurance (often prevents patients from obtaining needed medications)

Reading/writing abilities of the Stanleys (to determine which written materials are appropriate)
Normal diet patterns and sleep patterns of the family
Daily schedule
Ability of family to handle crisis situations
Degree of limitation on the patient's and family's functioning
Family's desires/needs to know about the illness or problem

The Identified Patient, the Health Problem, and Education Needs

Mr. Stanley summarized his problems briefly and succinctly:

Frequent episodes of "puffing"
Fatigue, sometimes with heart beating too fast

Mrs. Stanley added:

Poor appetite lately
Not sleeping well

Their nurse explained that poor appetite, rapid heart rate, and difficulty sleeping may be related to overuse or improper use of the inhaler and that she would help Mr. Stanley understand how to better manage his asthma at home.

Nursing Diagnosis and Educational Needs

1. Impaired Gas Exchange related to chronic airway obstruction
   Educational Needs: Instruct in proper use of inhaler; stress importance of eliminating smoking and review other bronchial irritants, including stress; help patient recognize warning signs and prevent exacerbations; stress danger of overuse of Serevent and Ventolin
2. Ineffective Airway Clearance related to reduced cough strength and slowed mucous transport
   Educational Needs: Teach controlled coughing and breathing techniques and ways to increase fluid intake; demonstrate proper use of inhaler; identify ways to avoid infection; identify signs and symptoms of infection
3. Activity Intolerance related to dyspnea
   Educational Needs: Learn how to manage activity and prevent excessive breathlessness
4. Altered Nutrition: Less than body require-

ments related to fatigue, weakness, and breathlessness
    Educational Needs: Reinforce planning of adequate fluid intake, small meals and frequent snacks with patient and wife
5. Anxiety related to episodes of dyspnea
    Educational Needs: Help patient and family express feeling of helplessness; discuss how to handle acute episodes to increase confidence and gain support; suggest methods of relaxation
6. Risk for Noncompliance with therapeutic program related to chronic nature of disease
    Educational Needs: Help patient develop an individualized program to integrate all facets of management; suggest a smoking cessation program and offer resources; offer suggestions that will help family cope with chronic illness

Mr. Stanley's primary nurse realized that she would have to pinpoint priorities for teaching and be organized so he could learn according to his physical ability.

She identified factors that would influence his learning.

Positive factors affecting behavioral change
    Has experience with disease and symptoms
    Has been smoke free for 10 months before resuming smoking
    Wants to be able to continue gardening
Negative factors affecting behavioral change
    Tends to delay seeking treatment for dyspnea
    Resumed smoking
    Both patient and family exhibit anxiety

Summary

The process of patient education is an integral part of nursing care. Although the steps of the process are always the same (assessment, planning, implementation, evaluation), the nurse must tailor practice to meet the needs of patients and the constraints of the patient care setting. Assessment, using an assessment guide, is as detailed and thorough as possible to determine accurate nursing diagnoses and factors that will affect patient and family learning. Thus, assessment reflects both process and product. Case studies

were offered in this chapter to illustrate assessment and nursing diagnosis.

The case of Mrs. Dawe shows how the home visit can be used to assess problems related to behavior management of chronic problems. The watchful and astute nurse noted that the home environment and lack of family knowledge posed obstacles to adherence to the diabetic, low-fat diet.

Mr. Stanley's case illustrated that even with limited time for assessment of a newly admitted patient, nursing diagnoses and educational needs can be formulated and later refined as more detailed information is gathered.

In both cases, assessment highlighted problems commonly encountered when patients and families face chronic conditions. There is an ongoing need for education. The nurse assesses the patient's and the family's basic knowledge about the problem and its management. The nurse also looks for educational needs to help the client cope with the recommended treatment plan and solve problems that arise at home.

Patient education involves much more than simply sharing the medical information we have with the patient by communicating it in a vocabulary he can understand. We recognize the importance of assessing individual situations to see the patient as he sees himself. Only then can we assist the patient in recognizing and overcoming obstacles that prevent the desired behaviors. This requires a skilled approach to patients for which health professionals must be prepared.

Strategy for Critical Analysis and Application

1. Using the Patient and Family Education Assessment Guide, conduct a home visit. Write up a summary of your assessment similar to the summary of Mrs. Dawe, illustrated in this chapter.

REFERENCES

Andrews, M., & Boyle, J. (1995). *Transcultural concepts in nursing care* (2nd ed.). Philadelphia: J. B. Lippincott.

American Hospital Association. (1984). *Guidelines for discharge planning*. Chicago: Author.

Bash, K., & Jones, F. (1994). Domestic violence in America. *North Carolina Medical Journal, 55*(3), 400-403.

Brown, G., & Runyan, D. (1994). Diagnosing child maltreatment. *North Carolina Medical Journal, 55*(9), 404-408.

Carpenito, L. (1992). *Nursing diagnosis: Application to clinical practice* (4th ed). Philadelphia: J. B. Lippincott.

Chez, N. (1994). Helping the victim of domestic violence. *American Journal of Nursing, July,* 33-37.

Deakins, D. (1994). Teaching elderly patients about diabetes. *American Journal of Nursing, April,* 39-42.

Eggland, E., Heinemann, D. (1994). Nursing documentation: Charting, recording, and reporting. Philadelphia: J.B. Lippincott.

Eliopoulous, C. (1987). *Gerontological nursing* (2nd ed.). Philadelphia: J. B. Lippincott.

Erikson, E. (1963). *Childhood and society*. New York: W. W. Norton.

Gragg, S., & Rees, O. (1980). *Scientific principles in nursing*. St. Louis: C. V. Mosby.

Horton, T. (1977). Conceptual basis for nursing intervention with human systems: Families. In J. Hall, & B. Weaver (Eds.), *Distributive nursing practice: A systems approach to community health* (pp. 101[a], 104[b], 105[c], 112 [d]). Philadelphia: J. B. Lippincott.

Kleinman, A., Eisenberg, L., & Good, B. (1978). Culture, illness, and care: Clinical lessons from anthropologic and cross-cultural research. *Annals of Internal Medicine, 88,* 251-258.

Leininger, M. (1978). *Transcultural nursing: Concepts, theories, and practices*. New York: John Wiley & Sons.

Lewis, J. (1976). *No single thread* (pp. 206-207). New York: Brunner-Mazel.

MacVicar, M., & Archbold, P. (1976). A framework for family assessment in chronic illness. *Nursing Forum, 15,* 180-194.

Maslow, A. (1970). *Motivation and personality*. New York: Harper & Row.

McAfee, R. (1994). Physicians' role in the fight against family violence. *North Carolina Journal of Medicine, 55*(9), 398-399.

McAfee, R. (1993, April). Doing something about violence. *Ross Roundtable Report-Family Violence* (pp. 1-12).

Orgue, M., Bloch, B., & Monroy, L. (1983). *Ethnic nursing care: A multicultural approach*. St Louis: C. V. Mosby.

Otto, H. (1963). Criteria for assessing family strengths. *Family Process, 2,* 329-337.

Redman, B. (1992). *The process of patient education* (7th ed.). St. Louis: Mosby-Year Book.

Richardson, B. (1982). The real world of diabetic noncompliance. *Nursing, 12*(1), 68-73.

Robinson, L. (1974). Patients' information base: A key to care. *Canadian Nurse, 10*(12), 34-36.

Tanner, C., Benner, P., Chesla, C., & Gordon, D. The phenomenology of knowing the patient. *Image - The Journal of Nursing Scholarship, 25*(4), 273-280.

8

Planning: Shared Goals for Patient Education

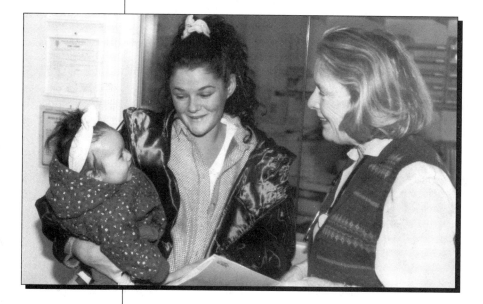

OBJECTIVES FOR CHAPTER 8

After reading this chapter, the nurse or student nurse should be able to:

1 Describe three characteristics of the adult learner.

2 Discuss the importance of constructing learning objectives before developing learning interventions.

3 Briefly define each of the following domains of learning:
  a Cognitive
  b Affective
  c Psychomotor

4 Describe how the Health Belief Model can be applied to goal setting with the patient.

Goal Setting: Targeting Outcomes for Learning

Once nursing diagnoses are formulated and validated with the patient and family, the nurse incorporates them in the patient care plan. If a computerized care planning system is used, the nurse tailors a critical pathway based on the problem or the diagnosis-related group to reflect the needs of the patient. The planning process can now begin. Nursing diagnoses or functional problems must be reviewed, and critical learning needs associated with resolving each problem are considered. Learning needs are ranked in order of priority by asking the question, "What is most critical to the safety of this patient?" Then, short- and long-term goals are negotiated. Finally, specific behavioral objectives for patient education help the nurse and other health care providers work with the patient and family to make the learning experience outcome oriented. Care maps, which are discussed in Chapter 13, also help providers and patients to sequence learning goals within an estimated length of stay as part of the diagnosis-specific critical pathway.

Patient learning occurs during the goal setting process, as the proposed treatment plan is reviewed and the patient's readiness to learn is assessed. Thus, teaching is not a separate intervention but is an integral part of every aspect of nursing care. Assessing readiness continues to be important. If patients are in denial about their problems, they are unable to participate in goal setting. Trends in the provision of patient education in the context of managed care attempt to dictate the teaching schedule. Readiness is a variable that must be considered in individualizing patient education although in some cases, it is necessary to proceed even when the patient does not seem ready because teaching and coaching are embedded in expert nursing care and are not limited to formal, planned teaching sessions (Benner, 1984). An exemplar of an expert nurse, included in Benner's work, offers the following illustration of

capturing a patient's readiness, which led to the goal setting process.

> He made it very clear that he was ready. He was asking a lot of questions. He had a regular ileostomy a couple of years ago and had finally been persuaded that a continent ileostomy was going to be the greatest thing for him. Earlier I thought he was feeling helpless about the operation he had just had. He looked as though he felt crummy. Physically, he was sort of stressed looking, nervous looking. Furthermore, he was treating the whole thing physically very gingerly. He didn't need to be that gentle with it. So by the time he started asking questions he was feeling better physically, feeling like there was some hope that he would learn how to deal with this. (Benner, 1984)

Using Data From the Assessment

In Chapter 7 we discussed the process of assessment. The more comprehensive the assessment, the more aware we will be of the needs and problems involved. This awareness facilitates our counseling of clients and helps us to provide them with learning experiences, through which they may gain knowledge, attitudes, and skills to promote health.

Assessment provides us with information about what the patient and the family know and what they want or need to know. The learning needs we identify relate to their right to know and prepare them to make informed choices. The definition of learning needs also involves dealing with barriers to behavioral change and expanding knowledge, attitudes, and skills related to diagnosis, complications, management, prognosis, prevention, and resources for assistance. We encourage the active involvement of patients and their families in assessment. Our task is to help them articulate their perceptions of their needs and problems.

Skills Needed by the Nurse

The process of planning for patient education is a responsibility shared by the nurse with the patient and family. It is, however, directed by the nurse who is ultimately responsible for determining priorities, sorting out "need-to-know" versus "nice-to-know" facts, and helping clients master skills critical to their future safety.

Patients expect nurses to exhibit certain strengths in this process. We interviewed many of our patients to determine how they would describe a nurse who is an excellent teacher, and then we used these descriptions to teach our nursing students. Patients were articulate in accounting the teacher-learner relationship. We extracted four characteristics of excellent nurse-teachers from these conversations (Box 8-1).

BOX 8–1. The Four Characteristics of the Excellent Nurse-Teacher

Confidence
- Selects what to teach
- Alleviates the patient's anxiety
- Provides appropriate learning environment
- Prepares appropriate teaching plan and material

Competence
- Decides what is important to teach
- Ensures the patient's safety
- Provides individualized written instructions
- Teaches home management of special problems

Communication
- Gives clear directions
- Uses simple pictures or models
- Speaks the patient's language

Caring
- Has empathy
- Recognizes patient concerns
- Provides encouragement
- Ensures adequate time
- Sensitive to patient's mood

---

1. *Confidence.* Nurse are experts about what to teach and are able to identify the main points of information they are communicating. They also "speak the patient's language" and often use simple pictures or models. They are organized and can alleviate the patient's anxiety. They instill confidence.
2. *Competence.* Nurses decide what is most important and give clear directions. They are concerned with the patient's safety. They provide good instructions and often give individualized written instructions about what to do at home. They tell the patient what to do if specific problems should arise.
3. *Communication.* These nurses speak well and listen well. They do not need to be a "long-winded lecturer." They get to the point. They involve the patient by finding out what the individual already knows, and they use these experiences or problems as examples when they teach. They stop and ask questions to be sure the patient understands the instructions. They use a "show-and-tell" approach. They are comfortable talking to the patient's family and involve them in teaching. They teach the patient who to call for help once at home. They review what the patient is told by his doctor, dietitian, and physical therapist.
4. *Caring.* These nurses can put themselves "in the patient's shoes" and consider how the person might feel. They understand that patients worry about pain, safety, appearance, and financial costs. They address these concerns. They are gentle but firm when the patient makes mistakes during the learning process. They are encouraging and provide enough time for the patient to be successful. They notice when patients are sad or troubled and help the patient confide any concerns.

Understanding Patient Concerns During Hospitalization

Although nurses are placing greater emphasis on discharge teaching, we must also be aware that patient concerns during hospitalization often interfere with discharge teaching. The nurse must anticipate patient concerns and address these rather than ignore them or underestimate their importance. Examples of thoughts, fears, and concerns of great importance to patients and families are:

Am I going to be all right?

What is going on; what are they planning to do to me?

Is this going to cost me my job? Will I be fired?

My wife will be worried to death. Who is going to tell her?

Do these doctors know what they're doing? My own doctor knows my condition, but what about all the other doctors?

Am I going to be in a lot of pain after this surgery?

There are so many staff here. Who is really in charge of me?

Fear often poses barriers to learning, and the ability to lessen anxiety is always a goal of patient education. It is important to remember that the patient and family may interpret the seriousness of the illness differently from the nurse and may experience one or more of the fears listed in Box 8-2.

Patients and families may also feel guilty for how they have related to one another in the past, angry about becoming ill or the problems the illness brings on the family, or helpless and unable to cope with the illness (American Hospital Association, 1983).

During the planning process, the nurse must attend to the issues causing greatest con-

---

BOX 8–3. Critical Learning Needs: Preparing For Discharge

1. What potential problems are likely to prevent a safe discharge?

2. What potential problems are likely to cause complications or readmission?

3. What prior knowledge or experience does the patient and family have with this problem?

4. What skills and equipment are needed to manage the problem at home?

---

cern for the patient and family. What to expect, how to get help, and how to manage pain are questions addressed through patient education.

Critical Learning Needs: Preparing for Discharge

Nurses also bring pressing concerns to patient education encounters. They are aware that there are many things patients must know and do correctly to survive independently of the health care team, and these things must be learned before discharge. The nurse must determine what learning is critical by asking the four key questions listed in Box 8-3.

Ensuring patient safety through teaching is not just an ethical necessity but also a legality. For example, hospital lawyers caution us not to overlook discharge teaching about drugs. Patients must be warned about the adverse reactions of any medications they have taken or have been prescribed, especially if the drugs can impair mental or physical ability. Otherwise, any injury resulting to that patient or a member of the public may result in a negligence lawsuit (Northrop, 1986).

Goals of Patient and Family Education

Goals for patient and family education must embrace the concerns of client and nurse.

BOX 8–2. Potential Barriers to Learning

Patient Concerns During Hospitalization

- Fear of pain
- Fear that the illness cannot be cured
- Fear of scarring or deformity
- Fear of being a burden on others
- Fear of dying
- Fear of cost of hospitalization

The nurse must be sensitive to the patient, yet must also provide direction and firm priorities for discharge teaching. Patients have told us they depend on nurses to do this. Therefore, goal setting is shared with the patient and family. Goals will target patient education to address survival skills, teaching the patient to recognize problems and helping the patient and family develop decision-making skills (Fig. 8-1). Every patient who enters into the health care system should know why he is there at that time. This may seem obvious, but we discover that patients often know their symptoms but not how they relate to a diagnosis. Patients often do not know how a group of symptoms relates to the current problem. By learning why they are "here, in this place, at this time" patients gain perspective on health management. Patients and family want simple explanations about the diagnosis, in terms they can remember and repeat to other family and friends. Even before they are ready to engage in formal learning activities, they want to know what will be expected of them when they are discharged. They want to know how to tell that they are in trouble and how to get emergency care (Box 8-4).

Goals are accomplished by mastering learning objectives that refer to the patient's ability to demonstrate or perform learning behaviors. Setting goals is an important step in the nursing process, but it is often ignored. Goals and objectives help the nurse focus on what is critical and keep patient teaching on track. Throughout this chapter, the nurse will learn how to negotiate goals with the patient and family and how to work together. We will demonstrate how learning objectives are constructed and how they determine the entire learning process. We will also outline the components of a learning contract and discuss its use as a motivator for learning, a mechanism for communication, and a source of standards for evaluating the teaching and learning process.

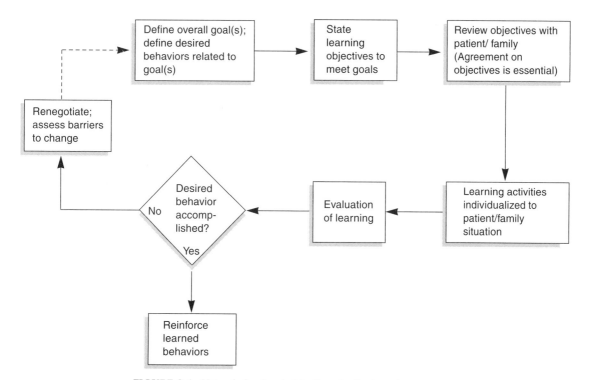

FIGURE 8-1. Using behavioral objectives in the learning process.

BOX 8–4. Goals of Patient and Family Education

- Survival skills
- Recognizing problems
- Decision-making

The importance of goal setting is better appreciated in light of the principles of adult learning. We begin by discussing the characteristics of an adult learner and considering how a negotiation of learning goals sets the stage for learning activities.

Characteristics of the Adult Learner

The question most commonly asked by nurses attending workshops we have conducted on patient education is, "How can I motivate patients to learn?" Nurses realize from their experience that the learners must play an active role in the teaching process— that nurses cannot *make* them learn, but they can *help* patients learn. What, then, prompts learning?

We can use several sources to arrive at a better understanding of the adult learner. We have chosen two that we have found to be most helpful in the patient education area. One of these is our own experience as adult learners, and the second is the work of Malcolm Knowles (1970), the father of *andragogy* (adult learning).

Many nurses teach patients and their families in the way they were taught as children. The learner assumes a passive role, and the nurse lectures and demonstrates to him as the teacher did in the grammar school setting. If the nurse tries to imagine herself as an adult student seated in a fifth grade classroom, she will understand why the adult patient needs a different environment. She might imagine herself feeling anxious about what the teacher expects, concerned that the material may be repetitious and boring and that the class schedule is rigid and her chair

uncomfortable. She knows that she is not allowed to speak without permission. She feels that her past experience is not important and that she may have to learn things that are not relevant to her interests.

When the nurse considers her own positive learning experiences as an adult, she is likely to recall an environment of physical and psychological comfort in which she felt accepted, valued, and encouraged to contribute her thoughts, ideas, and past experiences. The subject matter was of interest to her and would help her in her job or her role (e.g., as a spouse or parent). With help, she defined her own learning goals and then evaluated the result of the learning activities. There were opportunities for role playing or trying out new behaviors. She felt free to ask questions without fear of embarrassment.

Adult patients have similar needs as learners. Physical and emotional comfort and active participation in defining their own needs and goals motivate patients to learn. Nurses who are aware that adult patients and their family members learn best in the same kind of environment that would be personally comfortable for the nurses themselves tend to provide such an environment for patient education.

Malcolm Knowles contributes four reasonable assumptions about adult learners that distinguish them from children (see following section). Readers are strongly encouraged to read his book, *The Modern Practice of Adult Education*, for more information on the role of the adult educator and on strategies for helping adults learn (Knowles, 1970). We outline his four basic assumptions and some major points that apply to the patient education process. In Table 8-1 applications of each of the four assumptions to patient and family teaching are made.

Knowles's assumptions about the adult learner are as follows. As a person matures . . .

1. His self-concept moves from dependency to self-direction. He sees himself as capable of making his own decisions, taking responsibility for their consequences, and managing his own life.

TABLE 8–1. Application of Adult Learning Theory to Patient and Family Education

Assumptions About Learner	Applications
Self-concept moves from dependency toward self-direction; sees self as capable of making own decisions, taking responsibility for consequences, managing own life.	Acknowledge learner's desire to articulate own needs, make choices, and gain respect for own ability to manage life; create psychological climate that communicates acceptance and support; help learner to feel comfortable taking chances, expressing his thoughts and ideas without fear of shame or embarrassment; remember that adults are motivated to learn when they realize that they have a need to learn.
Growing reservoir of life experience is a resource for learning	Use past experiences as a resource for learning; remember that adults experience positive feelings of support and recognition when their experience is acknowledged; relate new learning to old; have adults teach other adults in a group setting; be aware that negative past experiences may pose barriers for learner and teacher.
Readiness to learn is strongly influenced by social roles and developmental tasks	Recognize social role of patient (e.g., father, mother, husband, wife, worker) and developmental tasks; relate learning to ability to become, to succeed in these roles.
Time perspective changes; orientation to learning shifts; needs immediate application of new knowledge and problem-centered learning	Give adults practical answers to their problems; help them to apply new knowledge immediately through role play or hands-on practice (i.e., return demonstration); remember that adults are particularly motivated to learn at times of crisis or when problems arise; prioritize learning activities by immediacy of need and patient-family perception of need; reinforce learning and promote problem-solving skills.

Adapted from Knowles, M. S. (1970). *The modern practice of adult education.* New York: Association Press.

2. He accumulates life experiences that are an increasing resource for learning.
3. His readiness to learn is increasingly oriented to his developmental tasks and social roles.
4. His time perspective changes and his orientation to learning shifts. He needs immediate application (rather than postponed application) of knowledge, and his learning is problem centered rather than subject centered.

The following points made by Knowles offer additional guidance in goal setting with the patient and family:

1. Adults see themselves as producers or doers and derive self-esteem from their contributions.
2. Adults have a need to be perceived by others as self-directing.
3. Adults respond in an informal and friendly environment, where they are known by name and valued as individuals.

To summarize, adults are performance centered and seek information that helps them in their daily lives. Patients listen for the "bottom line" and want health professionals to tell them what they "need to know" versus what is "nice to know." Patients rarely want a detailed description of anatomy and pathophysiology related to their body systems. They want to know how to perform a prescribed regimen of survival skills once they go home and how to adapt current life-styles to include health behaviors. Perceived benefits that encourage these behaviors are often related to performing roles as spouse, parent, and worker.

Because, as Knowles suggests, the adult's readiness to learn (thus, motivation to try out new behaviors) is influenced by developmental tasks, the patient educator will want to be familiar with Erik Erikson's writings on the eight stages of man (Erikson, 1950). Table 8-2 briefly outlines the eight stages as Erikson identifies them.

TABLE 8–2. Erikson's Eight Stages of Man

STAGE	ISSUE
Oral-sensory: birth to 1 y of age	Trust vs. mistrust
Muscular-anal: ages 1–2 y	Autonomy vs. shame
Locomotion-genital: ages 3–5 y	Initiative vs. guilt
Latency: age 6 to puberty	Industry vs. inferiority
Puberty, adolescence: puberty to late teens	Identity vs. role confusion
Young adulthood: late teens to mid twenties	Intimacy vs. isolation
Adulthood: variable	Generativity vs. stagnation
Maturity: variable	Ego integrity vs. despair

In Erikson's first stage, trust versus mistrust is the development issue; this stage lasts from birth to 1 year of age. Meeting the child's needs for physical care and for receiving love influences future trust of people and the world.

In the second stage, children strive for autonomy, building mental and motor skills and gaining a feeling of independence and control.

In the third stage, children continue to master skills and take initiative. They need freedom to gain independence without guilt.

During the fourth stage, children learn how things are made and how they work. They need encouragement for this industry and a sense of accomplishment as opposed to feelings of inferiority and failure.

In Erikson's fifth stage, during adolescence, identity emerges with the integration of roles as a student, son or daughter, wage earner, athlete, and so forth. Role models and peer pressure are strong influences in this stage.

Early adulthood, the sixth stage, is a time when intimacy, courtship, and beginning one's own family are issues. Roles as a spouse or parent are developed.

In the seventh stage, adulthood, productivity and contribution to society are valued. A sense of accomplishment from caring for others is pursued.

Maturity is Erikson's eighth stage. It is a time of reflection, looking back on life's accomplishments. Pride in family and children adds to self-esteem. Dealing with death and dying is characteristic of maturity (Kaluger & Kaluger, 1975).

The Health Belief Model Applied to Goal Setting

The Health Belief Model is also helpful in understanding patient motivation to adopt health behaviors and follow a treatment plan. As explained in Chapter 3, this model was constructed in the 1950s by a group of social psychologists at the U.S. Public Health Service to predict health behaviors (Hochbaum, 1958). It provides a tool for understanding the patient's perception of disease and his decision-making process in the consumption of health care services. Although the Health Belief Model was originally designed to predict the likelihood of patients' taking recommended preventive action, such as obtaining screening tests and annual checkups, it has been the basis for other models adapted to consider the consumption of health care services in the presence of chronic illness (Kasl, 1974; Janz & Becker, 1984). Although its application as a model in research is often for compliance prediction, it is also useful for gaining a better understanding of the patient's motivation for seeking and obtaining services. In the case of pediatric patients, the model can be applied to understanding parents' motivation to consume services.

The Health Belief Model predicts that an individual is likely to consume health care services if the following situations exist and the patient experiences the following:

1. Perceives that he has a disease or condition or is likely to contract it
2. Perceives that the disease or condition is harmful and has serious consequences
3. Believes that the suggested health intervention is of value
4. Believes that the effectiveness of the treatment is worth the cost and barriers he must confront

Additionally, demographic variables such as age, gender, ethnicity, and socioeconomic status, as well as cues to action, are considered modifiers of the individual perception that the disease or condition is harmful (Janz & Becker, 1984). Cues to action include mass media campaigns, advice from others, newspaper articles, or illness of a family member or friend. The Health Belief Model suggests that understanding the process of patient reasoning and sequencing provider-patient interactions to support it promote patient engagement in the patient education process. Table 8-3 outlines how the steps of the model can be applied to goal setting.

It is clear that gaining the patient's commitment to learn health behaviors and adapt them into daily life should precede patient education interventions such as skills training. Nurses should not approach patients as passive learners who are obligated to change their behaviors based solely on direction. The Health Belief Model illustrates that patients will calculate their perceptions of a "return on investment." Performing health behaviors commonly involves cost, discomfort, shifting of time and priorities, social isolation, and breaking of long-standing habits. By following the model in the goal-setting process, nurses can help the patient to see how benefits can outweigh these costs. Ongoing support and assistance from family and health care providers can be an important benefit that helps patients to "tip the scale" in favor of performing health behaviors. The process may reveal that the patient is unwilling to

change or perform some behaviors. Smoking is often an example of a behavior a patient is unwilling to change despite evidence presented by the health care system.

A review of research testing the Health Belief Model suggests that barriers and costs a person confronts are the most salient reasons for either engaging in preventive health behaviors or behaviors related to the illness regimen (Janz & Becker, 1984). Susceptibility to and severity of an illness were not as powerful predictors of behavior as barriers and costs, except for persons who already have an illness, such as coronary artery disease. To achieve better outcomes, nurses must encourage patients to discuss perceived barriers and identify possible resources to confront these barriers. If a patient cannot afford to purchase the prescribed medication, financial assistance or a less costly medication are needed. If the patient has been unsuccessful with a therapeutic diet because it is too confining, negotiation of the list of "forbidden foods" and helping the patient's entire family to change the way they prepare meals will set the stage for more effective patient teaching. Resources for cooking and preparing good-tasting food may also break down barriers to long-term health behaviors (Polin & Giedt, 1993). Furthermore, American Diabetes Association (ADA) diet planning for diabetic patients has shifted to updated guidelines that provide more flexibility for patients and less strict calorie restrictions. Because many patients with diabetes also have heart disease, the diet must target blood sugar levels as well as low-fat intake (Gershoff, 1994).

Another problem with patient education programs may come to light as we discuss with the patient the need to change two or more behaviors simultaneously, such as diet, exercise, smoking, medications, or treatments. Patients are often unsuccessful because they cannot make such profound changes. Nurses realize when they examine their own health behaviors, such as smoking, exercise, nutrition, sleep, and medications, that few of us "practice what we preach" for that reason. Setting priorities and establishing long-term plans of support, follow-up, and reinforce-

TABLE 8–3. The Health Belief Model Used in the Interview to Identify Patient Goals and Decisions

Steps	Application
I. The patient perceives that he has a condition or is likely to contract it.	I. a. Discuss the problem and symptoms. b. Explore patient's prior knowledge and experience. c. Assess obstacles to understanding (anxiety, fear, misconceptions).
II. The patient perceives that the disease or condition is harmful and has serious consequences for him.	II. a. Patient's perception of consequences (includes life-style) b. Discussion of prognosis c. Beliefs and attitudes; trust of providers and health care system d. Experiences of family/friends with similar problem
III. The patient believes that the suggested health intervention is of value to him.	III. a. Understanding of proposed treatment plan (includes medications) b. Discussion of what may happen with or without proposed treatment. c. Is this a cure? d. Financial costs, life-style changes, side effects discussed
IV. The patient believes that the effectiveness of the treatment is worth the cost and barriers he must confront.	IV. a. Contracting (agreement) with the patient on the treatment plan b. Provider responsibilities outlined c. Patient responsibilities outlined d. Patient education plan for developing needed knowledge, attitudes, and skills

The Health Belief Model was constructed to predict health behaviors. It provides a tool for understanding the patient's perception of disease and his decision-making process in the consumption of health services. In each of the four steps, family members and significant others should be considered.

References
1. Hochbaum, G. M. (1958). *Public participation in medical screening programs.* (U.S. Public Health Service Publication No. 572). Washington, DC: U.S. Government Printing Office.
2. Rosenstock, I. M. (1975). Patient's compliance with health regimens. *Journal of the American Medical Association, 234,* 402–403.
3. Rankin, S.H., Stallings, K. D. (1990). *Patient education: Issues, principles, and practices.* Philadelphia: J. B. Lippincott.

ment are critical for patients with many recommended changes. Realistic approaches and sequencing of learning, combined with support extending beyond the hospital or clinic walls, can enhance the patient's commitment to engage in patient education interventions, and promote self-efficacy in the management of health and illness (Strecher, DeVellis, & Becker, 1986; Bandura, 1982).

One way nurses at Boston's Beth Israel Hospital engage in goal setting with cardiac patients is by sharing a list of eight topics of common concern, including how the heart works, activity restrictions, sex, medications, and diet. The nurse uses the list to begin discussion; the patient may add to the list, based on what he expects to achieve. The nurse then serves as a clinical expert, pulling out the patient's knowledge, concerns, life-style, and past experience (Miller, 1985).

Focus groups or advisory groups of patients who have experienced a particular health problem can teach health care providers how to make goal setting patient centered. In Chapter 13, an example of cardiac education is described based on a product line model that follows the patient across various settings. By looking at what patients need and want to know at each stage, learning goals and objectives can be accomplished at the times that they are most important to patients. An added benefit is that information overload is avoided, retention is accomplished, and learning is tied to patient readiness (Hanisch, 1993).

Goals and Objectives

Adult learners are motivated to learn when they recognize a gap between what they know and what they want to know (Knowles, 1970). Assessment provides us with information about where the patient stands with respect to the knowledge, attitudes, and skills important to self-care. Goal setting is an activity whereby the patient educator contracts with the patient for what he wants to accomplish. The readiness of the patient and family to learn is especially important to consider. Their ability to participate in this step is influenced by their degrees of physical discomfort, denial, grieving, and dependency needs. At no time should teachers force their own goals on the patient and family. They should instead try to meet them on their own ground, encourage whatever participation they can, and consider ways to support and reinforce strengths.

The learning experience is directed by goals and objectives. *Goals* are the desired outcomes of learning. An example of a goal might be: Mrs. Murphy will follow her low-fat ADA diabetic diet. *Objectives* are specific statements related to the goal. They describe in more detail the behaviors that will be performed to meet the goal. The following are sample objectives: Mrs. Murphy can outline breakfast, lunch, dinner, and snack menus for one day using her ADA diet plan; Mrs. Murphy will keep weekly clinic visits with the nurse for weight checks and review of daily food intake; Mrs. Jones will record the foods she eats in a notebook each day and bring this notebook to clinic visits. Both goals and objectives must be clearly stated and agreed on by the patient, the family, and the teacher if patient education is to have a focus.

Rationale for Using Goals and Objectives in Patient Education

We have stated several times that patient education is a process of influencing behavior rather than of only giving information. For instruction to be successful, it must be directed toward accomplishing behavioral change. We must justify that what we teach will help the patient perform the desired behavior (Kaluger & Kaluger, 1979). Setting specific goals for patient education ensures that learning interventions will be tailored to the situation and to the client's needs. Goals also offer criteria for evaluation of patient education (see Fig. 8-1). Did the patient and family successfully meet the goal? Mager, a well-known author and educator, highlights other outcomes of goal setting that can be applied to patient education (Mager, 1975).

When goals and objectives are clearly stated, the learner knows what his role is and what is expected of him. He can organize his energies toward accomplishing the goal. Occasionally, goal setting itself is the only intervention necessary to motivate the patient to change behavior. He is motivated by articulating what he can presently do and what he wishes to be able to do.

The teacher also knows her role when goals and objectives are stated. Both teacher and learner know how the results will be measured. Written documentation of goals ensures the patient's straightforward communication with the health care team.

What happens when objectives are not clearly stated? There is then no sound basis for nursing intervention. We do not know which learning activities are appropriate or what the roles of the teacher and learner will be. A common result is that the patient and family receive information but fail to understand how to use it in their own environment and individual circumstances. They may acquire information, but they do not learn new skills.

Many health care professionals have not had experience in writing behavioral objectives and, therefore, have difficulty with constructing objectives, even though they understand the rationale for doing so. Learning to articulate behavioral objectives is not difficult and is outlined in this chapter. With practice, skill in writing objectives increases.

Another concern identified by health professionals is the problem of setting priorities for what is to be taught first. The following section considers the setting of teaching and learning priorities.

Considering Teaching and Learning Priorities

A common mistake made by health professionals is that of trying to teach too much during a short period of time. We have seen this occur most often in the inpatient setting, where patients are overwhelmed with instructions before discharge. Reinforcement and evaluation of learning are often neglected. We contend that, for a number of reasons, patient and family learning needs should be carefully prioritized and creatively met in a variety of settings. Although teaching about chronic illness often occurs in the hospital setting, it must be followed up and reinforced in the home or in the outpatient clinic. This shows the importance of the efforts of nurses to use telephoned or written communication to inform nurses and physicians in health departments, offices, clinics, and nursing homes about the teaching plan and the patient's progress. Learning overload also occurs in outpatient settings, where patients are given many instructions related to self-care and prevention. Review and reinforcement are often lacking when the patient attempts to integrate the learning into changes in daily behavior.

Nurses who teach diabetic patients, for example, struggle with priorities because so much content must be taught and skills must be learned in a short period of time. One nurse offers the following advice from his experience as a staff nurse in a diabetic clinic:

Before you start your teaching, consider your patient's needs. You may be ready to begin teaching him about the pathophysiology of diabetes when all he wants to know is whether he'll be able to return to work. If you're pressed for time, concentrate on survival skills—injection techniques, the signs and symptoms of hypoglycemia and hyperglycemia, basic dietary instruction, the importance of regular exercise.

He emphasizes that further teaching can be done when the patient is followed as an outpatient (Lumley, 1988).

A certified diabetes educator in another agency offers additional tips for teaching patients about insulin when "the clock is ticking" (Hurxthal, 1988).

- Assess the patient's strengths, resources, and daily schedule.
- Call in the family to learn even the most basic skills.
- Teach survival skills.
  - How to draw up insulin and inject it
  - How to self-monitor blood glucose
  - How to manage hypo- and hyperglycemia
  - What and when to eat in relation to insulin timing
  - When and how to call for help
- Formulate the follow-up plan.

When caring for elderly diabetic patients, Deakins (1994) reminds us of the importance of repetition in patient teaching. Patients must learn about the disease and master specific skills, as well as integrate the cornerstones of management—medication, activity, and diet—into their daily lives.

The following four points support the importance of prioritizing learning needs and setting attainable goals in each patient situation. They also highlight the need for cooperation among professionals in many health care settings.

1. Length of hospitalization has shortened dramatically in recent years due to rising health care costs, bed shortages, improved technology, and the advent of prospective payment systems. Patients are discharged when they are physiologically stable rather than when teaching is completed. Patients are often acutely ill during most of the hospital stay and have physical and emotional restrictions that prevent learning. They may leave the hospital having had little opportunity to practice skills, review information, or ask questions. Nurses are often informed of the patient's discharge with only a few hours' notice, and they worry that the client has not been taught enough to manage self-care.

2. Patients who are overloaded with learning materials and activities feel a sense of frus-

tration and failure when they cannot perform all behaviors successfully. This makes them feel powerless, defeated, and dependent. Many adults would rather deny failure than admit to it, and they will revert back to old behaviors instead of asking for assistance.

3. Patients need to know what self-care activities are most important in their individual situations. When time and energy are at a premium, they need to know what learning must be achieved for survival.

4. Health professionals also have limited time and energy. Setting priorities for teaching helps to structure their time for its best use and ensures that acute learning needs are met. Professionals can discharge patients more confidently when they know that learning will be continued and reinforced.

The prioritization of learning needs is helped by considering the individual within the context of Maslow's hierarchy of needs (see Fig. 7-3 in Chap. 7). Because five different levels of needs exist, we recognize that needs lower on the hierarchy must be at least partially met before needs on the next level can be satisfied. This helps us to order learning needs and to recognize the patient's reliance on others to help him satisfy higher needs.

Prioritizing Patient Learning Needs

In acute and chronic illness, patient education is often limited to physiologic and survival needs (Box 8-5). To assist in prioritizing learning needs, ask the following questions:

- What are the most acute needs of this individual?
- What does he already know? What behaviors can he perform?
- What learning needs are unmet? Which are life-threatening problems?

The potential scope of learning needs in level one (physiologic and survival needs) for

BOX 8–5. Basic Needs of Patients

Physiologic and Survival Needs

Care and use of oxygen

Recognition of health problems, danger signs, and how to respond to them

Knowledge of nutrition and hydration

Comfort with sexuality

Management of pain

Recognition of depression and how to deal with it

Administration of insulin and other medications or treatments

Care of ostomy or Foley catheter

Safety and Security Needs

Poison prevention for parents

Ability to hold job

Competence in handling hazards on job or in environment (e.g., toxins, dangerous machinery, stress)

Ability to deal with family violence

Financial capabilities in meeting basic needs of food, shelter, medication

Affection and Belongingness Needs

Adaptation to peer pressure

Maintenance of family role

Ability to contribute to family, work group, community

Need to feel lovable and desirable despite illness or problem

Ability to deal with body image, disfigurement

Esteem or Recognition Needs

Need to succeed

Need to make choices, control own destiny

Need to be recognized as a valuable individual

Need for privacy, dignity

Ability to deal with lack of respect, abuse, ill treatment on job or in family

Self-Actualization: Self-Determining Needs

Success through own definition of what is desirable

Ability to meet developmental milestones

Independence in meeting lower needs

acute and chronic illness encompasses knowledge, attitudes, and skills related to all the categories in the list in Box 8-6. Use the list as a framework for assessing individual patient learning needs and educational goals.

Stating Goals and Objectives

Learning connotes a change in knowledge, attitudes, or skills as a result of an educational experience. *Behavioral objectives*, also referred to in the patient education context as learning objectives, guide the planning of learning activities and the measurement of learning outcomes. They should state what the learner will *do* as a result of patient teaching (see Fig. 8-1). A common mistake of nurses is to define learning objectives in terms of the nurse's behavior rather than that of the patient. For example, they might state "Review with the patient four signs of a hypoglycemic reaction." Instead, the objective should state that the patient will describe or list four signs of a hypoglycemic reaction. Objectives referring to knowledge are often referred to as *cognitive*; objectives describing attitudes are called *affective*; and objectives outlining skills may be referred to as *psychomotor*.

Cognitive refers to rational thought, including basic facts and concepts. Being able to describe a health problem in his own words, list signs and symptoms associated with the problem, and outline steps in a procedure are examples of the cognitive domain of knowledge. Cognitive learning moves from simple to complex concepts, so that the patient can apply facts to different situations. Understanding basic anatomy and physiology addresses the cognitive domain of learning.

Affective refers to feelings, reactions, appreciation of costs and benefits, and a willingness to change. Helping patients explore options, gain support of significant others, and explore the relationships of values, culture, and beliefs promotes affective learning.

Psychomotor refers to musculoskeletal movement, the ability to perform a procedure, skill, and the dexterity to manipulate objects or

---

BOX 8–6. Scope of Patient Education Needs in Acute and Chronic Illness

1. Diagnosis: explained in ways understandable to patient
   a. Etiology
   b. Contagiousness, malignance, premalignance, heredity
   c. Anatomy, physiology involved (limit to basic facts)
2. Complications: provide meaning to patient symptoms or possible symptoms
   a. Causes
   b. Prevention
   c. Early signals
3. Management: "big picture" of treatment plan, including discussion of patient self-care behaviors needed after discharge
   a. Surgery
   b. Radiation
   c. Diets
   d. Exercise, relaxation programs
   e. Medication
   f. Behavior modification and controls
   g. Environmental control
   h. Counseling
   i. Appliances (e.g., pacemaker, braces, crutches, traction)
   j. Consultation and referral
   k. Soaks, hot packs, dressings, treatments
4. Aggravating factors
   a. Foods
   b. Tobacco
   c. Drugs, alcohol
   d. Schedule of work and rest
   e. Interpersonal relationships
   f. Environmental aspects
5. Prognosis
   a. Short term
   b. Signs of trouble, complications
   c. Long term
6. Prevention of recurrence of acute problems
7. Resources for assistance
   a. Continuing care plan
   b. Economic, transportation
   c. Self-help groups
   d. Printed patient education materials
   e. Patient videotapes
   f. Group or community classes

Adapted from Society of Teachers of Family Medicine. (1979). *Patient education: A handbook for teachers.* Kansas City, MO:

parts are included in this domain of learning. Mastering psychomotor learning usually involves the need for demonstration, practice, and more practice until the skill is ingrained. Periodic rehearsal or review is needed when skills are not required on a frequent basis.

As described by Mager (1975), a behavioral objective has three components: performance, conditions, and criteria. To write clear learning objectives for patient education in the domains of cognitive, affective, and psychomotor, nurses must follow the three steps.

Performance states any activity in which the patient will engage; it describes what the learner will do. It uses an action verb and denotes an activity that can be measured. The activity may be visible, such as writing a list, or invisible, such as solving a problem. Examples of action verbs are: choose, collect, compare, compute, define, demonstrate, describe, discuss, identify, list, locate, measure, name, practice, prepare, recognize, record, report, test, use, write.

Verbs such as believe, understand, value, and know are not measurable and should be avoided when performance is being described.

When choosing an action verb, the teacher should ask, "Can I measure whether or not the learner is able to do this?" The verb should be simple enough that the learner will be able to understand how he is expected to show his competence. Each learning objective should reflect only one behavior.

Conditions state what special circumstances will be included in the learner's performance. Examples of conditions follow:

- Time of day
- Sterile technique
- Equipment, tools
- Place
- Calorie restrictions
- In the presence of particular symptoms

Criteria offer a component of evaluation. They state *how* the teacher and learner will know when the learning has been accomplished. A criterion states how long or how well the behavior must be performed. Examples of criteria are:

- Score or speed
- Weight
- Quality
- Number of times
- Accuracy
- Frequency

Sometimes it is difficult to distinguish between a condition and a criterion. For example, consider the following behavioral objective: Mrs. Jones will draw up and administer 22 units of insulin using sterile technique at 7:00 AM on 3 consecutive days.

The criteria used in measurement include the number of units of insulin, the time, and the frequency of administration. Yet the time of day is a condition as well as a criterion because it describes a circumstance under which the behavior is performed. Criteria are especially important when teaching psychomotor objectives, such as walking with crutches. How many times does the nurse want to observe a return demonstration to be confident that the patient has mastered the skill? What degree of error or variation in performance is acceptable? For example, when teaching a patient to take his pulse, within how many beats of the nurse's measurement must the patient measure to be considered successful?

Mager states it is important for both the teacher and the learner to answer the questions in Box 8-7 related to the behavioral objective. These three questions are the components of a learning objective and are intended as a help to the writer designing an objective (Mager, 1975).

1. What does the learner have to do to show he has achieved the learning? (What is the learner able to do?)
2. Under what conditions will he do it? (Will he use special equipment or do without an aid?)
3. How will he know when it is done well enough? What is the performance standard? (How well must it be done?)

The nurse should make learning objectives specific, measurable, and attainable. A well-constructed behavioral objective is specific, and the learner knows what is expected. The

---

BOX 8–7. Three Components of a Learning Objective

- What is the learner able to do?
- Under what conditions will he do it?
- How will we know when he has accomplished it? How well must it be done?

For example, the patient will

1. draw up and administer 22 units of insulin,
2. using sterile technique,
3. from 7:00 to 7:30 AM on 3 consecutive days.

---

behavior is measurable, achievement can be evaluated, and the standard is attainable. This requires an understanding of the patient's view of what he wants to achieve. Although the learner's ability should not be doubted, it is important that goals are not set too high. Learning should be a positive, supportive experience, in which the learner gains confidence and self-esteem. Learning should begin with activities in which the patient will succeed and should move from simple behaviors to those that are more complex. Also, learning objectives that are critical for safety (three or four critical behaviors) should be identified as such and should be reviewed and reinforced throughout the patient's stay.

Learning objectives keep patient education focused on outcomes. For that reason, nurses should relate the objectives to nursing diagnoses and limit the number of learning objectives. We have witnessed exhaustive lists of objectives (with 30 or more!) that look scholarly and polished but are useless to nurses and patients. To cover the objectives, patient education has become an exercise of rapid-fire teaching and little practice on the part of the patient. In light of shorter lengths of stay, the number of objectives should be based on what is feasible for a patient to learn in a given phase or setting. Nurses should avoid the temptation of simply teaching the same amount in a fraction of the time.

Getting the Patient and the Family Involved

The involvement of the patient and family in setting learning goals affirms their willingness to participate. Criteria for evaluation should be acceptable to them and valued by them. For example, working an hour in the garden without breathlessness or being able to care for a grandchild may be more meaningful outcomes to them than 22 respirations per minute or a 10-lb weight loss. The behavioral change involved for these, however, may be the same and could satisfy both the provider and the patient. It is important that patients express their own goals verbally or in writing. The patient educator should encourage them to talk about the changes they would like to make and help them to state these in objective form.

Health professionals must honestly share with the patient their goals for him. We must be willing to revise these goals and objectives if they are not agreeable to him. The patient may understand the hazards of smoking but may not be willing to give up his evening cigarettes. The patient may understand the need for weight reduction and want to lose weight but be unwilling to sacrifice ice cream. A measurable reduction in smoking or a measurable weight loss using a modified diet plan may be a workable compromise.

Some strategies for getting the patient and the family involved include asking them for their perceptions of the patient's problems and what they would like to change. Share your view of the problem and ask the patient if he would like help in working on the identified problems. Discuss the priority of needs with the patient and write behavioral objectives using his input. Working together, contract for what you will teach, what the patient will learn, and what your respective responsibilities will be.

The Learning Contract

The learning contract is a tool used to formalize the agreement between the teacher and learner. It clearly states learning behaviors, the responsibility of the teacher and the learner, and the methods of follow-up and evaluation. The contract is renegotiated as learning is accomplished and new goals are defined. If the patient changes his mind or finds the goals too difficult to achieve, the objectives can be revised. We have used learning contracts with a high degree of success in the hospital, home, and clinic settings (Fig. 8-2).

Designing a Learning Contract

Figure 8-3 illustrates the essential components of a learning contract. We have found it helpful to type a standard contract form on hospital or clinic stationery and complete it with the patient. We keep a copy in the nurses' station or in the patient record and give a copy to the patient. A bonus clause has been used to denote additional resources available to the patient (e.g., self-help groups, classes, and other health professionals). As behaviors are accomplished, we find it essential to include a *reinforcement* as an intervention to support the patient when the contract is revised. The reinforcement may be weekly weight checks in the clinic, an occasional home visit, a telephone call, or a referral to the public health nurse or office nurse.

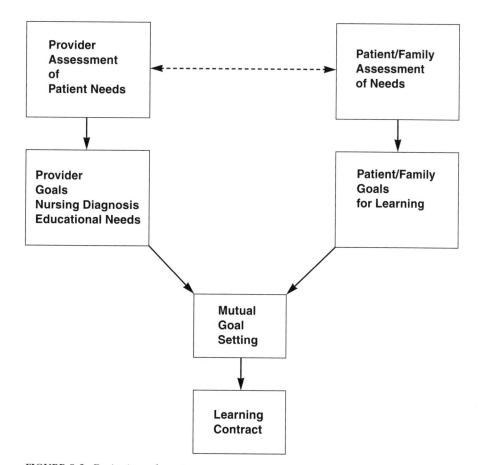

FIGURE 8-2. Designing a learning contract based on client goals for patient education.

Learning Contract

Goal:

Learning Objectives:

Provider/Teacher Actions:

Patient/Family Actions:

Method of Measurement:

Length of Contract:

Bonus Clause:

Signatures:

Date:

FIGURE 8-3. Sample learning contract used in patient education.

Benefits of the Learning Contract

The contract is often a *motivator for learning* for both patient and staff. Through the contract, goals and objectives become specific, achievable, and clearly defined. The contract provides a *mechanism for communication* by formalizing conversation. There is a time limitation for renegotiating the contract, which outlines the responsibilities of members of the health care team and the community resources that may be of assistance to the patient. It provides *standards for evaluation* of learning by specifying desired behaviors, conditions, and criteria and also provides opportunity for measurement of behavioral change.

❑ CASE STUDY

Mrs. Dawe's Diabetic Teaching Involves a Learning Contract

In Chapter 7 we introduced Mrs. Dawe who was struggling with her daily management of hypertension and diabetes. Mrs. Dawe identified her greatest problems as her weight and her high blood pressure. She agreed that she would like to work on these problems. She stated that her shortness of breath would decrease if she lost weight and she felt that she would be better able to follow her exercise plan. She described the low-fat, diabetic ADA diet she had been prescribed 5 years ago as "too restrictive," but agreed to an ADA diet that included one-half cup of ice cream each week. She felt that her weight increase and blood pressure problem were closely related. She also saw her shortness of breath as a problem and stated, "I would be happy if I could keep my granddaughter for the day without getting sick."

We shared our perceptions with Mrs. Dawe. They were similar to her own about her obesity, hypertension, and shortness of breath. We reinforced her knowledge of her health problems and her positive behaviors of checking her blood glucose and examining her feet regularly. We complimented her dependability in keeping her appointments and taking her medications. A diet was planned to help her lose weight and lower her blood pressure. She was in agreement with our suggestions. We would continue a discussion of her diabetes management at her clinic visit scheduled for the following week. Mr. Dawe was present during the discussion but was silent. We stressed the importance of family support in improving the overall nutrition and health exercise for both partners because the recommendations for healthy eating and well-planned exercise are important for everyone. The family's focus on healthful eating after a spouse or parent has a heart attack is critical. When all family members make changes to lower fat in their diets they show the patient that he is not alone and that they want him to stay around. That kind of support can be instrumental in helping the patient make necessary changes in the long run (Russell, 1994). Membership in the local chapter of the American Diabetes Association and a subscription to *Diabetes Forecast*, a monthly magazine for people with diabetes, were also recommended to the Dawes to help establish a "new start" to the treatment plan.

Learning goals and objectives related to her problems with obesity and hypertension were mutually negotiated. By 24-hour recall, Mrs. Dawe's current intake was estimated at about 2200 calories/day. She agreed to an appointment with the dietitian to learn about the new dietary guidelines and plan sample menus. She agreed to limit her salt and fat use in cooking.

NURSING DIAGNOSIS: Altered Nutrition: More than Body Requirements related to nonadherence to diabetic low-fat diet

Goal: Mrs. Dawe will follow a low-fat, high fiber diabetic diet by 6/1/95.
Educational Needs: With the dietitian, outline food exchanges for breakfast, lunch, and dinner using her ADA diet plan. Describe how one-half cup of ice cream is worked into the weekly meal plan.
Behavioral Objectives: Mrs. Dawe will record in notebook all foods eaten during the week. She will state why weight control is especially important in the management of diabetes. Mrs. Dawe will attend the diabetic patient luncheon at County Hospital.
Goal: Achieve systolic blood pressure below 160 mm Hg and diastolic blood pressure below 90 mm Hg by 6/1/95.
Educational Needs: Review high-sodium foods and ways to avoid them.
Behavioral Objectives: Mrs. Dawe will omit salt in cooking and name 10 high-sodium foods that should be avoided. Mrs. Dawe will eliminate canned foods from the diet during the week and substitute fresh fruits and vegetables, recording them in notebook.

Mrs. Dawe was willing to keep specific records in a notebook that she would bring to her next office visit. We wrote up and signed a contract that she kept at home (Fig. 8-4). When we returned to the office, we documented our agreement in the progress notes section of her chart and made an appointment for her with the dietitian; this had been suggested so she would have an opportunity to explore variations in her diet and receive cooking suggestions. Mrs. Dawe would return to the family practice clinic for a visit 1 week later. Prioritizing problems was not difficult because the problems were closely interrelated physiologic needs. An effort to set achievable goals increased the probability of attaining success and developing a positive self-image. Mr. Dawe was willing to help by supporting Mrs. Dawe's renewed effort to follow her diabetic diet and to limit her salt intake. He remarked, "It would help me to cut down on my salt, too, and I can use some at the table."

❑ CASE STUDY

The Riley Family Confronts Creutzfeldt-Jakob Disease

Mr. Frank Riley is hospitalized with Creutzfeldt-Jakob disease (CJD), a rare but fatal disease characterized by rapidly progressing dementia. CJD is characterized as a subacute spongiform viral encephalopathy. Transmissibility of the disease is still under study, and clustering within families has been reported. Mr. Riley, a 69-year-old retired farmer, presented with forgetfulness, depression, and difficulty sleeping. Myoclonic jerking was also noted. Manifestations of this disease are similar to those of Alzheimer's disease, but behavior changes progress more rapidly. Mr. Riley was admitted to the neurologic unit of the hospital with difficulty swallowing, about a month after the initial diagnosis of CJD. He is unsteady on his feet and progression of neurologic changes is found on his electroencephalogram.

The primary nurse caring for Mr. Riley found information in the *Journal of Neuroscience Nursing* to help her plan Mr. Riley's care (Neatherlin, 1988). She learned that death commonly occurs within 1 year of diagnosis and is usually a result of respiratory complications or infection as well as severe degeneration of the brain. CJD has no specific medical treatment and no cure. Patient education efforts are focused primarily on the family and center on home management of the patient, if discharged to his home as in Mr. Riley's case. Priorities are to maintain function and to prevent potential complications. In addition, general blood and body fluid precautions should be followed when handling excreta and secretions.

Mr. Riley's primary nurse interviewed his wife and sister about their plans for home care and the assistance they thought they would need. She then formulated nursing diagnoses, described educational needs, outlined goals, and formulated learning objectives for family education (Neatherlin, 1988).

NURSING DIAGNOSIS: Risk for Injury related to ataxia and myoclonic jerking

Goal: Prevent injury due to falls.
Educational Needs: Instruct family in safety measures for home care.
Learning Objectives: Mrs. Riley will demonstrate how to use bed side rails. Mrs. Riley will demonstrate how to restrain husband with a sheet around his waist while he is up in a chair.

NURSING DIAGNOSIS: Altered Mobility related to myoclonic jerking

Goal: Prepare family to safely respond to patient's decreased mobility.
Educational Needs: Instruct family to perform passive range of motion exercises and to use proper body mechanics for patient and self.
Learning Objectives: Mrs. Riley will correctly perform passive range of motion exercises with her husband. Mrs. Riley and Mrs. Griffith (Mrs. Riley's sister) will demonstrate proper body mechanics as they transfer Mr. Riley from chair to bed.

NURSING DIAGNOSIS: Altered Thought Processes related to disease

Goal: Orient patient continuously to day, date, time, and place. Adjust care and precautions based on observed behavior changes.
Educational Needs: Instruct family to provide consistency in environment and to use reorientation techniques with Mr. Riley.
Learning Objectives: Mrs. Riley will explain importance of orienting Mr. Riley to day, date, time, and place. Mrs. Riley will describe how to use signs and pictures in the home to aid orientation. Mrs. Riley will list behavior changes that may be expected and describe how to adjust care based on each one.

NURSING DIAGNOSIS: Risk for Aspiration related to difficulty swallowing

Goal: Prevent aspiration.
Educational Needs: Instruct family about potential for aspiration and measures to prevent aspiration.
Learning Objectives: Mrs. Riley and Mrs. Griffith will list four signs and symptoms of aspiration. They will also list three danger signs to look for while Mr. Riley is eating or drinking.

NURSING DIAGNOSIS: Fear of Family related to lack of understanding of low potential for infectivity

Goal: Decrease fear and increase comfort of family in care giving.
Educational Needs: Instruct family in effective handwashing and use of gloves to handle body fluids.
Learning Objectives: Mrs. Riley and Mrs. Griffith will discuss low risk of transmission of CJD. They will touch patient and participate in bathing and mouth care. They will demonstrate effective handwashing and proper use of gloves.

NURSING DIAGNOSIS: Anticipatory Grieving related to outcome of disease

Goal: Family will talk about their feelings related to Mr. Riley's diagnosis and prognosis and participate in discharge planning.
Educational Needs: Help family talk about feelings about CJD and how it has affected them as a family. Assist family to obtain home health or hospice consult.
Learning Objectives: Family will discuss diagnosis and prognosis of CJD. Family will explore how they will handle this family crisis and what types of assistance are needed.

Mr. Riley's primary nurse noted that Mrs. Riley stated she was most fearful of Mr. Riley "choking and falling" when she took him home. Teaching began on these diagnoses first. The nurse knew that as her relationship with the family developed, other diagnoses, including anticipatory grieving, would also emerge as priorities.

FAMILY MEDICINE CENTER

<u>Learning Contract</u>

Objectives:
To lose 6 lb during the next 2 months.
To achieve systolic blood pressure below 160 mm Hg, and diastolic blood pressure below 90 mm Hg.

Learner Actions:
Record in notebook all foods eaten each day. Follow recommendations of American Diabetes Association (ADA) diet. Limit ice cream to half-cup serving per week. Take medications daily and record in notebook. Eliminate salt in cooking and at meals. Record intake patterns in notebook. Eliminate canned foods this week. Return for clinic visit next week.

Teacher Actions:
Supply diet outline for 1200-calorie ADA low-fat diabetic diet.
Check weight and BP weekly.
Label reading models—will review with Mrs. Dawe at clinic visit 4/7/95. Instruction in reading labels on canned foods done today in the home.

Method of Measurement:
Weight
BP
Patient record in notebook

Length of Contract:
2 months

Bonus Clause:
Diabetic luncheon at County Hospital
ADA diet plan and instructions for caloric intake and meal spacing
Booklet: "Your Diabetic Diet"
Appointment with dietitian scheduled for 4/7/95

Signatures:

_____   _____

_____   _____

Date: 3/31/95

FIGURE 8-4. Learning contract with Mrs. Dawe.

❏ CASE STUDY

Mary Andrews Prepares for Diagnostic Tests

Mary Andrews is 26 years old. While on vacation in Paris 2 years ago, she experienced tingling sensations in her legs. They have recurred periodically since then. Last month she also began experiencing "double vision," while working at a computer terminal in her job as an insurance claim representative. Last week she fell down three steps when her legs "gave out." Mary's doctor has ordered diagnostic tests to rule out multiple sclerosis. The clinic nurse talked with Mary about the test schedule and found Mary frightened and nervous about the tests she was to undergo (McBride & Distefano, 1988). She stated, "I've had so many surprises. I'm frightened about what's happening with my body and about having so many tests."

The clinic nurse outlined the following guide to patient education:

NURSING DIAGNOSIS: Anxiety related to lack of knowledge about diagnostic tests and test results

Goal: Allay fear by helping patient anticipate procedure for each of tests she is having.
Educational Needs: Explain each test in detail—what will be done, what it will feel like, and what can be determined by the test.
Learning Objectives: Mary will discuss each of tests: the procedure, sensations she may experience, and the purpose of the test.

1. Myelogram
2. Cerebral spinal fluid examination
3. Magnetic resonance imaging

❏ CASE STUDY

Cindy Benjamin Must Manage Bipolar (Manic-Depressive) Illness

When 32-year-old Cindy was admitted to the acute care psychiatric unit, she exhibited classic symptoms of a manic episode. She was dancing, loud, unable to sleep, and impulsive. She resisted limits set by the staff; she responded with even more inappropriate and promiscuous behavior. The milieu was not therapeutic: other patients became more angry, and she responded with more aggression.

The patient care plan reflected the following approach to Cindy's care. The first step was to reduce the stimulation by confining Cindy to her room with hourly, supervised breaks. She was supervised to take care of basic grooming. A written contract was used to help her take responsibility for her own limits. She had to be reminded to follow the plan, but she did follow it. The plan was explained to the other patients at community meetings so they would reinforce the plan and understand that less stimulation would help Cindy focus on her behavior.

As the manic symptoms decreased, Cindy spent more time out of her room. Eventually the staff saw a mood shift to depression: less activity, loss of appetite, and neglected grooming. Then a new plan of care supported and encouraged Cindy to spend more time out of her room.

Like most patients with bipolar (manic-depressive) illness, Cindy began drug therapy to be used long term. Nursing diagnoses in her care plan included:

Aggression, Inappropriate
Manipulation
Manic Behavior
Depressive Behavior
Alteration in Thought Process
Self Care Deficit: Feeding, Hygiene
(McFarland & Wasli, 1986)

As Cindy's nursing diagnoses were resolved, the care plan was altered to place priority on:

NURSING DIAGNOSIS: Knowledge Deficit related to nature and management of manic-depressive disorder

Goal: Patient will accept her illness and take responsibility for her own treatment (including ongoing drug therapy and outpatient psychotherapy).
Educational Needs: Instruct Cindy about the nature of the illness, its course and symptoms, the treatment, and how to manage it. Include Cindy's fiance and roommate in teaching.
Learning Objectives: Cindy will state the diagnosis and describe what it is; describe symptoms of manic and depressed states and of relapse; outline the treatment plan she will follow after discharge; state reasons to contact her psychiatrist; describe the drug therapy to be used, including dose, schedule, and periodic blood levels; discuss reason to avoid alcohol; and state the importance of notifying other health care providers about the medication she takes (Brenners, Harris, & Weston, 1987).

Summary

Client goals for patient education are derived from nursing diagnoses and associated educational needs. We must also consider the common concerns or fears of the patient and pressing needs of the nurse to ensure a safe discharge. Adult learning theory emphasizes the goal directedness of adults and the importance of setting goals for patient education. Learning objectives, related to goals, were described for the three domains: cognitive (knowledge), affective (attitudes and understandings), and psychomotor (skills). It is important to identify the three or four objectives that are critical to the safety of each patient and reinforce these in each encounter with a patient. Box 8-3 in the chapter summarized the four questions a nurse can ask to determine which learning needs are critical for a safe discharge. Four case studies illustrated how nurses develop learning goals and objectives in a variety of situations.

Strategies for Critical Analysis and Reflection

1. Imagine that you are diagnosed with a rare illness that will require a lifetime of treatment. You are hospitalized after arriving in the emergency room following a fainting episode. What fears or concerns are you experiencing that may influence your readiness to learn? List your three most pressing questions.

2. You are working as a nurse on the mother-baby unit of the hospital. Six years ago, when you began work on the unit, you participated on a patient education committee that developed the postpartum teaching plan. This plan was based on a 3-day length of stay. Your average patient stay following a routine vaginal delivery is now 12 to 24 hours. How can the number of patient learning objectives be reduced? Which three or four critical objectives could serve as a basis for teaching survival skills?

3. Using the case study of Cindy Benjamin at the end of this chapter, develop a learning contract using the format in Figure 8-4.

REFERENCES

American Hospital Association. (1983). *Teaching patient relations in hospitals: The hows and whys* (pp. 88-92). Chicago: Author.

Bandura, A. (1982). Self-efficacy mechanism in human agency. *American Psychologist, 37*, 122-147.

Benner, P. (1984). *From novice to expert: Power and excellence in clinical nursing practice.* Menlo Park, CA: Addison-Wesley.

Brenners, D., Harris, B., & Weston, P. (1987). Managing manic behavior. *American Journal of Nursing, 87*(5), 620-623.

Deakins, D. (1994). Teaching elderly patients about diabetes. *American Journal of Nursing, April,* 39-42.

Erikson, E. (1950). *Childhood and society.* New York: W. W. Norton.

Gershoff, S. (Ed.). (1994). Rethinking the diabetic diet: The `rules' ease up. *Tufts University Diet and Nutrition Newsletter, 12*(6), 3-6.

Hanisch, P. (1993). Informational needs and preferred time to receive information for phase II cardiac rehabilitation patients: What CE instructors need to know. *Journal of Continuing Education in Nursing, 24*(2), 82-89.

Hochbaum, G. (1958). *Public participation in medical screening programs.* (U.S. Public Health Service Publication No. 572.) Washington, DC: U.S. Government Printing Office.

Hurxthal, K. (1988). Quick! Teach this patient about insulin. *American Journal of Nursing, 88*(8), 1097-1100.

Janz, N., & Becker, M. (1984). The health belief model: A decade later. *Health Education Quarterly, 11*(1), 1-47.

Kaluger, G., & Kaluger, M. (1979). *Human development: The span of life.* St. Louis: C. V. Mosby.

Kasl, S. (1974). The health belief model and behavior related to chronic illness. *Health Education Monographs, 2*, 433-454.

Knowles, M. (1970). *The modern practice of adult education.* New York: Association Press.

Lumley, W. (1988). Controlling hypoglycemia and hyperglycemia. *Nursing, 18*(10), 39.

Mager, R. (1975). *Preparing instructional objectives.* Belmont, CA: Fearon Publishers.

McBride, E., & Distefano, K. (1988). Explaining diagnostic tests for MS. *Nursing, 18*(2), 68-72.

McFarland, G., Gerety, E., & Wasli, E. (1992). *Nursing diagnoses and process in psychiatric mental health nursing* (2nd ed., pp. 192-193). Philadelphia: J. B. Lippincott.

Miller, A. (1985). When is the time ripe for teaching? *American Journal of Nursing, July,* 801-804.

Neatherlin, J. (1988). Creutzfeldt-Jakob disease. *Journal of Neuroscience Nursing, 20*(5), 309-313.

Northrop, C. (1986). Don't overlook discharge teaching about drugs. *Nursing, 16*(11), 43.

Polin, S., & Giedt, F. (1993). *The Joslin diabetes gourmet cookbook.* New York: Bantam Books.

Russell, B. Family matters. (1994). *Tufts University Diet and Nutrition Letter, 12*(8), 6.

Strecher, V., DeVellis, B., Becker, M. (1986). The role of self-efficacy in achieving health behavior change. *Health Education Quarterly, 13*(1), 73-92.

Implementation: Interventions for Patient Education

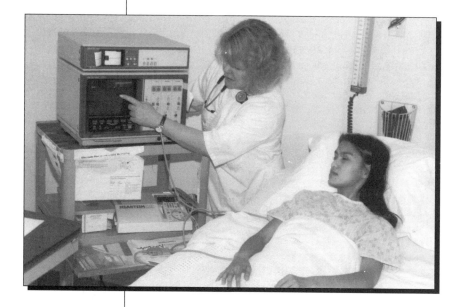

OBJECTIVES FOR CHAPTER 9

After completing this chapter, the nurse or student nurse should be able to:

1 List benefits and drawbacks for each of the following teaching formats: individual, group, and self-directed learning.

2 Discuss how a teacher can use each of the following instructional methods to achieve different types of learning objectives: lecture, discussion, demonstration, role play, tests, programmed instruction.

3 List guidelines for developing effective written patient teaching tools, such as handouts and one-page discharge instructions.

4 Describe ways to increase the effective use of patient education videos.

5 Discuss how to individualize a standard teaching plan that is part of a managed care system.

6 Describe strategies that encourage active patient involvement in patient education interventions, both for individual and group teaching programs.

Interventions for Patient Education

Individualized goals set the course for patient education interventions. Between the time goals are agreed on and the time learning activities begin, decisions must be made about content, staff, teaching methods, and teaching tools. The nurse often coordinates this planning through team planning conferences, contact with the patient's family, and a significant knowledge of hospital and community resources. A nurse may also serve as case manager, promoting patient education as an integral part of the total plan of care.

This chapter offers practical advice and frameworks for making decisions about the design and implementation of educational interventions. Characteristics of a learning environment are outlined, teaching and learning styles are discussed as they relate to program design, and the selection of instructional methods and media is explored. Emphasis is placed on making patient education realistic based on length of stay and focused on survival skills. Included are suggestions for developing and evaluating both printed patient education materials and educational videotapes. This chapter begins by discussing interventions for individual patients and includes case studies to illustrate practical applications. Chapter 10 will address how to design interventions for groups of patients and will also describe two such programs that we developed.

Scope of Teaching and Learning

Planning interventions that assist learners in achieving their goals involves making decisions about setting, content, resources, and instructors. Although learning interventions must be tailored to each patient, teaching programs planned for target populations (e.g., patients with newly diagnosed diabetes) provide guidance and standards for care. We strongly support the development of these programs within hospitals and other health care agencies, tightly linked to case manage-

ment and quality improvement systems. A patient education coordinator, hospital-based educator, clinical nurse specialist, or patient care coordinator may organize task forces composed of physicians, nurses, dietitians, pharmacists, physical therapists, and so forth, to derive teaching plans for special groups. Teaching plans should be viewed as an integral part of the design of patient care services, taking into account case management tools, quality processes, and the patient experience that crosses service or department lines. This approach tends to gain support from physicians and other health providers who will feel confident about the quality of the intervention and the preparation and knowledge of staff. Established teaching programs encourage a consistent approach among staff, facilitate a planned interdisciplinary format, and provide populations to be studied so that we may gauge the effectiveness of patient education. We encourage nurses to investigate programs that have been developed in their institutions and to become involved in promoting them. Programs often provide written and audiovisual teaching tools for the learner as well as teaching guides for health professionals, such as care maps. (Chapter 13 offers additional information about care maps.)

In institutions where teaching programs are not developed, the nurse may wish to consult with other health care agencies to see what approaches they have applied to specific populations. Information about teaching programs may also be obtained from organizations such as the American Hospital Association, the National Institutes of Health, the American Cancer Society, and the American Diabetes Association (ADA). Another valuable resource for planning patient education programs is a series of Clinical Practice Guidelines developed by the Agency for Health Care Policy and Research (AHCPR) and published by the U.S. Department of Health and Human Services. These interdisciplinary patient care guidelines address a wide variety of health care problems to assist practitioners in the prevention, diagnosis, treatment, and management of clinical conditions, with a focus on patient outcomes. For each clinical practice guideline developed under the sponsorship of AHCPR, several documents are produced to meet different needs. These guidelines contain background information, research findings, a literature review, and bibliography. A patient's guide (or parent guide for pediatric problems) is also available in English and Spanish, providing information to increase patient involvement in health care decision-making. A strong feature of the AHCPR guidelines is their recommendations for patient education. Guidelines are available on-line through the National Library of Medicine. For a listing of AHCPR guideline products, you may call the AHCPR Clearinghouse toll-free at 1-800-358-9295 or write to: AHCPR Publications Clearinghouse, P.O. Box 8547, Silver Spring, MD 20907.

Patient teaching programs must be continually evaluated to validate that patient outcomes are achieved. Program objectives and interventions for inpatient programs should be realistic based on the length of patient stay and should consider mechanisms for follow-up and continuity of care. Patient education programs can become outdated within a few months of being developed, due to dramatically changing delivery patterns for health care. For example, a new program to teach parents of pediatric bone marrow transplant patients at a large academic medical center became outdated within a few months of its creation when the care shifted from the hospital to outpatient setting. We encourage the development of programs that cross settings and providers, focusing instead on patient outcomes, and the flexibility to address patient needs wherever the patient may be. These are often called product-line models.

Determining Content

Many nurses feel confident about the content of material they should teach patients and their families. However, some nurses may be unsure of the content and survival skills that need to be taught. Consequently, essential content may be missed, incorrect information may be given, or learning activities may be inappropriate. Some nurses also tend to react to their lack of preparation by avoiding teaching situations and hoping that someone else will meet the patient's learning needs. Nursing management and staff development must ensure the quality of patient education by preparing all nurses to teach and developing patient care standards that include patient education. Resources such as handouts that support learning should be available for patients, and coaching and modeling should be available to help all nurses become capable teachers. Clinical nurse specialists can help others to become experts at determining what to teach by leading patient care conferences, evaluating video and written materials for possible use, and being available as resources for difficult teaching situations. Textbooks, reference books, drug handbooks, nursing journals, and books addressing special patient groups provide valuable pointers for determining content.

Setting Priorities

Consideration of the patient's ability and readiness to learn will help the teacher to set priorities in initiating learning activities. Priorities in the teaching plan are influenced by what the patient and the family see as important, the level of their anxiety about a particular topic or skill, the level of need (e.g., survival skills), and the time period available for implementing teaching and learning activities. When issues surrounding pain management preoccupy a patient's attention, frequently the case with cancer patients, this topic should be a priority for education (McCaffery, 1994). In general, learning should progress from familiar to unfamiliar and from simple to complex. Printed materials, intended for patient use, often lend guidance in introducing concepts and relating these concepts to self-care. Great care should be exercised to select the three or four most important learning objectives and to use these as a basis for evaluation, remembering that the three goals of patient education are to help patients gain survival skills, the ability to recognize problems, and the confidence to make appropriate decisions that benefit health status.

Selecting Instructional Methods and Instructional Media

Instructional methods encompass the format chosen for teaching (e.g., self-directed, individual, small group, large group) and the learning activities used (e.g., lecture, demonstration, discussion, role play). *Instructional media* are tools used by the teacher to help the learner to retain, compare, visualize, and reinforce learning. Often too much emphasis is placed on media, and instruction is insufficiently personalized. An excuse often offered by health professionals for lacking patient education interventions is the lack of funds to purchase videotapes, television equipment, computers, and so forth. Although the effectiveness of instructional media's contribution to learning has been emphasized in patient education literature, and expensive equipment impresses the public, media must be tailored to individual situations in planned intervention. If funds are not available for investments in software (e.g., videotapes or computer-assisted learning programs) and hardware (e.g., video monitors or computers), effective learning can still occur in inpatient and outpatient settings. One-on-one teaching using a clear list of discharge instructions can often provide patient outcomes that are missed when patients are overwhelmed with information from a variety of formats during a short length of stay.

Nurses recognize that low or absent literacy skills pose challenges to the safety and effectiveness of patient instructions (Dixon & Park, 1990). This chapter also offers tips to improve the effectiveness of written discharge instructions and patient education videos by evaluating them from the patient's perspective.

Creating a Climate for Adult Learning

Adult learners have special needs as they engage in teaching and learning activities, just as they had in the goal-setting process. When these needs are met, learning becomes satisfying and effective. If the teacher fails to acknowledge the learner's needs, barriers arise that slow down or prevent the learning of new behaviors.

A climate that promotes adult learning considers the physical and emotional needs of the learner. It uses problem-centered learning, in which the nurse relates material to the patient's life situations and addresses concerns. The learning activities include opportunities for an exchange of ideas between the teacher and learner and for applications of learning in simulated or real exercises. We discuss these needs in more detail and offer tips for fulfilling them.

Physical Comfort

Obvious barriers to learning exist when pain or anxiety interferes with the exchange of ideas or the ability to listen. Patients who are in the hospital or bedridden in the home may depend on others to assist them with bathing, elimination, dressing changes, medication, and ambulation. The thoughtful teacher will be sensitive to these needs and help the patient to be as comfortable as possible. The teacher will consider whether the patient is physically able to tolerate an hour-long teaching session, for example, or to participate in group learning. She will encourage the learner's participation by making certain he has his eyeglasses or dentures and is positioned comfortably. The teacher should be mindful of the basic human needs of all patients and recognize that they may become hungry, thirsty, restless, or uncomfortable and that they need to be recognized and treated as individuals. The nurse may capitalize on the time spent helping patients to meet their basic needs by teaching content and skills related to their care. She might teach the patient and family members about medication while administering it and then ask them to repeat the information the next time she administers it. The teacher may talk through the procedure while changing a patient's dressing and ask him to direct her the next time she changes it. She may discuss the function of insulin with the patient at the time he administers his insulin or discuss insulin reactions with him after he experiences such a reaction.

Emotional Needs

Many patients perceive a mystique surrounding the roles of doctors and nurses. Especially in times of illness or change, patients often desire to be taken care of or to find someone who will perform "magical" acts to restore a previous state of health, erase pain, or remove conflict. Too often, health care personnel have perpetuated this desire by encouraging dependence or by not taking the time to encourage patient learning and participation in medical management. Patients may be hesitant to participate at a later time, feeling incapable of learning the proper skills or of managing aspects of their own care. Later, they may worry that they will be deprived of necessary help and unable to meet their own needs.

It is important in patient education to acknowledge each patient's support needs and his anxiety about learning new health behaviors. Patients should know that they will receive necessary help and teaching until new skills are mastered and that they will be supported by medical personnel. Patients may be afraid to disclose their lack of knowledge or to make mistakes. The patient educator can confront these barriers by remaining mindful of the patient's need to be recognized as capable and as an individual. She will structure learning to proceed from simple to complex, so that the patient will feel successful, and she will make herself available for support and advice as the patient tries out newly learned behaviors. She will understand that in times of crisis or stress the patient may need greater support and may test her willingness to help him. In light of short hospital stays, patients

and families frequently feel ill-prepared for discharge. Some report that they were given "too little information, too late." On the contrary, other patients and families report that they were given "too much information, too soon," causing them to be overwhelmed, insecure, and unable to manage. The key to successful patient education is to focus on three or four critical learning objectives and teach survival skills. In addition, all patients should know how to recognize problems and how to reach help after their hospital discharge.

Two examples illustrating emotional needs in patient learning follow.

The first patient, Mr. Benton, was a 53-year-old man who had been an insulin-dependent diabetic for 6 years. He made frequent visits to the clinic with a variety of minor complaints but left the clinic much improved after each visit. He lived alone and depended on the clinic staff to support him. He called the nurses' station almost daily, occasionally stating, "I just can't seem to get going, give myself my insulin, and get to work." Through our teaching and review, we knew that he had mastered the necessary skills to do so. The clinic's social worker was called on to help Mr. Benton get involved in the local chapter of the ADA, thus increasing his support system. In addition, the clinic's nurses scheduled regular, monthly, one-half hour visits, during which they would support Mr. Benton and occasionally ask him to share his expertise in insulin injection with patients who had newly diagnosed diabetes.

The second patient, Mrs. Hester, had received prenatal care at the clinic and was looking forward to breast-feeding her baby. She had read many books on infant care and attended prenatal classes. Although the classes stressed the importance of being flexible in planning labor and delivery, Mrs. Hester was determined that she would have a natural childbirth. A breech presentation, however, necessitated cesarean section. Mrs. Hester successfully nursed her baby in the hospital and had good support and teaching from the hospital staff. Two days after discharge, Mrs. Hester called the clinic's nurse. She was crying, stating that she felt like a failure because the baby "would not take her milk." After supporting her on the telephone, the nurse suggested that Mrs. Hester come to the clinic and feed her baby in the examination room where the nurse could offer assistance. The patient happily agreed. When she arrived, the nurse realized that Mrs. Hester's anxiety and fatigue were causing her difficulty with nursing. Together they reviewed the progressive muscle relaxation exercises done in prenatal classes. Mrs. Hester then became relaxed before nursing her baby, and the baby nursed successfully. The nurse complimented Mrs. Hester on how well she was caring for the baby, weighed the baby so the patient could verify that he was gaining weight, and offered additional visits of this nature if needed. She also reminded Mrs. Hester to nap when the baby napped and drink plenty of fluids. The patient agreed to call the nurse the next day and let her know how the breast-feeding was progressing. When she did, the report was a positive one. Mrs. Hester remarked, "It was just so good to know I could call you if I needed help."

Problem-Centered Learning

Learning activities should be centered around potential problems that the patient may face. The teacher will want to assist the learner in recognizing the problem, knowing what to do, and feeling competent in performing the necessary behavior. Patients should be able to describe their diagnosis or health problem and how their symptoms relate to it. Patient education should help the patient who is experiencing an acute episode answer the following questions: "Why am I here at this time...and what could I have done to prevent it?" Patients often bring problems or concerns with them to the learning session. Breast-feeding problems are a good example. Similarly, expectant parents may express the following concerns:

How can I deal with the pain of labor?
How will I know if the baby is sick?
What do I do if the baby doesn't stop crying?

Preoperative patients also want information:

What will it be like in surgery?
What will they do to me?
Will I be in pain?
What will it be like when I wake up?

Diabetic patients and their family members also often have questions:

Why are the shots needed?
How should the shots be given?
What is an insulin reaction?

Some patients will mention their problems and concerns freely, whereas others hesitate to do so. Occasionally, patients with newly diagnosed problems do not know what to ask. It is the teacher's job to encourage the patient to verbalize concerns and then to address those concerns in learning activities. If the patient and the family need help describing concerns, teachers may begin, for example, by saying: "Patients who are pregnant often have questions about labor and delivery and want to know what to expect. I wonder if you might have concerns about that?"

Application of Learning

Learning activities are structured to provide opportunities for the application of learning. Although teaching may include lecture and discussion, it should also propose problems and give the learner a chance to react to them. Application should be as immediate as possible, and the learner should be able to receive support and ask questions when trying out new behaviors. Simulated situations in the health care setting aid in resolution of life problems. An example of this would be a mock labor and delivery used in prenatal classes.

Participative Learning

Participation must be encouraged at the onset of learning activities if the learner is expected to build confidence. Some patients are more comfortable than others in voicing concerns and attempting new skills. Others are reluctant and anxious and may need special attention to prepare them for learning activities. Participation can be gained from even the most reluctant learner with adequate support and realistic, limited learning goals.

Nurses are frequently unable to evaluate patient learning because participation has not been accomplished and they have not observed the application of learning. This problem may arise when adequate time is not allowed for teaching and learning, when learning activities are restricted to lecture and demonstration, when learning is assumed to be accomplished by media alone, when the nurse is not comfortable with the teaching role, or when the nurse does not like to teach. These problems are alleviated by careful selection of learning activities and preparation of staff members who will serve as teachers. Frequently alternating instruction with return demonstration is also an effective strategy. This allows the patient to see incremental learning, receive immediate feedback, and learn through repetition.

The Teacher-Learner Relationship

Learning is a shared experience requiring openness on the parts of both the teacher and the learner. The teacher must be willing to establish a relationship with the individual learner, to be dependable, to encourage the learner until goals are met, to be flexible enough to negotiate, and to provide support and reinforcement. She commits herself in an agreement, a *learning contract*, whether verbal or written. She is responsible for recognizing her own learning needs and is willing to admit it when she does not have an answer. She is eager to continue her own learning.

As in all therapeutic relationships, the teacher-learner relationship takes time to develop. By giving the patient an opportunity to "tell his story," the nurse and patient become acquainted. Assessment and problem identification begin. The learner begins a

testing phase, in which he considers the willingness and ability of the nurse to understand his needs, to help him, to support him, and to commit herself to mutual goals. Eventually, the teacher and learner establish a working relationship and engage in activities together. The teacher provides experiences through which the learner tries out new behaviors (Kreigh & Perko, 1979). The teacher must instill in the patient the confidence that he can learn to participate in his health care and perform survival skills. To do this, the teacher uses repetition, focuses on a limited number of priorities, and helps the patient relate teaching to everyday life. The teacher respects the patient's cultural and religious beliefs and acknowledges his right to choose.

Styles of Learners

Patients approach learning in a variety of ways determined by individual life-style, personality, and past experience. The patient educator will want to identify characteristics of the learner's style to aid in planning teaching interventions. Although one patient may read extensively about the health problem and vocalize many questions, another patient may want to know only the basic facts, saying, "Just tell me in a few sentences what is wrong with me and what I need to do." Some patients are comfortable in classroom lectures and others are not. Although one patient may be enthusiastic to return demonstrate a procedure he has been taught by the nurse, another may hesitate and ask the nurse to review the procedure several times. One patient may freely discuss his difficulty and confusion, but another may deny problems unless he knows they are observed. The patient may play the informed expert and offer the nurse a challenge while she assesses his learning needs. Still another patient may hold back what he knows, wishing to be taken care of rather than to assume responsibility in his health management. Patients also learn at different rates depending on age, intelligence, motor skills, degree of impairment, anxiety, and past experience. Each teaching and learning activity must be adapted to the style and need of the learner.

Styles of Teachers

Just as learners have characteristic styles, so too the nurses who teach them have particular teaching styles. Some are comfortable with an "expert" role in telling or showing; others encourage constant involvement from the patient in a give-and-take fashion. Some may have difficulty dealing with the patient who sees himself as an expert; others may feel comfortable allowing the patient to direct the teaching while they clarify, correct, and supplement knowledge. These same nurses may have problems working with a passive, dependent, or depressed patient.

The approach of the nurse in patient education must be flexible because she must respond to the style of the learner despite her own preferred style of teaching. For example, a nurse with high-control needs as a teacher may compete with the expert patient, in which case the learning experience will become frustrating and unproductive. A passive, dependent patient, however, will also learn little if he is only taught according to the needs he verbalizes. For these reasons, a nurse involved in teaching patients should consider her own teaching style and may require training to overcome difficulties adapting to particular learning styles. In addition, the compatibility of the teacher with the learner is an important consideration when selecting patient teaching staff.

We are familiar, for example, with a situation in which a controlling nurse was assigned to teach tracheostomy suctioning to a patient who had a radical neck dissection and glossectomy. The patient was attempting to control his environment in response to his multiple losses and refused to accept any teaching from the nurse who communicated little empathy. His discharge from the hospital was delayed until a new nurse, who understood his attempts to exert control, was assigned as his primary nurse.

Preparing Staff for Teaching

It is important to provide a planned, consistent approach in patient education, while at the same time, avoiding unnecessary repetition and confusing presentation of material. The nurse should not overload the patient and family but must include ample opportunity for review and practice. In addition, the contributions of other members of the health care team (e.g., physical therapists, dietitians, pharmacists) must be considered as part of the teaching plan. Collectively, teaching "to" the patient by all of these professionals can be overwhelming. Thus, in a short hospital stay, patient education may be more effective if carried out by one or two professionals who are responsible for the entire teaching plan.

In the midst of other patient care planning, few of us are afforded the luxury of time needed to construct such approaches. We have discovered, however, that teaching protocols may be established in cooperation with other members of the team and then adapted to patient situations. The protocols are targeted toward specific patient groups as part of case management (Lindberg, Hunter, & Kruszewski, 1994). Provider responsibilities are outlined, and staff members are trained in the use of the care map and teaching activities. This type of planned team approach saves time, alleviates confusion, and directs the selection of staff.

Responses to the following questions will also aid in selecting staff members best suited to carry out patient education interventions:

Does the staff member have ample opportunity to interact with the patient and family?

Does the staff member understand the goals, objectives, and learning style of the patient?

Does each staff member understand his role and the other providers' roles?

Does the staff member have adequate preparation and knowledge to perform patient teaching?

Who will coordinate the teaching plan?

It is important to repeat that interdisciplinary care planning does not require that every member of every discipline teach every patient. The team should plan and focus on the overall key learning needs of the patient based on the prognosis and distill this into one set of discharge instructions.

Staff development efforts should support staff involvement in patient teaching, eliminating barriers perceived by nurses such as inadequate knowledge of the content to be taught or lack of preparation to carry out teaching activities (Marchiondo & Kipp, 1987). Suggestions are offered in Chapter 2.

Instructional Methods and Instructional Media

In Chapter 8, we referred to three types of learning behaviors: *cognitive* (knowledge and information), *affective* (attitudes and values), and *psychomotor* (skills and performance). Learning in each of these three areas contributes to behavior change.

For example, in education of a patient with newly diagnosed diabetes, the following patient behaviors are desirable:

1. Cognitive
   a. Can describe what diabetes is and name three things a diabetic patient should do to manage his care
   b. Can state that insulin reactions may be caused by the following:
      The wrong amount or kind of medication
      Late or omitted meals or snacks
      Failure to follow diet plan
      Increased activity
2. Affective
   a. Can discuss why it is important for the diabetic patient, his family, his physician, and other health care professionals to work together in his medical management
   b. Can state why he should tell his friends and coworkers that he is a diabetic, explain to them the signs and symptoms of insulin reactions, and tell them how to help if reactions occur

3. Psychomotor
   a. Can make food choices to plan one breakfast, one lunch, and one dinner within guidelines of an ADA high fiber, low fat diet
   b. Can demonstrate proper technique for daily washing and checking of feet

Learning objectives must be categorized into these three areas to prepare for the selection of teaching and learning formats, methods, and media best suited to patient education needs.

Teaching and Learning Formats

Teaching and learning formats are chosen to accomplish patient education objectives. The teacher considers, for example, whether learning can be accomplished in a large group or whether it is better suited to an individual teaching situation. In many instances, a combination of formats can be used to provide learning experiences, add variety, and meet different types of objectives. We will look at three teaching and learning formats: individual teaching, group teaching, and self-directed learning.

Individual Teaching

Often called one-on-one teaching, individual instruction is ideal for continued assessment of the learner and technical skill training, such as urine testing, insulin injection, and self-catheterization. It promotes sharing of confidential information and problems, tailoring of teaching plans, and learning by persons with a low literacy level, physical impairment, cultural barriers, anxiety, or depression. Individual teaching is often used as an initial intervention, through which basic knowledge and skills are achieved and the patient's confidence in self-care is increased. Advantages of this format include an active learner role that builds motivation, an opportunity for consistent and frequent feedback, and flexibility to create an unstructured, informal atmosphere. "Teachable moments" can be capitalized on with one-on-one learning. The teacher can respond to the learner's problems and needs in a timely fashion and can help the learner to build problem-solving skills. Preoperative teaching, initial diabetic teaching, and diet teaching are often performed using the individual format. The obvious disadvantages of individual teaching are a lack of sharing with and support from other patients and their families and the high cost of staff time for instruction. However, especially in ambulatory settings, one-on-one teaching is often most productive because it is intensive, highly individualized, can occur spontaneously during every patient encounter, is culturally sensitive, and provides repetition and review.

Group Teaching

A group-teaching format may be selected for patient education. There are three distinct advantages to group learning: it is economical, it helps patients learn from one another and teach one another through their own experiences, and it fosters positive attitude development. Even though group members may have slightly different learning goals, a needs assessment can be done in patient advisory or focus groups or at the time of group teaching by asking patients what they want to learn. Teaching content can be tailored to meet learner objectives. Small groups (2–5 patients) may be able to offer some of the advantages of individual teaching. Nurses in psychiatric acute care settings find small groups an effective format for medication teaching, activities of daily living teaching, and discussion about postdischarge concerns. Medium-sized groups (6–30 patients) may be used effectively for prenatal care, pediatric care, stress reduction, safety, diabetes review, or self-help and support groups. Large groups (30 or more patients) are appropriate for lectures and videos but should be interspersed with small group experiences or discussion. A medium or large group format is generally unacceptable for skill training and reduces patient-teacher feedback. It is difficult in these groups to evaluate whether individual learning goals have been met. Patients who are physiologically or emotionally unstable are poor candidates for group teaching. The teacher of a group must be aware of the characteristics of patients who are present and must be flexible in her approach. The group format is ideal for teaching patients and their families together.

Self-help groups are gaining the recognition of professionals and patients. They offer mutual assistance to patients with common health-related learning needs. The groups are often led by patients themselves and may be sponsored by community agencies or health care organizations. Some self-help groups are begun on the grass-roots level by lay persons who recognize the need for mutual support in dealing with prevention, management, and adaptation to chronic illnesses. Some physicians are uncooperative or indifferent toward the self-help movement, demonstrating reluctance or refusal to refer patients to such groups. However, as health care costs rise and hospitals face greater barriers to providing free services, health care professionals, especially physicians and nurses, are reconsidering their attitudes toward self-help groups. They are beginning to recognize that many active self-help support groups play an important role in educating patients and their families and that they encourage appropriate use of health care services. Due to public interest and demand, most hospitals now sponsor a variety of self-help groups open to the community. We have found that nurses are generally more aware than physicians of community groups and that nurses tend to make more referrals to them.

Combining Individual and Group Formats

In health care delivery systems, the management of patient education encompasses not only individual teaching of patients but also group teaching. Institutional leadership and management of such programs has become a recent focus. Although teaching plans have continued to develop and patient education is incorporated into critical paths and care maps that guide the sequence and timing of patient progress in many agencies, these structures are not in place to support the delivery of patient education in all settings (Redman, 1993).

An increasing number of hospitals and health care agencies have developed systematic patient care maps for educating patients with specific diseases or problems. They use individual and group formats, including self-instruction, and prescribe specific approaches and teaching roles. Patients and their families are taught through use of a standard outline, including basic information components that are then tailored to the individual situation. Nursing diagnoses guide the nurse in selecting the kind of teaching needed by a particular patient. Some items may be deleted, for example, and others may be expanded on to address the patient's personal barriers to behavioral change. Such care maps generally include teaching about pathophysiology, treatments, medications, diet, diagnostic tests, procedures, recommended activity, and self-care skills. The benefit of using care maps is that hospitals can tailor patient instruction to the specific procedures relevant to the patient's experience in that institution. Patient learning outcomes are tied to each phase of the patient's course based on an estimated length of stay, thus improving efficiency and quality, and potentially decreasing inpatient days. The New England Medical Center (Etheredge, 1989) promoted some of the first programs integrating managed care and patient education, which will be described further in Chapter 13.

Staff members are trained through classes and tutoring to use the teaching formats and strategies. The roles of various providers are outlined according to subject matter and areas of expertise. Specific provider responsibilities are described with respect to the teaching and learning process. Although nurses often perform the initial assessment, many providers are involved in intervention, evaluation, and documentation of teaching and learning.

Teaching materials should be selected based on the patient's interests, abilities, and cultural background. Time required for teaching segments of the content is estimated, and resources are suggested to help patients meet the learning goals. Content, teaching strategies, and activities suitable to meet the goals are preselected and defined by a planning committee when the care map is established. A combined format of individual and group teaching may be involved as well as referral to community resources for support after discharge. Teaching aids, such as audiovisuals and printed matter, may be purchased by the health care institution to enhance patient teaching. In addition, the care map specifies what types of information should be documented in the medical record and where it will be located. Measures for evaluation of patient learning are offered.

We believe that care maps should blend the use of formats in systematic patient learning experiences. We do caution that all teaching plans must be individualized to meet patient needs and that an assessment of readiness and barriers to learning is an essential preliminary step in any patient education approach.

Learning Activities

Whether the format for teaching is individual, group, self-directed, or a combination, the principle of patient inclusion applies. At the outset, the teacher should introduce each patient to the three or four critical skills they need to learn. By providing this "big picture" or "bottom line," as some patients describe it, the patient acknowledges the need to participate actively in the process of patient education.

Learning can be enjoyable. Knowing how to use a variety of learning activities to meet educational objectives can make patient education more interesting, challenging, and effective for both the teacher and the learner. The patient educator will want to choose learning activities thoughtfully, so that they will be suitable for particular patient objectives. We offer a guide for selecting activities conducive to cognitive, affective, and psychomotor changes (Box 9-1). Notice that

BOX 9–1. Selecting Learning Activities for Patient Education

I. Cognitive (Knowledge)

A. Learning facts
Lecture
Demonstration
Independent study format
Tests
Discussion—questions and answers
Practice
Simulation

B. Visual identification
Demonstration
Simulation
Tests
Practice
Independent study

C. Understanding and applying knowledge
Demonstration
Practice
Role play

Discussion—questions and answers
Independent study
Simulation
Tests

II. Affective (Attitudes and Appreciations)

Discussion—questions and answers
Role Play
Simulation

III. Psychomotor (Skills and Performance)

Practice
Role Play
Simulation
Demonstration
Tests
Independent study

some learning activities are appropriate for more than one type of learning objective. Brief descriptions of the major types of learning activities are offered with suggestions for effective and appropriate application.

Self-Directed Learning

Computer-assisted instruction (CAI) and self-directed learning workbooks are often the first methods of self-paced patient learning that come to mind. CD ROM and videodisk formats have also become popular resources for patient learning. A growing trend in health care settings is the creation of patient and family education resource centers, small libraries containing books, videotapes, and pamphlets that discuss health and illness topics. For example, the Cancer Resource Center located at the University of North Carolina Hospitals serves about 100 patients and families each month with answers to questions about cancer, information about support groups, and tips on coping with cancer treatment. Professionals

who staff the center report that when patients are first diagnosed with cancer, they usually have numerous questions about the illness, treatment, and prognosis. They are concerned about their insurance, how they will be affected by surgery or treatment, and how to talk to their children about the disease. But most important, they are concerned that as their questions continue to arise, they will have somewhere to turn for answers. This center offers much more than facts. It offers assistance based on the patient's expressed needs and information about support groups in which experienced facilitators can help patients learn about treatment options, nutrition, coping with cancer, survivorship, and insurance. It even offers a program that pairs newly diagnosed patients with other patients who have the same diagnosis. Such resource centers are responsive when patients are ready to learn and bridge the gaps often experienced by patients as they receive care in multiple settings from multiple providers. Resource centers are viewed as especially valuable by patients and families who are coping with chronic health problems.

Lecture

Lecture is the method most often used by nurses instructing or transmitting information to patients. It is an effective method of teaching cognitive behaviors and is more efficacious when used with discussion. Lecture is enhanced by use of handouts, pictures, and visual aids (such as overheads and slides) that promote identification. Material presented in a lecture should be prepared according to the learners' level of understanding, and learners should have an opportunity to ask questions. Lengthy lectures may cause loss of attention; patients become bored, distracted, or anxious about the material presented. Learners may be eager to contribute or to try out or apply knowledge; this eagerness may be stifled by a formal lecture approach in which the teacher is the expert. Long lectures may also create the impression that the patient's problem is so complicated that he will be unable to manage it. It is important to remember that lectures can be highly effective for influencing cognitive behaviors but will not be effective in achieving affective or psychomotor learning objectives. For example, a lecture is often used to give initial knowledge about pathophysiology to diabetic patients but is ineffective when used alone to teach insulin injection. Lectures may be given in person, televised, or audiotaped. In individual teaching, the amount of total teaching time should include a minimum of lecture and should focus on building survival skills needed to ensure patient safety after discharge.

Group Discussion

Discussion requires two or more people to exchange ideas. It differs from lecture in that it is an excellent method of actively involving patients in the learning process. This learning activity promotes understanding and application of knowledge (cognitive behaviors) as well as developing certain attitudes (affective behaviors). It is frequently directed by the teacher, who asks specific questions or proposes problem situations. Discussion facilitates learning from the experience of others, fosters a feeling of belongingness, and reinforces previous learning.

Demonstration

Demonstration is useful for cognitive and psychomotor learning. It is most often used to teach skills and to present standards for performance. Demonstration may be done in person or in videotaped programs. The sense of sight is used in learning from demonstration, but hearing, smell, and taste may also be stimulated. Demonstration should be performed slowly, and the teacher should be certain that the learner can see and hear well. This strategy shows the learner that the behavior is possible and increases his confidence that he will be able to perform it. For example, when teaching insulin injection, the nurse may demonstrate injection on herself or on a model using sterile water before the patient actually performs an insulin injection. When demonstration is used to teach discharge skills, the actual type of equipment or supplies to be used at home should be used for teaching. Repetition and return demonstration are needed for teaching procedures with multiple steps.

Role Play and Return Demonstration

Both role play and return demonstration involve doing or practicing. They help the learner to apply knowledge or skills, usually after demonstration. When used appropriately, role play and return demonstration tailor the learning to the patient's past or present life experiences while the teacher is there to offer guidance and feedback.

In role play, the learner acts out his own situation or that of another person. This is highly effective in meeting affective objectives. Return demonstration follows exhibition of a skill by the teacher; the patient performs the skill one or more times. In both cases, clear instruction must be given to the learner about what to do and how to do it. Enough practice time should be allowed for the learner to repeat the exercise until he has mastered it. Role play and return demonstration are effective strategies for teaching cognitive, affective, and psychomotor behaviors. Role playing helps patients learn to recognize and handle problem situations, such as a hypoglycemic reaction or cardiac arrest, with which they have no first-hand experience. Also, for patients who experience complications or readmission, return demonstration can be used as a way to assess skill deficits that may contribute to exacerbations of a chronic condition. For example, nurses in one rural community hospital assessed through return demonstration that there was a high readmission rate for patients with chronic obstructive pulmonary disease (COPD) who were previously discharged with metered-dose inhalers. Even though the patients had been taught during hospitalization, the return demonstration identified improper technique using inhalers as preventing patients from getting the prescribed doses of medication at home. Then priority in patient teaching was placed on practice and coaching to develop proper technique for using inhalers.

Tests

Tests may be valuable learning experiences because they relate where the learner is and where he wants to be to the progress that he has made toward meeting his goal. Tests are helpful when used to guide patients and give feedback. They are effective in meeting cognitive and psychomotor objectives but are obviously inappropriate for affective learning because attitudes and values are not measured with a "right-versus-wrong" approach.

Patients may become anxious about testing because of past school experiences. The nurse should introduce tests positively in patient education and should use the results to reinforce progress toward the learning goal. Tests may use a written, oral, or skill format. They may be used in assessment to determine the patient's initial level of understanding or skill and in evaluation after the lecture or demonstration.

Programmed Instruction

Patients can learn by independent study or by using specially prepared workbooks, textbooks, audiotape, and computer programs. Many commercially prepared programs are available; however, teachers may choose to prepare their own. Programmed self-study units allow learners to work at their own pace for mastering cognitive and psychomotor behaviors. Frequent testing and review are offered during instruction. Knowledge about chronic illness and management, preventive health topics, and diet teaching are commonly offered in programmed instruction packets. The teacher should be aware of the level of motivation or readiness of the learners, their literacy levels, and visual and hearing abilities because these factors are crucial in evaluating the appropriateness of such programs for individual clients. When programmed instruction is used, it must be suited to patient needs and situations. The nurse should set the stage by introducing the three or four critical things the patient needs to learn, and then follow up teaching with review to ensure that the patient has achieved those outcomes. Patient readiness, physical ability, intellectual and language ability, and patient interest should be considered before programmed instruction is selected for discharge teaching.

Media

Media are usually used to enhance the previously mentioned learning activities. Media should not be used in place of the teacher but can effectively promote all three types of learning when used in combination with other strategies. A health care professional should be available to discuss, demonstrate, and clarify concepts introduced by media. This role should not be neglected or left to lay volunteers. Media should be carefully selected and should be consistent with instructional objectives.

Media Uses in Teaching and Learning

Having cautioned our readers that media should not be used carelessly in patient education, a question that may arise is, "What then is the advantage in using media?"

Media help to deliver a message. A variety of media can be creatively used to help patients learn more, to help them retain better what they have learned, and to encourage the development of skills (Brown, Lewis, & Harcleroad, 1973). Nurses seldom have formal training in media selection and application, and they consequently look for guidance in these areas. We attempt to provide an overview of the types of media suited to patient education. We begin by offering guidelines for media use so that nurses may avoid some of the common pitfalls of inappropriate or unsuccessful use of media.

The teacher must follow three steps when using media in instruction: preparation, presentation, and review. To *prepare*, it is necessary to preview the material to be used. A plan for using a medium is constructed including how it will be introduced, followed up, and related to other learning experiences. The environment also needs to be prepared. This includes obtaining physical facilities and equipment needed to display the medium. The learner must be informed of what to expect from the medium, (i.e., significant points or upcoming discussion). *Presentation* of media requires care so that projection and materials are clear, sound is adjusted, and, in general, the message can be received. *Review* involves follow-up of the learning experience and evaluation of whether learning objectives were met. Several generalized principles can be applied to all types of media.

1. No one medium is best suited to all purposes. For example, in some instances visual identification is best accomplished with a picture, cartoon, or slide, but in others three-dimensional images, such as films or videotapes, are most effective.
2. The application of media should be consistent with learning objectives. Just as learning activities promote certain types of behaviors, media are also chosen to coincide with objectives.
3. The teacher must be familiar with the content of the media. A common mistake made by nurses is to use materials unknowingly that are inappropriate in message, presentation, or educational level. Media must be previewed and evaluated.
4. Media must be compatible with learning formats. To illustrate this point, videotapes may be used in a large group (provided that they can be projected adequately) but audiocassettes should not.
5. Media must be selected with the capabilities and learning styles of the audience in mind. Printed booklets with few illustrations are poorly suited to the patient who is unable to read or who dislikes reading, and the message will fail to reach him.
6. Physical conditions influence the effectiveness of media. Improper acoustics, lighting, or seating, distractions, and room temperature may all interfere with the delivery of the message.

Posters, Displays, Flipcharts, and Bulletin Boards

Visual displays using drawings and illustrations do not have to be works of art to deliver a message. They do need to be aesthetically appealing, using contrasting colors and large lettering. There are many advantages to choosing posters, displays, flipcharts, and bulletin boards. They are inexpensive, require little time to prepare, and attract interest. They clarify information, simplify concepts, and summarize teaching. Contributions from participants can be written on flipcharts or chalkboards during a teaching session. Bulletin boards in waiting rooms or hospital corridors can spark curiosity about health care issues and problems.

Use of these types of media is inappropriate in large groups unless the displays are enlarged. They are not well suited to teaching in which movement needs to be demonstrated.

Graphics

Graphics include graphs, charts, diagrams, cartoons, and maps. They can be used to show proportions and relationships that are difficult to understand when presented only by spoken or written material. They emphasize the most important points of a presentation. Drawings and cartoons can deliver a message to patients with limited reading and vocabulary levels as well as to children. For example, picture pages are often used to teach insulin injection techniques to newly diagnosed diabetic patients. Cartoons can make learning fun and present thoughts in a humorous but effective fashion. Graphics highlight sequence and also convey general information and key concepts. Some of the main advantages of using graphics for patient education are their abilities to attract attention and to deliver information economically. The graphics may be prepared by the patients themselves or by patient educators, or they may be produced commercially.

Overhead Projection

Overhead transparencies are popular for use in teaching both large and small groups. They require an overhead projector and a screen or white wall. Overheads encourage verbal and visual creativity and allow the teacher to control the materials shown and their timing. They can present ideas in a colorful sequence and help the learner to focus on thoughts and ideas. The instructor can add interest by writing or underlining on the transparencies during the presentation. Overhead transparencies are easy to make and can be prepared ahead of time in a copy machine or thermofax. Each overhead should present one idea or topic and have a limited word count. Overhead projectors are relatively light in weight and can be easily transported. Overheads can be used in a well-lighted room as long as there is dimmed light near the screen; this makes overheads more desirable than slides for keeping learners awake and attentive. When preparing or purchasing commercial transparencies, the teacher will want to consider whether the message comes across clearly and encourages learner participation. Two cautions are offered when using overheads. First, print should be large and details kept to a minimum. Second,

the teacher must be careful not to use overhead transparencies as a temptation to present too much material. A few overheads used to bring out the main points and provide review of what patients need to remember will be most helpful.

Photographs and Drawings

Patients enjoy pictures and learn from them. Visual images promote understanding of facts and ideas by helping the learner to imagine real situations and reflect on past experiences. Still pictures may be presented in printed matter, on slides, or on videos. They may encourage discussion when the learner is asked to describe what he sees.

Pictures can attract and maintain the patient's interest. They also help the patient to remember what has been said. Generally, color pictures appeal to learners more than do black and white pictures. The color should be accurate and portray a realistic image. Images should be relevant to the learners, reflecting a familiar environment, similar age of patients, a variety of gender and cultural backgrounds, and familiar geographic locations.

Slides can be prepared rather easily and portray situations related to actual patient experiences. They may be commercially prepared as well. They require only a projector and screen and can be easily transported.

Slide-tape programs include a tape recording to accompany the images. The recorded message explains the picture, and magnetically imposed sounds direct the synchronized program of still pictures and speech. An inexpensive cassette tape player or a slide projector are used to deliver this medium. Slide-tape programs may be ideal for self-instruction as well as for group teaching. They are produced commercially or by the teacher and are well suited to teaching illiterate patients if the text is concise, simple, and clear with vocabulary restricted to one- and two-syllable words.

Audio Materials

Audiotapes, usually cassette tapes, offer a distinct advantage for some patient teaching occasions. They are small and easy to transport, and they require only an inexpensive recorder for use. They are available on a variety of topics, are economical, and can be used almost anywhere. Audiotapes can be made by the teacher and tailored to the individual situation to reinforce facts, directions, and support. Patients may use them in the home, car, or office as well as in the hospital or clinic. Study kits with printed text or pictures are available to accompany the audio component.

Audio materials are helpful in delivering a message to patients who enjoy radio and who benefit from repetition and reinforcement. Relaxation and stress reduction exercises are also well suited to delivery by audiotape. For patients suffering from retinopathies secondary to diabetes, audiocassettes may be the only practical media.

Videotapes

Television's popularity and pervasive use among American households promotes learning in many spheres and influences knowledge, attitudes, and skills. It is entertaining as well as educational. Videotapes present experiences, places, and situations that can recreate life situations, thus encouraging patients to explore attitudes and understandings. Videotaped programs also teach basic facts and how to handle problems. They may be effective for patients with limited reading abilities.

The use of television and videotaped recordings has become an attractive teaching and learning activity in the school, office, and health care setting. Many groups have made significant investments for the purchase of programs (software) and equipment (hardware). Videocassette recorders (VCRs) are now widely used in all types of health care settings as well as in patients' homes. It is important to consider how suitable this medium is for specific learning objectives and to understand how television is best incorporated into patient education.

Television is best used when the program is carefully selected (see Appendix B), introduced, and followed up as part of patient teaching. It should not be expected to replace the teacher. Hospitals with cable distribution systems may wish to concentrate on video programs because they can be broadcast throughout the hospital and reach more people. Videotapes may be purchased commercially or prepared by audiovisual departments and teachers.

Videotapes are often a good basis for discussion. They must, however, be carefully previewed and selected. The teacher will want to evaluate the film with consideration of the patient group's actual life situations, levels of understanding and literacy, and learning needs. Films 15 to 20 minutes in length are ideal for most situations; those longer than 30 minutes are difficult for many patients to sit through. Discussion time should be planned and the presentation reinforced. The videotape should be well suited to learning objectives, and key points should be covered. The teacher may wish to use a handout highlighting these key points so the patient can follow these points as the videotape progresses.

It is critical to remember that skills must be taught with active learner involvement in return demonstrations. A videotape cannot provide this. Because we are concentrating patient teaching efforts on survival skills, videotapes must be carefully balanced with other formats to avoid overloading the patient with too much information. Making and duplicating your own videos has become a frequently used strategy to combat the pressures of early discharge by supplementing teaching in the patient's home. Sending a video home with the patient may be one of the best applications for this medium because it can continue coaching, provide for continued affective learning, and prevent feelings of isolation. Many situations that patients are instructed to handle may not be experienced until the patient goes home. For example, baby care and feeding are often learned best after discharge with the help of a video, provided the patient has a VCR and an interest in using it. Many hospitals are also using videotapes for preadmission teaching and preoperative teaching. For example, Saint Mary's Regional Medical Center in Reno, Nevada, developed a series of videotapes for home care, including the titles "After Your Mastectomy," "Ostomy Care at Home," "Realities of Chemotherapy," "Birth Day Preparation," and "Your Role in Surgery." Each video includes self-care instructions by health professionals and realistic accounts by individual patients with the same diagnosis. They demonstrate self-care, outline warning signs that necessitate physician contact, and answer patients' most common questions. Patients can review a demonstration of self-care procedures as often as needed, along with family members. Saint Mary's Hospital advertises the following outcomes achieved through the use of patient education videos: increased patient satisfaction; increased physician satisfaction; assistance with meeting the requirements of the Joint Commission on the Accreditation of Healthcare Organizations; reduced risk of malpractice, negligent discharge, and inappropriate readmissions; and enhanced community image and cost savings.

Electronic Media

Computer-assisted instruction is now common in hospitals, physicians' offices, and homes. Many software programs are available to help patients learn how to adopt healthier life-styles and manage health problems. There are six types of CAI: drill and practice, tutorials, problem-solving, simulation, gaming, and testing. CAI is frequently accompanied by printed materials, such as workbooks, and visuals, such as slides or videotapes.

Drill and practice lessons help patients learn or review facts and offer question-and-answer formats to assess understanding. Tutorials use branching options to individualize lessons to the knowledge and needs of the patient. Problem-solving, simulations, and gaming help patients gather information and make decisions in hypothetical situations. Testing can be done with CAI as part of tutorials, simulations, and practice to assess knowledge and attitudes, and feedback can also be provided (Thomas, 1988).

Software for CAI programs can be developed by a skilled designer, but it is also readily available commercially. It should be compatible with hardware and evaluated based on each programs' instructional objectives and how well the objectives can be met by the CAI lesson (Bolwell, 1988). An index to CAI software is offered by the text, *Nursing Informatics: Where Caring and Technology Meet* (Ball, Hannah, Jelger & Peterson, 1994). Christine Bolwell, editor of a newsletter and author of a directory of educational software, provides information about the many programs and vendors of CAI for patient and nursing education in one of the text's many valuable chapters.

Another valuable resource for information about electronic media for patient education is Scott Stewart, who has complied and updates a directory of such programs, including CAI, videodisk, and CD-ROM applications (Box 9-2).

Just as with other media, electronic media lessons should be previewed and evaluated, giving consideration to patient needs, the patient's actual life situations, level of understanding, and literacy. Key points should be reviewed by the nurse. Patients vary in comfort and experience with computers, and some may be anxious about or disinterested in CAI. Other patients, especially teenagers and young adults, may be reached effectively with CAI lessons on such topics as pregnancy prevention, birth control, drug abuse prevention, and wellness.

BOX 9–2. Primary Contacts for Patient Education and Electronic Media

Christine Bolwell, RN, MSN
Diskovery: Computer-Assisted Healthcare
  Education
1620 Saratoga Avenue, Suite 214
San Jose, CA 95129
(408) 741-0156

Scott Stewart
Stewart Publishing, Inc.
6471 Merritt Court
Alexandria, VA 22312
(703) 354-8155

In the next decade, experts expect computers will be used much more creatively for patient education. Computer programs can already help diabetic patients adjust insulin dosages and plan meals, track data about glucose levels, offer self-paced instruction about knowledge of diabetes, and offer nutritional analysis of foods. It is predicted that home computers and video will provide increasing opportunities in the near future for providers to observe and instruct patients at home and to link home and provider information systems (Redman, 1993).

Objects, Models, and Demonstrations

Having actual objects available during patient teaching helps the learner to become actively involved and to apply knowledge and skills immediately. The patient may observe, handle, manipulate, display, discuss, assemble, and disassemble objects while the teacher provides feedback. For example, breast models are often used to teach patients to examine their breasts, and pelvic models are used to show patients how to insert a diaphragm. The teacher usually demonstrates the use of the objects or models, and the patient repeats the performance. Some models, such as the Resusci-Annie used to teach cardiopulmonary resuscitation (CPR), are expensive. Others, such as the plastic female pelvic area, may be supplied free of charge by pharmaceutical companies. Through creative experimentation, many nurses find that they can make their own models for teaching a variety of skills. One nurse who was unable to purchase an expensive breast model made her own from a nylon stocking stuffed with cotton socks. She simulated a breast mass in another stocking by adding Styrofoam particles and used the two "breasts" to teach breast self-examination.

Displays can be used to encourage patient participation. For example, teaching about infant safety becomes more effective when it is accompanied by a display of actual infant car seats. In one-on-one encounters, demonstration and return demonstration can often be performed by the patient without the use of models. Examples of this are blood glucose monitoring, breast examinations performed in the privacy of the patient's room, dressing changes, and baby bathing. Furthermore, these teaching and learning opportunities can occur even if funding for teaching aids is lacking.

Community Resources

Health departments, health agencies, businesses, and professional groups such as fire and police departments offer learning experiences for patients. Valuable support and information can be gained through such resources as diabetic groups, ostomy clubs, hospital health nights, bicycle safety programs, and community infant car seat programs. The patient educator can benefit from knowledge of and referrals to teaching programs that offer skills training. In one outpatient clinic we saw many patients and their families in the rehabilitation phase after myocardial infarction. We wanted to give family members CPR training but were unable to do so because we did not have enough staff to offer the teaching or the finances to purchase equipment. Many of the family members were unable to pay registration fees for CPR classes at local schools. We discovered that a local fire department offered CPR classes free of charge, and we referred our patients to them.

Games and Simulations

Games can be used to involve the patient in teaching and learning. Instructional games can introduce information and offer practice in simulated situations. One of the advantages of using games as learning experiences is that actual situations can be viewed in a condensed time span. During a game, the patient can take a course of action and look at the consequences in a nonthreatening way. Problem- solving can be incorporated into the game. Commercially prepared games should be evaluated for use with individual patients. The patient should be able to succeed, yet be challenged, in the exercise. Games may use flash cards, pictures, or computer programs. They may be modifications of popular games such as Bingo or crossword puzzles. With the exception of computer games, most games are relatively inexpensive to purchase or make. Simulations include planning lowfat meals, using food models, and shopping for low-sodium foods in a mock supermarket.

Printed Materials

Pamphlets and information sheets are among the most common teaching tools. Printed materials can help to explain common health problems and their management and make the public more aware of health risks and prevention. Some printed materials are ideal teaching tools because they have large print, use language appropriate for the patient audience, emphasize important points, and reinforce learning. Distributing written information seems, at first glance, to be a quick and easy way to teach without requiring the health professionals' time in talking with patients. This is a misconception held by many physicians and nurses. Handing out written materials does not ensure a transfer of knowledge. Many patients are anxious about the information contained in the literature or are unable to understand it. Even when printed matter is evaluated and used appropriately, taking into account interest and reading level, the message may not be received. Many well-educated patients do not enjoy reading or retain what they read.

Printed patient education materials may be used effectively to enhance participative learning. An individualized teaching plan, designed to use patient assessment data, will guide educators in the appropriate use of books, pamphlets, and information sheets. Specific suggestions for evaluating printed patient education materials are offered in Appendix A. We have found printed materials especially helpful in contraceptive counseling. After receiving basic teaching in the office, patients may take a booklet home to consider the various methods of contraception. Patients then frequently return for the next visit prepared to ask questions and willing to take responsibility for choosing a method. Although many patients initially come to an office visit with a particular method in mind, we have discovered through assessment that the decision has usually been based on the experience or on the advice of friends. A combined approach of one-on-one counseling and written patient education materials promotes enlightened choices.

The use of written materials requires assessment of the readability of each booklet, pamphlet, or handout. The teacher must be certain that the wording and sentence complexity are compatible with the patient's level of understanding. Many formulas can be used to predict readability or the grade level at which patient education materials are written. One of the most popular formulas is the SMOG formula (National Cancer Institute, 1981), as shown in Box 9-3. This formula requires time to count words, sentences, and syllables and to do simple computations. Word processing software for the computer, such as Wordperfect 6.0, also tests reading levels of text. Another method we have used when time has been limited involves having the patient read aloud the first paragraph in the booklet and then tell us, in his own words, what it means. In this manner, we learn whether eyesight and ability to read are adequate and whether the content is understood. We have discovered that patients frequently display less comprehension than would be expected from their highest grade of school completed.

The One-Page Instruction Sheet

Patients should *always* be given written discharge instructions to outline medications, treatments, follow-up appointments, and emergency guidelines.

Many nurses find it helpful to organize instructions chronologically. For example, a handout outlines what to do before breakfast, before leaving for work, at lunch, before bed, and so forth. Often instructions are given to both the patient and another family member. They are always reviewed with the patient before discharge. It is common hospital policy to have the patient or family member sign at

BOX 9–3. SMOG Readability Formula

1. Count off 10 consecutive sentences near the beginning, in the middle, and near the end of the text. If the text has fewer than 30 sentences, use as many as are provided.

2. Count the number of words containing 3 or more syllables (polysyllabic) including repetitions of the same words.

   a. Hyphenated words are considered as one word.

   b. Numbers that are written out should be counted. If written in numerical form, they should be pronounced to determine if they are polysyllabic.

   c. Proper nouns, if polysyllabic, should be counted.

   d. Abbreviations should be read as though unabbreviated to determine if they are polysyllabic. However, abbreviations should be avoided unless commonly known.

3. Look up the approximate grade level on the SMOG Conversion Table below:

Total Polysyllabic Word Count	Approx. Grade Level (+1.5 Grades)
0-2	4
3-6	5
7-12	6
13-20	7
21-30	8
31-42	9
43-55	10
56-72	11
73-90	12
91-110	13
111-132	14
133-156	15
157-182	16
183-210	17
211-240	18

Adapted from McLaughlin, G. (1969). SMOG grading: A new readability formula. *Journal of Reading, 12*, (8), 639–646.

the bottom of the instruction sheet, indicating that they received the information. A duplicate copy is placed in the patient record.

With the widespread use of computerization, nurses are finding it helpful to prepare basic instructions for patients with a particular diagnosis-related group (DRG) or nursing diagnosis. These standard instructions can be tailored for each patient and printed out on the nursing unit. We caution that *only* information pertinent to the patient should be given, and instruction lists should be only as long as necessary. The suggestions in Box 9-4 are offered for evaluating your individualized handouts.

Brief patient emergency instructions can be printed on refrigerator magnets along with a telephone number. Also patients should be encouraged to post their one-page instructions at one or all of the following locations: on the refrigerator, by the telephone, and at the workplace. Instructions are ineffective if the patient cannot find them or has difficulty remembering the self-care regimen when he is away from home.

Patients benefit from instructions that use short, nontechnical words of two syllables or less, give simple definitions, and are written in the active voice. Tell readers only what they need to know and do.

BOX 9–4. Patient Instruction Evaluation Checklist

- Are sentences and item length as short as possible?
- Is unfamiliar jargon avoided?
- Are instructions limited to "must-know" facts?
- Is information organized in a logical way?
- Is a shopping list provided for equipment and medications?
- Do patient and family know how to identify problems, what to look for?
- Do patient and family know what to do if problems arise?
- Who is to be called if problems occur?
- Is emergency plan included?

Special Challenges: Patients With Low Literacy Skills

Nurses must consider that nearly 20% of Americans (one of every five) lack the necessary literacy skills to benefit from even our simplest handouts or videotaped programs. They are functionally illiterate. When they enter our agencies as patients, we have difficulty reaching them in patient education encounters. Despite our attempts to simplify our written materials from the typical ninth or tenth grade (or greater!) reading level to an improved sixth grade level, the patient with low literacy skills is still lost.

The special challenge of patient education with these adults is presented comprehensively in the book by Doak and colleagues (Doak, Doak, & Root, 1994). This text is a must for all nurses. It helps us understand such patients, how to test their comprehension, and how to test their ability to read current materials; it teaches us how to write and rewrite materials and how to use audio and visual aids. Another valuable resource is a free publication from the U.S. Department of Agriculture entitled *Guidelines: Writing for Adults With Limited Reading Skills* (U.S. Department of Agriculture, 1988). The authors tell us that videotapes are not a quick answer for these patients. Illiteracy is not just the inability to read. Illiterate adults and those with low literacy skills process information differently than do readers. They may have limited vocabulary, may not understand abbreviations, and usually do not ask questions. Yet they may have average IQs and speak articulately. Identifying many of these individuals can be difficult because they have learned to cope in varying degrees and can hide their limitations from others.

A patient with limited reading skills often has a short attention span, thus the message should be short, direct, and specific. He may depend on visual cues to clarify or interpret words; therefore pictures, illustrations, and graphics must work in conjunction with words. A patient with low literacy skills also has difficulty understanding complex ideas. Information should be broken down into basic points with examples that apply the material to real-life situations he is likely to encounter.

For teaching patients with low literacy skills, guidelines are offered to help us adapt our existing methods and materials for these adults (Box 9-5).

Many of the tips for working with patients with low literacy skills should be used with *all* patients but are often overlooked. For example, what is critical when the patient is given a medication prescription? Should he know how to spell the name of the medication? Or is it more important that he knows what the medication is for, what it looks like, when to take it, and possible side effects? To keep the messages in our instructions as simple as possible, we must ask:

- What should the patient be able to do?
- What should the patient change or do differently?
- What one or two points are most critical for the patient to understand?

We may consider it critical that an elderly patient take his diuretic medication at the beginning of the day to avoid sleep disturbance from increased urination. The patient should weigh himself daily and record weight. He should report any dizziness, falls, rapid weight loss or gain, swelling in ankles or fingers, bleeding, bruising, or muscle cramping.

The nurse uses simple messages, familiar words, and pictures. She organizes text in

---

BOX 9–5. Guidelines for Teaching Patients With Low Literacy Skills

- Focus information on the core of knowledge and skills patients need to survive and to cope with problems.
- Teach the smallest amount possible.
- Make points vivid. Put important information either first or last.
- Sequence information logically, for example, step-by-step (1, 2, 3...), chronological (a time line), or topical (using 3 or 4 main topics).
- Have the patient restate and demonstrate.
- Review.

small sections with headings: Your Fluid Pill, Every Morning..., and Call the Doctor If....

Other suggestions for developing useful instructions include:

- First list what the patient should do; limit the number of don'ts.
- Avoid mixing the sequence of do's and don'ts because this may confuse patients.
- When giving instructions for medications, list the exact times the medication should be taken. Avoid language such as "take three times a day."
- For PRN medication, list each one separately with the instruction "take for _____," being specific about which symptom. Also, mention how often it can be taken, how long between doses, and how may times in 24 hours it can be taken. What should the patient do if the symptom is not relieved?
- List any symptoms for which the doctor should be notified immediately.

Table 9-1 shows a sample medication instruction sheet.

A safety hint that can be applied to all patients is to give a complete list of all medications to be taken after discharge. Patients may have old prescriptions at home or PRN medications that should not be part of the current treatment plan. This discharge list helps to reinforce the medication plan.

Testing the readability of patient education materials before patient use continues to be an important and simple step. It is also important to have patient education materials reviewed by actual patients, followed by an assessment of their comprehension of the material and suggestions for making the content more "patient friendly." Most nurses believe that every patient who is given printed matter should be asked to read a portion aloud and explain to the nurse what it means in his own words. They believe that this is the final and most critical test for readability.

Making written patient education materials more readable and effective is only a partial solution. Many patients cannot or will not read written material at all. This includes not only patients who are functionally illiterate, but those with physical handicaps or language barriers. For these patients, individual teaching, demonstration, coaching, involvement of family and significant others in the community, as

TABLE 9–1. Medication Instructions

Use	Rather Than
Take once daily	Take daily
Take at about 8 AM and 8 PM	Take twice daily
	Take every 12 h
Take at about 8 AM, 2 PM, and 10 PM	Take 3 times daily
	Take every 8 h
Take at about 8 AM, 1 PM, 6 PM, and 10 PM	Take 4 times daily
	Take every 6 h
Take 30 min before meals on an empty stomach	Take before meals
Take during meals 3 times a day	Take with meals
Take every _____ h as needed for (symptom)	Take as needed for (symptom)
Do not exceed _____ in a 24-h period	
DO NOT USE	
Take for (symptom)	
Take as directed	

well as novel approaches with "wordless" patient education materials can improve comprehension of instructions and patient safety (Feldman, Quinlivan, Williford, Bahnson, & Fleischer,1994). Pictorial care maps designed for patients are also described in Chapter 13.

Designing a Patient Education Program

This section is designed to answer questions about choosing from among the possible options in teaching formats, learning activities, and media. Nurses involved in patient education are asked to make these choices every day, whether they are answering to individual patient and family situations or designing larger, agency-wide programs.

Many variables influence the design of a patient education program. Among these are the numbers and types of staff, monetary resources, types and needs of patients, type of health care setting, proximity to instructional design and audiovisual experts, and the availability of hardware and software suitable for use in patient teaching. Thus, there is no one prescription we can offer for designing interventions (patient education programs) that is practical for every situation. Instead, we look at the questions asked by nurses as they select instructional formats, learning activities, and media, and we offer suggested courses of action.

Selecting an Instructional Format

Group teaching seems to be a good way to provide economical patient education, yet doctors and patients often tell us they prefer individual teaching. How can we encourage clients and physicians to accept the value of group teaching?

All patients should be provided with some individual teaching to help them understand and accept their diagnosis and understand their own role in the management of their health. Every patient in every setting should know why he is there, what he can contribute to managing his health, and what he can expect to learn from health care providers that will enable him to do this. Provided that an assessment of the patient and family learning needs is made, group teaching can then be as effective as continued individual teaching for cognitive and affective learning. Skills are best taught in small groups (2–4 patients) or in one-on-one formats. Important considerations in offering group classes include whether transportation and time are convenient and whether patients and their families are physically able to attend. Physicians may be more supportive of group teaching if they are introduced to the class objectives, content, and staff. Some physicians are interested in participating as teachers; this was our experience in the prenatal classes described later in this chapter.

Hospital-wide programs, for example critical pathways and care maps, seem to be the best way to teach patients with common health problems. Can this concept also be used in an outpatient clinic? If so, with which target populations should we begin?

Similar programs can be effective in an outpatient clinic or home health setting because they direct the coordination of the health care team through teaching protocols. Evaluating common learning needs of patient populations requiring ongoing teaching can be accomplished by using computer statistics that list the most common diagnoses. Nurses may also keep a log of patient education encounters for a 6-month period and make their own comparisons. We used this method in an outpatient clinic and discovered that the following situations are ideal for group teaching: weight reduction, hypertension, diabetes, prenatal care, and neonatal care. It may be helpful to start with those patient problems or diagnoses that are considered to be "high volume" or "high risk" in your practice setting.

Selecting Learning Activities

How does the nurse decide what learning activities are best for the situation? It seems that lec-

ture is the only learning activity used although others would be equally effective.

Lecture can be an effective way to teach basic facts. Remember that a combination of learning activities works best in each situation. It will help the patient and family to assume active roles in learning and to enjoy patient education if we keep the following points in mind:

- Match learning activities with learning objectives. Refer to the outline in the section above, Learning Activities, for those activities best suited to cognitive, affective, and psychomotor learning.
- Keep the patient and the family involved through discussion, role play, games, and media.
- Test the patient's new abilities to help him feel a sense of accomplishment. Try to build success and reinforcement into patient education.
- Make learning fun. Humor and support decrease the learner's anxiety and help him to learn at his own pace.
- Allow ample time to practice skills. Skill-building exercises should not be last on the agenda because they often determine how safely the patient will be able to perform new skills at home.
- Incorporate methods other than lecture alone to teach skills and develop the patient's attitude.

Selecting Media

Are there general guidelines that can be used to evaluate different types of media, whether they are written materials, videotapes, slides, or CAI?

Yes. Appendix A provides a checklist for evaluating written patient education materials. It is adapted from the Society of Teachers of Family Medicine, a group actively involved in promoting patient education. Appendix B is an evaluation guide used when previewing patient education videos.

What help can the hospital or nursing school library provide in locating patient education materials?

Many medical and nursing libraries participate in an interlibrary program that circulates videotape programs, including those on patient teaching topics. Taking the time to discuss patient education interests with the librarian often results in acquiring media on loan at no cost. Most hospital and nursing school libraries subscribe to the National Library of Medicine's on-line reference systems as well as computerized catalogues of patient information. These systems use computerized information retrieval programs that can contribute to the development of bibliographies and to the collection of materials on patient education.

What are the advantages of making your own media programs?

Larger hospitals often decide to make their own videotape programs once they have invested in a cable television system. If the hospital already owns videotaping equipment and has target populations that would benefit from a tailor-made program, video production may be beneficial. Smaller hospitals may have less expertise and different audiences and would therefore be better suited to commercially produced programs and less expensive VCRs. Slide programs can be produced easily and economically in large and small hospitals and other health care settings. A good camera and slide projector are necessary. Practitioners can take their own slides and construct the program. They can personalize learning by using scenery, equipment, and people familiar to the patients. Programs can be accompanied by pulsed audiotape if a cassette recorder with a built-in synchronized pulse capability is purchased. Printed patient education materials, such as booklets and information sheets, are easily made in house and may offer specific instructions for emergency care or hospital and office policies. With physicians and dietitians, we have coauthored several booklets that were better suited to our patient's needs than those commercially available. Perhaps the most basic and helpful of all media for patient education is the one-page interdisciplinary instruction sheet that is made in house.

I am unsure how to prepare to teach a patient education class. I have had a lot of experience with individual teaching but feel unprepared for group teaching. What should I do?

Advanced preparation and coaching are important before teaching a group. The first step is to define who the target audience will be, the estimated size of the group, the goals for the patient education session, and the amount of time available for teaching. Then, a variety of teaching methods may be combined, such as lecture and discussion, or perhaps a case study. Hospital staff development coordinators may be a valuable source of help in planning your program because they are experienced in planning classes using adult education models. Generally, group teaching is used to persuade patients to perform health behaviors. Information and facts are presented to help them understand the need to act a certain way and then examples are given to help patients understand what they need to do. These principles apply equally to health promotion or disease-specific management classes.

Knowing the facts about the health problems to be addressed is important. A review of the nursing literature and possible sources such as the AHCPR guidelines are a good place to start. Presenting information persuasively requires a confident teacher with a lively affect who can keep the learners' attention. It is helpful to observe others who are experienced in group teaching and witness first-hand group teaching techniques. Nurses are usually good group teachers because they are at ease with patients and families and are viewed as credible and sensitive. Still, it is important for nurses to realize that having an impact on patient opinion in a powerful way to influence behavior requires us to think as a patient would think. The Health Belief Model which is discussed in Chapter 8, outlines the four steps that lead to patient decisions about whether to perform health behaviors. We discussed in that chapter how the model was applied to individual situations to engage patients in the learning process. When organizing a group class, this model can be also be used as a guide. First, patients must believe they have or are likely to be affected by a particular health problem. Evidence that the patient has hypertension

or diabetes or is at risk can be provided, along with some facts about the prevalence of the problem. Patients should be able to understand in their own words a simple definition of the health problem. In the second step, they must believe the condition discussed is harmful and has adverse consequences. Patients frequently wish to talk about how this problem has or may affect their lives, families, work, and social roles. The third step necessitates an understanding of the proposed treatment plan or health promotion plan and what behaviors the patient is asked to consider integrating in his life. These should be stated clearly, with practical suggestions to help patients overcome barriers they might encounter, including learning skills, finding ongoing support, and perhaps acquiring financial assistance. In the fourth step, patients weigh the perceived costs and benefits of the proposed health interventions and make decisions about their further commitment to act.

It is important to appreciate that group teaching can call patients to act and thus can contribute self-care. Learning should be patient centered, with opportunity to ask questions and share experiences. Therefore, time must be allocated in group teaching for such activities, which may mean that content offered in lecture format must be limited.

Table 9-2 illustrates how group teaching can be organized following the steps of the Health Belief Model and can help you in selecting what information to share and deciding how to sequence learning activities.

❑ CASE STUDY

Mrs. Betts Learns Postoperative Cataract Care

Mrs. Betts is a 66-year-old widow and describes herself as very active. "I've been independent all my life; nothing slows me down." She lives alone. Mrs. Betts is going to have cataract surgery as an outpatient at the Eye Center. The day before surgery she went to the Eye Center for preoperative teaching; her daughter who lives two blocks away drove her.

TABLE 9–2. The Health Belief Model Used in Planning Patient Education Interventions

Steps	Application
I. The patient perceives that he has a condition or is likely to contract it.	I. a. Discuss problem and symptoms (to be prevented or treated).
II. The patient perceives that the disease or condition is harmful and has serious consequences for him.	b. Explore prior knowledge and experience of audience.
III. The patient believes that the suggested health intervention is of value to him.	c. Address obstacles to understanding (anxiety, fear, misconceptions, denial).
IV. The patient believes that the effectiveness of the treatment is worth the cost and barriers he must confront.	II. a. Describe potential consequences of the problem.
	b. Discuss prognosis.
	c. Explore common beliefs and attitudes.
	d. Describe experiences of individuals with similar problem (including life-style).
	III. a. Describe proposed treatment plan, health promotion activities, proposed behavior changes (includes medications).
	b. Discuss what may happen with or without proposed treatment.
	c. Is this a cure?
	d. Financial costs, life-style changes, side effects discussed.
	IV. a. Outline provider responsibilities.
	b. Outline patient responsibilities.
	c. Outline needed knowledge, attitudes, and skills.
	d. Suggest and provide resources for knowledge and skills development.

References:

1. Hochbaum, G. M. (1958). *Public participation in medical screening programs* (U.S. Public Health Service Publication No. 572). Washington, DC: U.S. Government Printing Office.
2. Rosenstock, I. M. (1975). *Patient's compliance with health regimens Journal of the American Medical Association, 234*(4), 402–403.
3. Rankin, S. H., & Stallings, K. D. (1990). Patient education: Issues, principles, and practices. Philadelphia: J. B. Lippincott.

The Health Belief Model was constructed to predict health behaviors. It provides a tool for understanding the patient's perception of disease and his decision-making process in the consumption of health services. In each of the four steps, family members and significant others should be considered.

Nursing diagnoses included:

1. Knowledge Deficit related to surgical procedure and discharge instructions
2. Potential for Infection
3. Potential for Injury due to limited depth perception and postoperative activity

The clinic nurse clarified Mrs. Betts' misconceptions about what a cataract is and what the surgical procedure for cataract extraction involves. Specific discharge instructions were discussed with the patient and her daughter. Both were given a one-page written instruction sheet listing the schedule for eye drops after surgery and specific directions to prevent injuries resulting from limited depth perception and intraocular pressure. Mrs. Betts was impressed with the need to slow down; to avoid straining, coughing, bending, and lifting; and to be careful not to rush or to hit the eye. She was also taught to hold onto bannisters and take care with pouring liquids and climbing stairs. She was given her appointment for the first postoperative visit 1 day after surgery.

The skills Mrs. Betts needed to clean her eye and instill eyedrops to prevent infection required demonstration and opportunity for her to practice. The clinic nurse used the model of an eye for this purpose and helped Mrs. Betts[*] practice the proper procedures on herself. She also gave Mrs. Betts two poster pages, How to Clean Your Eye and How to Put Drops in Your Eye, that gave large-print step-by-step reminders about the procedures. In bold print, at the bottom of each poster appeared: "Phone 511-1123 if you have pain or if blood soaks your eye patch"(Carver, 1980).

❑ CASE STUDY

Mrs. Fox's Fracture

Mrs. Fox is 70 years old. She is well-known on the medical surgical unit of the small community hospital. She has been admitted three times in the past year because her diabetes was "out of control" due to poor dietary habits. She is inactive, watches television and plays bridge for entertainment, and smokes two packs of cigarettes per day.

Her current admission was the result of a fall down the front stairs of her home. Mrs. Fox had a fractured tibia. A cast was applied in the emergency room. Because of poor circulation and immobility, Mrs. Fox was admitted overnight for evaluation. Her physician planned to discharge her within 2 days.

During the admission assessment, her nurse noted the following important information:

The Fox's live in a one-story ranch home with wood floors and area rugs.
Mr. Fox works evening shift as a security guard for the local shopping mall.
Mrs. Fox has not followed her diabetic diet.
Mr. Fox found Mrs. Fox asleep on the couch with a burning cigarette in her hand last week and is worried about a fire in the home while he is at work.

The nursing staff held a patient care conference to discuss what to do with Mrs. Fox. Considering the short time she would be hospitalized, the nurses were overwhelmed by what must be taught so Mrs. Fox could manage her care. Should they immediately get a dietitian involved to repeat diet teaching? What about the smoking and its hazards? They decided to first make a list of all nursing diagnoses and then worked together to set priorities:

1. Altered Tissue Perfusion in peripheral system
2. Impaired Tissue Integrity
3. Risk for Injury
4. Impaired Physical Mobility
5. Altered Nutrition: More than Body Requirements
6. Impaired Home Maintenance Management
7. Activity Intolerance
8. Pain

After careful consideration of survival skills and safety issues, the nursing staff confidently placed highest priority on Impaired Physical Mobility, Risk for Injury, and Altered Tissue Perfusion. Survival skills were crutch-walking ability and circulation checks on the affected leg. Goals for Mrs. Fox and her family were:

Properly maintain the cast with adequate circulation.
Assess the cast and the skin under the cast edges to determine skin condition four times daily.
Assess foot and leg for circulatory and neurologic impairment four times daily.
Walk safely with the use of crutches and appropriate gait.
Prevent axillary skin breakdown.
Administer medication as ordered.
Adapt home environment to prevent injury due to falls.
Provide at-home assistance with activities of daily living.

An excellent resource on teaching cast care and crutch walking is *Manual of Home Health Care Nursing* (Walsh, Persons, & Wieck, 1987). Skills such as these must be taught with active learner involvement and repeated practice. The nurse should accurately assess and document the patient's abilities in these areas.

The nursing staff caring for Mrs. Fox made the difficult decision to accomplish diabetic teaching and promote smoking cessation with post-hospital referrals. They decided to focus their immediate efforts on the problems posed by this injury. They also called a team conference with the physical therapist to coordinate therapy for crutch-walking skills, dietary for diet reinforcement, and the hospital social worker to work with the Foxes on the possibility of a home health referral and at home assistance to assure safety. Every nurse who entered Mrs. Fox's room for the next 24 hours demonstrated and reinforced circulation checks and crutch-walking skills and received return demonstration. Mr. Fox was also involved in teaching. A one-page instruction sheet reflected priority instructions regarding ambulation and circulation.

———————————————————————❑

Home Health Care to Meet Posthospital Needs

The field of home health care services is growing at a rapid rate to meet many different patient needs such as treatments, counseling and pain relief for cancer, high-technology services, and physical therapy. As a result of economic pressures from DRGs, patients are often discharged while still needing some level of professional health care.

Nurses must become familiar with this expanding area of care so they can assist patients with discharge planning. Nurses must anticipate the needs patients will have at home, what kinds of resources are already on hand, and what types of outside help they will need. The case study of Mrs. Fox illustrates critical needs, including patient teaching, that remain after discharge. A nurse works with the family to assess the physical layout of the home, how to adapt it if necessary, and how to add needed equipment, such as hospital bed, commode, or handrails. She helps the family assess whether the principal caregiver will need to involve other helpers to assist, pick up medications, run errands, and so forth. The nurse helps the family consider emergency procedures such as getting a portable generator to back up a ventilator in case of power failure. She must also know how to find out what the patient's insurance will cover, and she may consult others to determine this. For patients who qualify, third party payment will reimburse for at least part of home health care services. The way the nurse documents patient needs is important and can influence whether or not skilled nursing services are covered (Walsh et al., 1987; Eggland, 1987). The following suggestions are offered:

• Clarify the homebound status of the patient. The patient's condition prevents him from leaving home without help from others; therefore, leaving home is rarely feasible. Stress functional limitations.

• Emphasize acute episodes or acute exacerbation of the condition within the last 30 to 60 days, if possible.

• Chart "negatively" to reflect the level of current need. For example, size and appearance of wound should be documented rather than stating, "wound healing well." Give specific measurements whenever possible.

• Emphasize the need for reinstruction rather than for reinforced teaching. If family's ability to master learning is limited, this should be noted.

• Document that the patient's condition is unstable. Skilled nursing care to monitor medications or vital signs may not be reimbursed unless the patient's condition is unstable.

Home health care incorporates many types of agencies with which nurses should become familiar. They include home health care agencies (some hospitals have their own and are certified by Medicare), home health care services (private companies not certified by Medicare), hospices (for terminally ill patients with caregivers in the home), registries of nurses, and pharmaceutical home health care (specializing in total parenteral nutrition, intravenous antibiotics, feeding, and so forth).

In the case studies we presented of Mrs. Fox (this chapter) and Mr. Stanley (see Chap. 8), the patients may benefit from home health care services. We should not assume, however, that reimbursement will automatically follow. We did learn, for example, that Mrs. Fox's Medicare would cover skilled observation of her circulatory status with her cast every 2 to 3 days for a 2-week period because of her diagnosis of diabetes. We discovered that visits to assess Mr. Stanley's asthma and COPD would be limited to four visits but could be extended if chest physical therapy and postural drainage were ordered. Many acute care nurses are unaware that home care nurses must also focus on discharge planning at the time of admission and skillfully achieve patient learning outcomes rather than simply prolonging care.

Summary

We discussed the importance of matching learning objectives to appropriate learning methods and media to achieve positive results in patient education. Various examples were offered to illustrate the design of interventions based on nursing diagnoses, learning needs, goals, and patient learning objectives. Case studies illustrated interventions for individual patients, including tips for using home health care services to bridge the gap between hospital and home, and to ensure the patient's continuity of care. Valuable appendices for evaluating patient education materials and videos are provided at the end of the book.

Strategies for Critical Analysis and Application

1. Using the case study of Mrs. Fox, describe which instructional format and methods you would choose for discharge teaching, based on the patient's length of stay and priorities for patient learning. How would you coordinate your teaching with the physical therapist? Who else besides the patient should be included in teaching?

2. Select a sample patient education handout and a sample video addressing a topic of your choice. Evaluate them using Appendices A and B. What suggestions would you make for making them more patient centered? How could they be adapted to meet the needs of patients with low literacy skills?

3. If you were asked to teach a 1-hour class to fellow nursing students about the need for their own adequate nutrition and exercise, how could you prepare the class using the Health Belief Model as a guide?

REFERENCES

Ball, M., Hannah, K.J., Jelger U.G., & Peterson, H. (Eds.). (1994). *Nursing informatics: Where caring and technology meet* (2nd ed.). New York: Springer-Verlag.

Bolwell, C. (1988). Index to computer-assisted instructional (CAI) software for nursing education. In M. Ball, K.J. Hannah, U.G. Jelger, & H. Peterson, (Eds.), *Nursing informatics: Where caring and technology meet* (2nd ed., pp. 371-395). New York: Springer-Verlag.

Brown, J., Lewis R., & Harcleroad F. (1973). *AV instruction: Technology, media and methods* (4th ed.). New York: McGraw-Hill.

Carver, J. (1980). Cataract care made plain. *American Journal of Nursing, 80*(5), 626-630.

Dixon, E., & Park, R. (1990). Do patients understand written health information? *Nursing Outlook, 38*(6), 278-281.

Doak, C., Doak, L., & Root, J. (1994). *Teaching patients with low literacy skills*. Philadelphia, J. B. Lippincott.

Eggland, E. (1989). Nurses' guide to home health care. *Nursing, 17*(10), 75-81.

Etheredge, M. (1989). *Collaborative care: Nursing case management*. Chicago: American Hospital Association.

Feldman, S., Quinlivan, A., Williford, P., Bahnson, J., & Fleischer, A., (1994). Illiteracy and the readability of patient education materials. *North Carolina Medical Journal, 55*(7), 290-292.

Kreigh, H., & Perko, J. (1979). *Psychiatric and mental health nursing: Commitment to care and concern* (pp. 74-77). Reston, VA: Reston Publishing.

Lindberg, J., Hunter, M., & Kruszewski, A. (1994). *Introduction to nursing: Concepts, issues, and opportunities* (2nd ed., pp. 229-231). Philadelphia: J. B. Lippincott.

Marchiondo, K., & Kipp, C., (1987). Establishing a standardized patient educating program. *Critical Care Nurse, 7*(3), 58-66.

McCaffery, M. (1994). How to use the new AHCPR cancer pain guidelines. *American Journal of Nursing, July,* 42-46.

National Cancer Institute. (1981). *Readability testing in cancer communications*. (NIH Publication No. 81-1689). Bethesda, MD: Cancer Information Clearinghouse.

Neeson, J., & May, K. (1986). *Comprehensive maternity nursing*. Philadelphia: J. B. Lippincott.

Redman, B. (1993). Patient education at 25 years; where we have been and where we are going. *Journal of Advanced Nursing, 18,* 725-730.

Thomas, B. (1988). Educational software. In M. Ball, K.J. Hannah, U.G. Jelger, & H. Peterson (Eds.), *Nursing informatics: Where caring and technology meet* (pp. 301-307). New York: Springer-Verlag.

U.S. Department of Agriculture, Office of Information (1988). Guidelines: writing for adults with limited reading skills. Washington, D.C.

Walsh, J., Persons, C., & Wieck, L. (1987). *Manual of home health care nursing* (pp. 336-353). Philadelphia: J. B. Lippincott.

CHAPTER

10 Designing Patient Education Programs in the Community and in the Home

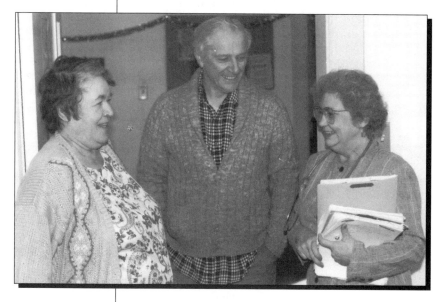

OBJECTIVES FOR CHAPTER 10

After reading this chapter, the nurse or student nurse should be able to:

1 Identify three challenges encountered when designing community-based patient education interventions.

2 Describe two ways to gain credibility in a community before beginning a community education program.

3 Discuss how family roles and expectations can affect learning in the home or community.

Patient Education: Issues, Principles, Practices, Third Edition, by Sally H. Rankin and Karen Duffy Stallings.
Lippincott–Raven Publishers, Philadelphia, © 1996.

Planning Interventions for Communities or Groups

Educating communities or groups of people is more difficult than educating one person or one family. The boundaries of communities are amorphous and not always clearly defined. When a needs assessment indicates that community education is desirable, the implementation process must proceed in a careful and organized fashion. Methods of evaluation must be included in the program design and the economic realities of undertaking such a program should be considered.

This chapter discusses two community patient education projects: prenatal classes and a program of discharge planning and home follow-up for cardiovascular surgery patients. We are including the prenatal classes as an example of community education because they were open to all pregnant members of the community, not just to clinic patients. The prenatal clients met the definition of a *group* because they were a group of people with common goals interacting independently. Additionally, the prenatal class met the definition of *community*: they were a specific population living in a defined area having shared institutions, values, and problems. The cardiac risk factor reduction and family support program is included in this chapter because the greatest part of the intervention occurred after discharge while the patient was in the home and community.

We present guidelines for establishing such community health education and health promotion classes. We include the philosophies of the programs, the objectives established for classes, the evaluation methodologies, and appendices that include outlines and appropriate materials to use. The protocol for the cardiac risk factor reduction and family support telephone calls is also included. Before we embark on discussion of the specifics about each set of classes, we mention the problems encountered when health education is attempted at the community level.

Observations Related to Community Health Education

Just as the client exists not in a void but rather as the sum of family, socioeconomic, educational, and cultural influences, so must the community be considered in relation to many interfacing systems. A community health education program cannot be created as if the community existed in a vacuum. Social, economic, organizational, and environmental influences must instead be considered (Green, 1980). Each community is unique. For example, a community venereal disease education program for teenagers in Beverly Hills should differ considerably from one planned for a small Appalachian community in West Virginia.

Just as a needs assessment is required for the patient, so may an assessment of the community's health education needs be performed. Any type of health education or health promotion program should be requested by the community. Hospitals may use community programs to promote goodwill, market hospital network services, or promote their image as invested in health promotion. As capitation (prenegotiated rates for providing all health care services needed by a patient) becomes the preferred method for insurance companies to contract with providers, prevention may be seen as a way to attract customers and maximize profitability by decreasing the need for illness care. Because it generally requires greater time and financial expenditure to plan and implement programs for a community than for one patient, and because the community as a whole, directly or indirectly, will probably pay for all or part of the program, it is essential that the community recognizes and expresses a need for the services. Needs of communities can be ascertained in various ways. An effective manner of gathering data pertaining to health education needs is to first approach medical personnel involved in the delivery of community health care. Public health departments are one obvious place to collect these data. Next, formal and informal community leaders should be polled about their perceptions of health education needs. Patient advisory groups, focus groups, or surveys can be used. Congruence between these two needs lists must then be determined. One of the greatest causes of past failures in community health education has been the imposition of programs, perceived by health care professionals as needed, on a population that neither perceives the same need nor desires the program.

Another factor that must be considered in planning community health education programs is the credibility of those teaching the material. One study found that an inner-city community preferred and better responded to health education offered by a nurse who was a member of the community than that offered by outside health care professionals (Dyson & Dyson, 1979). Another community health education project involved indigenous community leaders to act as lay health educators. The leaders were trained to facilitate health knowledge acquisition and to recognize health problems that needed professional attention (Salber, 1979). Such programs are especially successful in minority communities that have developed distrust of outside professionals, who they perceive as trying to impose their ideas on communities that they do not know or understand. We are aware of an effective program that prepared hairdressers to teach their female clients the importance of breast self-examination. Other programs aimed at health promotion were supported by and located at local churches. The North Carolina Division of Adult Health Promotion and African American churches teamed up to fight cancer in ten counties of the state. They targeted a goal of improving diet as one way to decrease the risk of cancer in rural North Carolina's African American adult population and were awarded a grant from the National Cancer Institute. Five churches of various sizes and denominations were recruited from each county to participate in the dietary behavior change project entitled "Black Churches United for Better Health." African Americans are underserved by the traditional health care system; thus,

health promotion messages may not reach them. Nontraditional health prevention programs must be used. The training of lay health advisors who have a tradition of being natural helpers, are sensitive to cultural norms, and are based at churches where people turn for everyday support and guidance had the greatest potential to affect health status (Cowan, 1994).

Credibility in highly educated and sophisticated communities must be maintained by using health professionals at similar educational and socioeconomic levels to those of the population being served. For example, a community hospital in a prosperous southern California community always uses physicians to present health education seminars to the public because the community would not be responsive to less highly trained professionals.

Another factor to be considered is financing of community education programs. In the case of the prenatal classes, charges for clinic patients were covered by the obstetric package fee; nonclinic patients were charged a moderate fee for five classes. The family-focused educational intervention (cardiac risk factor reduction and family support) was conducted by master's degree nurses employed as research assistants; there was no cost to the family. The telephone monitoring system is a low-cost intervention. Nursing costs, based on research assistant salaries of $8.50/hour ranged from $25 for the entire 8-week period for uncomplicated cases, to a high of $50 for complicated cases (Rankin & Gilliss, 1987).

Our experience has been that a community is willing to pay for the service when it wishes to participate in health education. When we are considering a group such as schoolchildren, however, monies usually come from foundation grants or federal or state governments. Obviously the state of the national economy is important to the funding of such programs. During recessions we see little federal funding for what is viewed by government as unessential. A good example of the economy's effects on health care delivery is the issue of nationalized health care. During the middle and late 1970s, many of us believed that nationalized health care was soon to become a reality. The advent of a new administration in the 1980s, however, repealed that expectation. The debate about nationalized health care continues in the 1990s. Managed care has taken firm hold in the health care delivery system and on the horizon is the trend toward capitation. These changes hold new opportunities for strengthening health promotion efforts if they can be demonstrated as cost effective or cost saving.

Another factor in the success or failure of community health education involves its general appeal. To succeed, community health education must be timely and well presented and able to attract the attention of many people. The advertising profession has accumulated a vast store of knowledge that enables businesses to sell their products. Unfortunately, we rarely use advertising research to sell health education. All too often, community health education projects are the ideas of single, well-meaning health care professionals who determine a need and decide to fill it.

Research on the usefulness of television's ability to affect health education indicates that although television does not produce behavioral changes, it will arouse interest and inform people of health matters (Richman & Urban, 1978). One specific evaluation indicated that a series of programs on alcoholism, broadcast on a public television network, heightened public awareness of alcoholism but did not stimulate corrective action (Dickman & Keil, 1977). Due to this finding, and to obvious cost reasons, the use of television in health education must be carefully considered for its limited yet valuable role in the process of health promotion.

Godfrey Hochbaum, a well-known health education specialist, suggests that we promote healthful practices by showing them to be pleasant and easy rather than by trying to scare people into healthy behaviors (Hochbaum, 1979). We cannot force health education onto a community any more than we can force a person to practice contraception. However, by using advertising technology and by promoting the positive aspects of health practices, we may enjoy more success in future community health education.

Examples of Two Community Health Education Projects

Both of these projects could be implemented in any community. We first discuss a community health education project followed by a home-based educational intervention.

Prenatal Community Education

A program of prenatal education was originally developed as part of a clinical practicum for a graduate nursing student. The classes evolved in response to an informal needs assessment conducted at the outpatient clinic of a university's family medicine residency training program. Faculty, residents, and nurses designated prenatal classes as the outstanding patient education need for clinic patients. The clinic served a group of prenatal families who were socioeconomically and culturally diverse. Teenage parents, unwed mothers, and international patients did not seem to be served by traditional couple-oriented approaches to childbirth education. The involvement of childbirth coaches was strongly supported, and these individuals included mothers, sisters, and friends, as well as spouses. When the Family Practice Clinic assumed the leadership of the prenatal classes, the following philosophy about the delivery of prenatal education was developed.

There is a strong agreement among staff at the Family Practice Clinic that education is an essential ingredient in the health care we deliver to our prenatal patients. Although there have been many attempts to provide this education in the past, it was not until recently that a commitment was made to offer prenatal classes to all of our patients on a regular basis.

We believe that prenatal classes should be attended as early as possible in pregnancy. There are numerous advantages to the patient, her family, the physician, and the nurse.

1. The mother's participation in her own care is essential, especially in the areas of nutrition and care of her body. The classes give

both parents the information they need to work in partnership with the physician and nurse.

2. Classes dealing with the labor and delivery processes give expectant parents an opportunity to verbalize anxieties or fears about childbirth.

3. Expectant parents enter a supportive relationship with other expectant parents.

4. Relaxation and breathing techniques are learned. This may make both routine obstetric examinations and the labor and delivery better experiences.

5. Expectant mothers and fathers are encouraged to communicate their feelings effectively with one another and to consider ways to keep the communication lines open during stressful events surrounding the birth of their child.

6. Parents gain knowledge about newborn care and helpful suggestions for dealing with the new baby's siblings and other family members.

7. The prenatal care curriculum offers a blend of general childbirth education and Lamaze techniques. We do not promote any one specific approach to the birth experience or child care. Our aim is to provide expectant parents with information that enables them to consider their own needs and wishes. We stress the importance of openness and flexibility in planning for labor and delivery and in considering each family's special circumstances.

8. We believe that expectant parents learn from us and from each other. As health care providers, we also learn a great deal from our patients in an informal group, in which all members are supported and encouraged to share their thoughts and feelings with one another.

9. A commitment to patient education is demonstrated by our willingness to become team members in health care with our patients. It is a statement of our respect for patients as consumers. Finally, offering an attractive prenatal care package is an important step toward enrolling new families in the practice.

Development of the philosophy continues the clinic's history of interest in the consumer. The philosophy is viewed as an attempt to specify and to advocate the rights of the prenatal client and her support system. Evolution of the philosophy preceded the establishment of behavioral objectives and methods of evaluating participants' satisfaction.

Care is taken to ensure continuity of the prenatal classes regardless of changes in clinic staff and residents. Guidelines and standards were developed to help each staff nurse who would serve as a prenatal class coordinator handle the logistics of the classes, as well as to allay anxiety she might have about the program.

After guidelines were developed, objectives were written for each class (see Appendix C). During the first class meeting, a learning needs assessment was filled out by each client and her significant other. These assessment data were then put into the general schema of classes. In this way the prenatal clients are able to set their own agenda (i.e., the class is taught to meet their needs not the health care professionals' needs). Data from the learning needs assessment were transferred to the client's chart, with her knowledge, so that during routine office visits the physician could discuss her stated concerns. The learning needs assessment included questions about previous pregnancies, who would attend classes and delivery with the patient, previous prenatal education, and what the patient was hoping to learn in the classes.

Classes were enlivened by group discussions and demonstrations. During the first class we enlisted the assistance of a couple who attended the previous set of classes and were willing to bring their infant to a new series of classes. The expectant parents always had many questions for the parent visitors and seeing the outcome of the prenatal period—a healthy baby—focused the class for everyone. We also separated the participants into smaller groups of five or six to discuss such topics as sexual activity during pregnancy and to play educational games related to nutrition. During the fourth class, which discussed the care of the newborn, a family nurse practitioner or a family medicine resident demonstrated physical assessment of a neonate. The couples were invariably amazed to see the newborn's range of behaviors. We feel this class helps them better envision their forthcoming infant and also helps them to lay the foundation for infant stimulation practices. During the class on contraception we obtain samples of all the different contraceptive devices and pass them around the room. The demonstration segments break the tedium that can occur with the lecture format and also allow the participants an opportunity to become acquainted with one another.

At the end of the last class each participant is asked to complete an evaluation form rating the classes and teachers and offering suggestions for improvement. Evaluations were useful in planning future classes and in giving specific teachers feedback on their performance in the classes.

Another evaluation format, a confidence survey, was used during the first class series to obtain information related to the participants' growth in confidence levels during the five class meetings. One of the purposes of any type of prenatal education is to instill confidence in the couple so that they will be able to manage self-care practices related to pregnancy and to care for the neonate. Confidence levels on 19 different items were determined on pre- and posttests (i.e., at the beginning of the class series and after the last class). When the data from a past class were tabulated, they showed that all clients had increased their confidence levels or remained the same on every item, except for three items on which 2 patients had decreased their confidence level. Any increase in confidence level as measured by this instrument would be accepted as an indication that the intervention had created a positive change. Using a control group that had not attended the classes would have been one method of verifying that the experimental prenatal patients had indeed increased their confidence levels as a result of the classes. The confidence level survey used in the classes is shown in Figure 10-1.

Another method of evaluation and feedback we used was asking patients to write a summary of their birth experiences. Patients were given a guide for writing the report (Box 10-1). This is a keepsake for the family as well as a process to help the mother work through feelings about such a powerful experience. Although not all patients are willing to write a report, most are eager to discuss the birth experience. This provided us with valuable pointers about how to improve childbirth classes to better prepare patients for labor and delivery.

Additions were made to the patient education offerings at the clinic due to evaluations of the prenatal classes. More in-depth classes were provided on breast preparation and breast-feeding for patients in the seventh to eighth month of pregnancy. A room at the clinic was also equipped for patients to view

---

BOX 10-1. Suggestions for Writing About the Birth Experience

Beginning of Labor

How and when did it begin? What did you do? How did you feel?

Admission to the Hospital

When were you admitted? What was it like?

Stages of Labor

How long did each stage last? Did you feel that the nurses kept you informed on your progress? Which "tools" helped the most? Which helped the least? Did you receive medication? If so, what kind, when, how effective was it? What kind of emotional support did you have?

Birth

What did the baby look like? How did you feel during and immediately after birth?

Postpartum

How long did you stay in the hospital? Describe how you felt during the first week you were at home following delivery. What problems did you have? What people or things were most helpful to you?

INSTRUCTIONS

We are interested in knowing how confident you feel about your knowledge associated with pregnancy, labor, and delivery. Please answer these questions carefully by circling the response that refers to your confidence level.
A sample question will help you understand how to fill out the questionnaire.
I know how to fill out this questionnaire.

VC   C   ?   I   VI

VC — I feel very confident and secure in my knowledge of this material.
  C — I feel confident that I can deal adequately with this material.
   ? — I have no particular feelings about this material; I do not know what this material means.
   I — I feel insecure, knowing that I would have a difficult time dealing with this material.
 VI — I feel very insecure, knowing that I definitely could not deal with this material at this time.

1. I know which foods a pregnant woman should eat and why.

     VC   C   ?   I   VI

2. I understand the changes in my breasts.

     VC   C   ?   I   VI

3. I know about the possible effects of alcohol on my baby.

     VC   C   ?   I   VI

4. I know how many pounds I can gain during my pregnancy.

     VC   C   ?   I   VI

5. I understand restrictions placed on me because of my job.

     VC   C   ?   I   VI

6. I know how to do a pelvic tilt.

     VC   C   ?   I   VI

7. I understand the reasons for frequent urination during pregnancy.

     VC   C   ?   I   VI

8. I know the danger signs to watch for during pregnancy.

     VC   C   ?   I   VI

9. I understand the fear—tension—pain cycle.

     VC   C   ?   I   VI

10. I know how to do breathing exercises to be used during labor.

     VC   C   ?   I   VI

(continued)

FIGURE 10–1. Prenatal confidence level survey.

11. I know what to expect from a newborn baby.

| | VC | C | ? | I | VI |

12. I understand the differences between bottle feeding and breast feeding for the mother and baby.

| | VC | C | ? | I | VI |

13. I know how to give a baby bath.

| | VC | C | ? | I | VI |

14. I know what kind of birth control to use while nursing.

| | VC | C | ? | I | VI |

15. I know what kinds of pain medications are available during labor.

| | VC | C | ? | I | VI |

16. I know at least three signs of beginning labor.

| | VC | C | ? | I | VI |

17. I know how to get my body into shape after delivery.

| | VC | C | ? | I | VI |

18. I understand the various forms of birth control and the ones best suited for me.

| | VC | C | ? | I | VI |

19. I know the types of equipment and clothing necessary for myself and my baby.

| | VC | C | ? | I | VI |

FIGURE 10–1. (Continued)

videotapes on cesarean delivery, basics of baby care, and postpartum fatigue and depression. A daily baby care "call-in" telephone hour was proposed to be offered at the clinic to provide information and answer patient questions before their first return visit to the clinic.

❑ CASE STUDY

The Vuong Family

Because this neighborhood health care clinic's surrounding community included a growing number of Vietnamese families, the nurses at the clinic were learning about that culture—the goals, beliefs, and attitudes surrounding childbirth. One patient, Vuong Mai, came for her first clinic visit when she was 12 weeks pregnant. She came to the visit alone. She was quiet and seemed withdrawn; therefore, the assessment of her learning needs about the pregnancy was difficult. Also time is limited during an outpatient encounter. A nursing student working at the clinic that day offered to conduct two home visits to help identify Mai's needs. She composed the following family assessment.

Family Profile

The family unit is composed of the husband, Tran, age 38, who works in a print shop; Mai, age 28, the wife, who works full time as a seamstress and is pregnant with their first child; and Li, age 28, who is Tran's sister and works in the same print shop as her brother. Mai is expecting her first child on March 17, 1995. She is receiving prenatal care and has had an uneventful pregnancy. She states she knows nothing about pregnancy, labor, delivery, or caring for a newborn child and denies having had any role model in these areas. Mai and Tran are both Vietnamese and immigrated legally from Vietnam in 1990 and 1988, respectively. Li had previously come to the United States as a refugee in 1986 with two other siblings. She then sponsored Tran in 1988. Mai was sponsored by a brother who had been a refugee in 1981. Tran and Mai knew each other in Vietnam but courted and married in San Jose, California. They have been married 14 months and have lived in San Francisco since marriage. Li has always lived with them. Prior to leaving Vietnam, Tran worked as a farmer. This was a difficult life, physically and economically. He came to the U.S. in hopes of a better and prosperous life. Mai did not complete high school; she left school to work and support her family after 1981. All three of them continue to financially support their parents, and Mai sends her brother, who lives in Texas, one third of her monthly salary.

Both sets of parents are supportive of the pregnancy. However, neither mother is able to come and help with the care of the newborn, a traditional role of Vietnamese grandmothers (Grosso, Barden, Henry, & Vieau, 1981).

Family System

The Vuong family is a warm, hospitable Catholic family with a secure sense of family loyalty, closeness, and strength. In Vietnamese culture the family is the fundamental social unit, the primary source of cohesion and continuity (Nguyen, 1988). Although separated geographically from most of their family, Li's living with them provides Tran and Mai with some of the traditional stability of living with extended family. She will have a significant role in caring for the newborn child, and because unmarried Vietnamese women never live outside of their family of origin, they provide family for her as well. Traditional Vietnamese families have a patriarchal structure where the senior man is the head of the household and the woman is dutiful and respectful toward her husband (Calhoun, 1985). In the Vuong family, Tran is the head of the family, as was evident in the way he often spoke for his wife and appeared to be her caretaker. Mai was dutiful to her husband in the way she respected his opinion and served him and their guest first. However, these roles were also flexible: all three members of this family shared the domestic duties of their small two-room flat. They were also emotionally supportive and mutually respectful of each other as was evident in the gentleness Tran and Li showed toward Mai

when she had difficulty understanding the questions of the English-speaking interviewer. They live among and work predominantly with Vietnamese immigrants and refugees. This may signal enmeshment within their ethnic community because they have few non-Vietnamese friends. Consequently, this results in their being limited in their awareness of community services (i.e., childbirth preparation classes). This also decreases their opportunities to assimilate into their new culture and improve their English language skills.

All three family members stated that they did not know what to expect with pregnancy and childbirth and portrayed concern regarding their lack of knowledge. They are presently receiving their knowledge from friends and neighbors because they have no family in the immediate area. This could potentially lead to confusion, fear, and unrealistic expectations of the course of the pregnancy and labor and delivery. Tran and Mai consider themselves to have strong emotional ties to one another. They are supportive of each other and agree that they seem able to communicate fairly well. Tran conveyed concern for Mai's moods of withdrawal and inability to verbalize her feelings of anger. Emotions are typically kept to herself. In Coughlin's work, one interview included the description of a good (Vietnamese) family as one that will treat a pregnant woman like a princess, pampering her and acceding to her every wish (Coughlin, 1965). Tran and Li seem to have formed an alliance in which they bond together to support Mai and relate to her gently. They did most of the speaking for her during the interviews and translated to clarify key questions. Although culturally understandable, this could foster her dependence on her family to meet her needs of effective communication.

Family Roles and Expectations

All three members of the family are anticipating the new baby with pleasure. Having been raised in traditional Vietnamese families, they respect their cultural heritage and believe the family to be important. When asked about raising their child in the American culture, Tran responded, "I think my baby was, born, okay I have to teach her. Sometimes we have to keep the Vietnamese idea in my family. I want to say no anything Vietnamese ideas very good, but I think American idea something very good. So we have to keep two of them in my family." Mai echoed, "together." In anticipating becoming parents,

Tran and Mai seem aware that their child will be raised in a different culture and have some understanding of the challenge before them. Another strength of the potential parent-child system is Tran's involvement in the pregnancy. He speaks about needing to move to a larger home and shopping for the baby's bed; he frequently speaks for Mai and asks questions related to her health. Mai and the other members of her family do not yet recognize her pregnancy as a child within her. Traditional Vietnamese belief is that the fetus attains a complete human form by the third month (Coughlin, 1965). The family feels once the baby moves (quickening) it will become more real to them and they will be able to continue in the tasks of pregnancy. Having no role models regarding pregnancy, childbirth, or the care of the newborn, the Vuong family has a knowledge deficit regarding the role changes and task realignment a new family member will bring into their home. In Vietnamese culture the fathers are not expected to participate in childbirth (Hollingsworth, Brown, & Booten, 1980); childbirth is regarded as a thing among women. Tran expressed feeling uncomfortable with entering the labor and delivery room. This may cause a conflict with the American expectation that fathers be involved in coaching the woman through labor and delivery. Mai very much wants a son. There is potential for her feeling like a failure if her first child is a daughter. Although all Vietnamese children are welcomed in the family and treated with equal tenderness, sons are definitely preferred (Coughlin, 1965). Due to a knowledge deficit regarding pregnancy, childbirth, and child care, Mai is at risk for difficulty in making the transition to the role of mother. Mai is reluctant to use her English language skills and has limited comprehension of the English language. This fosters dependency on her family and other members of her ethnic group to communicate for her. The family is interested in seeking out knowledge in the areas that they feel are lacking and are interested in the child preparation classes offered by the clinic. Because extended family is so important in the Vietnamese culture, having no grandmother in the same geographic location may make the transition of having a newborn more difficult for this family.

Recommendations

1. The family needs to be encouraged to participate in childbirth preparation classes. This will provide anticipatory guidance in relationship to the labor and delivery process. Li or another woman needs to accompany Mai to the classes even if Tran feels that he wants to be involved in the coaching of Mai's labor and delivery.

2. The family needs to find a trusted friend who might give them reliable information regarding what is normal in pregnancy, labor, delivery, and newborn care. They also need to ask questions of their physician and the clinic nurses.

3. Mai needs to learn to verbalize her feelings of anger in a culturally appropriate way to minimize future conflicts in interpersonal relationships.

4. The health providers of this family need to be made aware of the family's cultural differences and work with them within their cultural context. An example of this would be not to pressure Tran to be Mai's labor coach but rather allow a woman to be with her.

5. Mai needs to continue to hear from her family that it will be acceptable with them if she has a daughter rather than a son.

6. Mai needs to be encouraged to continue English classes and to use her language skills to decrease her dependency on others to communicate. The clinic should not rely on written learning materials to provide instructions to Mai.

As an outcome of this family assessment, Mai and Li did participate in the clinic's childbirth classes. They were also given needed attention when Mai came for her prenatal visits because the clinic staff was aware of her needs and appreciated cultural norms of the Vietnamese family. Most of the written teaching materials could not be used because of Mai's limited ability to read and understand English.

Childbirth is an important event in the lives of families, and cultural practices do affect how prenatal care is provided. Most nurses do not expect to be experts on all cultural groups and their beliefs about birth. Even if we could, variations exist even among people in the same cultural group. All nurses should be open and interested in learning about the needs and concerns of patients as influenced by culture. Suggestions are offered in Chapter 4. Nurses should respect each patient's background and through patient education help families form partnerships in prenatal care (Neeson & May, 1986).

The development of prenatal patient education materials to teach maternal nutrition has become a critical need in health care settings serving multilingual populations (Scharf, 1989). In addition to writing manuals in Lao, Vietnamese, Cambodian, and Spanish, work also includes the use of "nonlanguage" materials (Bruce, 1989).

Family-Focused Educational Intervention to Promote Recovery

The impact of diagnosis-related groups (DRGs) on hospital discharges is discussed in Chapter 1. Better discharge planning is noted as a possible device to prevent problems during the home recovery phase. In addition to discharge planning, the effectiveness of telephone calls by nurses to patients and their family members recovering at home after major cardiac surgery has been tested in two randomized clinical trials (Gortner, Gilliss, Sparacino, 1986; Gilliss, Gortner, Sparacino, 1989; Gortner, Gilliss, Shinn, 1988). This section of the chapter describes the clinical trial and interventions used to promote recovery of both the patient and family members after cardiac surgery. A case study is presented at the end of the chapter to illustrate the use of this patient education intervention with an elderly patient and his spouse.

A randomized clinical trial is a test of clinical interventions using subjects who are randomly assigned to either experimental or control status. Experimental subjects receive the intervention, and control subjects receive standard care. After the intervention has been completed, results from the two groups are compared to determine if there are differences between them.

In the two research trials referred to above, patients and family members assigned to the experimental group were prepared during the discharge teaching period and then telephoned at home by nurses who were clinically competent to counsel the patient and spouse using psychoeducational techniques. These psychoeducational patient education interventions involved three different phases.

The Psychoeducational Interventions

The *first phase* occurred in the hospital during the discharge teaching period. This phase included teaching risk factor reduction for the patient, skills such as dietary changes, appropriate exercise, cessation of smoking, and reduction or elimination of stressful life-style patterns. Slide-tape programs were used to teach the patient and spouse about risk factor reduction, resumption of sexual activity, and other common problems associated with the first 6 weeks of the home recovery period. The slide-tape programs, initially developed with nursing input, standardized the teaching and discharge preparation for all families and patients.

The combination of auditory and visual stimuli as a means of teaching patients and family members about risk factor reduction and resumption of activity expedited the teaching and assisted patient learning in situations where cognitive functions were not always completely intact. The slides and tapes also facilitated nurse follow-up because it was possible to refer back to the hospital teaching sessions and to reinforce the material taught in the hospital.

Phase two involved discharge teaching for the patient and family members and was oriented toward the emotional and psychological aspects of family recovery, as well as individual recovery. The work of Gilliss and Rankin has indicated that patients and family members may be at risk for disequilibrium after cardiac surgery with the reemergence of old conflicts and unhealthy behavior patterns not uncommon (Gilliss, 1983, 1984; Rankin, 1988). The stress of the surgical experience can reignite old problems and behaviors related to alcoholism, scapegoating of vulnerable family members, marital infidelity, and physical illness.

Because the care of the recovering patient usually is a family responsibility, and frequently a spousal task, the patient and spouse are sensitized during this discharge teaching period to the social and emotional issues frequently confronted during the first 6 weeks of home recovery. An original slide-tape program, "Working Together for Recovery," was developed for the project by Catherine Gilliss, a nurse, based on her earlier dissertation research and a college student whose father's experience with cardiac surgery had sensitized him to the problems encountered by families (Gilliss, 1983). "Working Together for Recovery" was formatted in slide-tape programs described in phase one and took 8 minutes to view. During phase two, patients and spouses are enlightened regarding common problems such as sleeplessness, anxiety, depression, overprotectiveness, and the medical regimen. Suggestions for coping with such problems are made in the slide-tape, and after the formal presentation, the nurse individualizes the session so that dilemmas particular to each couple can be discussed. For example, couples with young children are prepared for the children's needs for information.

During this session couples are encouraged to discuss their fears and to anticipate ways in which their relationship may be at risk for marital discord and disruption (Rankin & Gilliss, 1987). The nurse can use her own experience working with other couples to explain that fears related to recovery are universal. Indeed, the normalization of fears can be one of the most therapeutic aspects of this psychoeducational intervention.

The last aspect of this session is to offer various resources to the family to assist with the recovery period. In addition to information related to visiting nurses and home health aides, families are informed about the Mended Hearts self-help groups sponsored by the American Heart Association (AHA). Referrals to cardiac rehabilitation programs are made in consultation with the physician, and names of groups to assist in smoking cessation are also made available.

Phase three of the intervention involves telephone follow-up with the patient and spouse for a period of 8 weeks after discharge from the hospital. Intensive follow-up was deemed necessary for 8 weeks because it is during this period that most problems develop. This is compounded by the reality that length of inpatient stay has dramatically decreased. Most patients and family members have spoken of this 8-week period after discharge as the most difficult. As with many inpatient procedures, the patient and family contacts with the surgeon and other physicians decrease after discharge. During the first few weeks at home, patients and family members typically have many questions. Phase three allows for a reinforcement of phases one and two and is also an opportunity for the nurse to assist in early symptom identification and to reduce family strain. The protocol for phase three includes material from phases one and two and is intended to reinforce the earlier interventions (Gortner, Price, Rankin, 1985).

The model for the protocol used during phase three builds on the earlier work of a nurse in the Stanford Cardiac Rehabilitation program. Her work with patients and families after discharge enabled the research team to specify the protocol and make it appropriate to the special needs of recovering cardiac surgery patients and their spouses.

Nurses make their first telephone call to the family within 72 hours of hospital discharge. During this brief call the nurse ascertains the patient's health status and questions the family about any symptoms that might signify the need for a physician visit. The nurse also establishes the time and dates for future telephone calls so that the patient and spouse will expect telephone calls on a regular, ongoing basis. The form in Box 10-2 includes the questions and probes used by the nurse to monitor the recovery process, reinforce risk factor modification, and assist the patient and spouse with psychosocial issues related to recovery.

During the telephone calls, which occur weekly for 8 weeks, the nurse continues with symptom identification, reinforcement of risk factor modification, and referral when necessary to appropriate physician or, on occasion, mental health personnel. Patients and family members are typically concerned with their progress and the achievement of milestones indicating that recovery is pro-

BOX 10–2. Nursing Intervention to Monitor Recovery From Cardiac Surgery

Introduction: This is (interviewer's name) calling from the hospital. I am calling, as I said I would, to find out how you are doing. Is this a good time?

Concerns

1. How have you been since you came home (or, since I last spoke with you)? (Probes: How have you been spending your days? What do you do?)
2. What have been your major concerns since you came home (or, since I last spoke with you)? (Probes: Are there specific questions that have come up since you've come home? Are there specific situations related to the surgery that have come up since you've come home?)
3. What have you done about (the concern/question)? (Note: the nurse should explore each concern or question.)
4. How has that worked for you? (Note: the nurse should explore the effectiveness of each action.)
5. Do you think more action or a different action is necessary? (Probes: Have you been thinking about trying something else? Do you think you need additional help? From whom? What type of help?)

Recovery

6. How do you think you are recovering? (Probe: What makes you think that?)
7. You saw and heard a slide-tape presentation in the hospital about reducing risk factors associated with heart disease. These included stopping smoking, following a low-fat diet, getting daily exercise, reducing stress, and taking prescribed medication. Have you been trying to reduce your risks since you have come home from the hospital? (Probes: Which ones? Are there other things you have been doing which you think will help your recovery?)
8. Have you spoken to or seen your nurse or doctor since you have come home? (Probe: What did you talk about?)
9. How does she think you are recovering?

Spousal Involvement

10. How has your spouse been involved in taking care of you since you came home? (Probe: What sorts of things has your spouse been doing to help since you came home?)
11. How have you and (spouse's name) been spending your time together?
12. One of the slide-tape presentations you and your spouse saw in the hospital discussed both patient and spouse reactions to the stress of heart surgery. Some of the common reactions that were noted were feeling anxious, feeling depressed or blue, not sleeping well, arguing more with a spouse or family member, feeling irritable. Have any of these reactions occurred for you? (Probes: What have you been thinking about? How have you been behaving?)
13. Do you think (spouse's name) has been experiencing any of these reactions?
14. How have the two of you been handling these reactions together?
15. Have you thought of some (other) ways you might want to deal with the reactions? (Probe: What do you feel you need at this time?)

Conclusion and Summary

Mr./Mrs. I have no more questions, but I would like:

16. To know if you have additional concerns that you would like to discuss with me....
17. To go back to the concern you expressed regarding... (What you have said suggested to me that it might be helpful to describe the specific intervention suggested.)
18. To set up a time to talk on (date) at (time).

(continued)

BOX 10–2. *(Continued)*

Interviewer Recording

In addition to recording your interview notes, please complete the following regarding nursing diagnoses made during the interview and intervention used:

Problem/Nursing Diagnosis:

Intervention: _____ Provided new information relevant to current recovery

_____ Clarified information patient received in the hospital education program

_____ Reinforced information patient received in the hospital education program

_____ Provided comfort, reassurance, empathy

_____ Assisted patient/spouse in decision making

_____ Referred patient /spouse to _____ (person's name) for assistance

Reprinted with permission from Gortner, S., Gillis, C., Sparacino, P., (1989). *Improving recovery from cardiac surgery* (2R01-NR1031-03 Final Report). Bethesda, MD: National Center for Nursing Research, National Institutes of Health.

gressing as it should. Reassurances offered by nurses are helpful in maintaining the momentum of recovery and achieving the mastery needed to accomplish desired goals.

Spouses or other family members involved in caregiving are also contacted during the telephone calls. The form that is used to interview them is similar to that in Box 10-2. Frequently, they are more anxious than the recovering patient is but are afraid to voice these fears (Gilliss, 1984). Reassurance by the nurse that the patient is indeed progressing and that spousal fears are common helps alleviate some of the spousal emotional distress. During the calls, nurses often uncover physical and psychological problems related to recovery. For example, nurses have ascertained situations requiring referral to physicians related to iatrogenic hepatitis, postpericardotomy syndrome, congestive heart failure, and serious psychological disturbances Gillis, Tack, 1990).

Although patients and family members recalled the positive nature of weekly telephone calls from nurses, it was possible to demonstrate only slight differences in patient recovery for the experimental patients and no differences for the spouses during the first randomized clinical trial of 67 families. The second trial had a larger sample size (150 families), and statistically significant differences

were found between the control and experimental patients in terms of achievement of selected recovery milestones for both patients and family members. It may be that spouses in the experimental group are able to assist the recovering patient in achievement of these milestones.

The model for this psychoeducational patient teaching intervention is generic enough in its approach that it could be applied to many other surgical and illness situations involving protracted home recovery. For example, parents of newly diagnosed diabetic children have frequently spoken of their immediate concerns regarding diet and control of hypoglycemic episodes. Scheduled telephone calls to the family by nurses could provide assistance with such concerns. The nurse in this situation could troubleshoot potential problem areas such as the needs of siblings in families with a chronically ill child and the distinction between normal growth and development versus disease-related issues. The model has been successfully applied in other settings and is also being used in cardiac rehabilitation programs.

The combination of physiologic and psychological preparation of the nurse makes her uniquely qualified to help patients and families. Such assistance is also much more economical than visits to the doctor's office or hospitalizations resulting from late identification of problems.

❑ CASE STUDY

Fred Scott

Fred Scott is a 73-year-old man admitted to a northern California regional medical center for a double valve replacement and a coronary artery bypass graft of two arteries with lesions. Mr. Scott has a 55-year history of smoking two packs of cigarettes a day and a documented history of emphysema. Mr. Scott has been referred to the medical center from a small hospital in the mountains of eastern California.

Fred and Irma Scott have been married for 50 years and have two grown children, one of whom lives 75 miles away from her parents. Their son lives out of state and cannot be counted on for caregiving responsibilities. Mrs. Scott presently is managing their small 25-acre farm, on which they have a few head of cattle and three horses. Mr. and Mrs. Scott are high school graduates and can read and write English without problems.

The nurse first met the Scotts the day before he was discharged from the hospital. At this time she showed the Scotts and their daughter the slide-tape presentations prepared by the AHA that covered what to expect the first 6 weeks at home. After their daughter left the hospital, the nurse showed the couple "Working Together for Recovery" and together they discussed Mrs. Scott's tendency to be overprotective and Mr. Scott's frequent failure to communicate his feelings to his wife, which results in tension for both of them. The nurse who did all of the discharge teaching for cardiac surgery patients also instructed the couple regarding medications, diet, smoking and follow-up appointments.

The nurse telephoned Mrs. Scott within 72 hours of her husband's discharge and Mrs. Scott reported that her husband was doing well although he was very tired from the 6-hour drive home. In response to questions about how she had been involved in caring for her husband since he came home, Mrs. Scott admitted that she was actually looking forward to taking care of her husband because she had "always wanted to be a nurse" and also because she felt committed to her husband after 50 years of marriage. A time and date for the following call was established and Mrs. Scott was given a telephone number to reach the nurse in case of emergency.

A week later the nurse telephoned the Scotts and discovered that Mr. Scott was short of breath. After collecting more data related to Mr. Scott's symptomatology and medications, the nurse discovered that the couple was confused about the instructions they had received during discharge teaching regarding the administration of his medications, and Mr. Scott had not been taking them as prescribed. The nurse clarified the medication regimen and also collected data related to diet and exercise and how Mrs. Scott was coping in terms of caregiving. Both admitted to fatigue and feeling somewhat blue although they felt Mr. Scott was making progress.

The third call 2 weeks after hospital discharge found Mr. Scott taking small walks around the farm and generally feeling much better. Mrs. Scott seemed to be working hard on changing their diet to meet the recommendations made in the hospital, and she was also monitoring Mr. Scott's medications. The fourth and fifth calls were similar in nature to the third, and the couple and the nurse began to believe that Mr. Scott was "out of the woods." Risk factor modification was the primary theme of these three telephone calls. Both the patient and spouse responded to the nurse's questions by stating that they were sleeping much better and their dual anxieties and depressions had lifted.

The fifth week after discharge from the hospital the nurse discovered that Mr. Scott had been having more difficulty breathing. She suggested that Mrs. Scott take her husband to his local medical doctor and then call her with the results. Mrs. Scott followed the nurse's advice, driving her husband 25 miles on snowy roads to his doctor. Mrs. Scott called the nurse the next day to say that her husband was hospitalized and was having increasing difficulty breathing. The focus of the nurse's interventions shifted to provide support for Mrs. Scott and to reinforce the excellent nature of the home "nursing" she had been providing.

Six weeks after discharge from the first hospital Mr. Scott was still hospitalized although he had begun to respond to intensive antibiotic and respiratory therapy. During the seventh week after the original discharge after surgery, Mr. Scott returned home.

Mrs. Scott drew up a written schedule of medication times and dosages at the nurse's recommendation. She encouraged her husband to return to exercise routines with guidelines established by the nurse. Hypervigilance on the part of Mrs. Scott became a problem for the couple and interfered with Mrs. Scott's ability to obtain adequate rest. However, the nurse was able to decrease Mrs. Scott's anxiety through her reassurances and attempts to help Mrs. Scott voice her worries.

Although Mr. Scott was not as fully recovered at 8 weeks after surgery as many patients are, he had resumed light work on the farm, was taking all of his medications on schedule, and had regained 1.4 kg (3 lb) of the 4.54 kg (10 lb) he had lost after surgery. Mrs. Scott admitted that she continued to worry about her husband, but stated during the last scheduled telephone call that she felt comfortable calling the nurse for reassurance and advice.

Summary

This chapter discussed two community-based patient education interventions. The first described prenatal classes, initiated by the nursing staff of a family practice center to address the educational needs of their obstetric population. The program was designed to appeal to all patients in the prenatal practice and to encourage the development of labor coaches, especially among unmarried mothers. Methods of needs assessments were described, class objectives were offered, and evaluation strategies were suggested based on their successful use in the family practice prenatal program. A case study was presented to demonstrate the effects of culture and its impact on prenatal education needs for a Vietnamese family. It illustrated the need for a combined format of individual and group teaching. Also described were interventions for patient and family members after cardiac surgery, beginning in the hospital and reaching into the home through a telephone follow-up program. This patient education program encompasses three phases and each phase builds on the previous one. These interventions are referred to as psychoeducational patient education because they include teaching and psychosocial strategies to enhance the recovery of both the patient and family.

The case study of Fred Scott was presented to illustrate that although the recovery from cardiac surgery was stormy, the intervention improved the quality of the patient's life and also supported the primary caregiver. The nurse's early intervention and recommendation that medical care be sought during the patient's increasing respiratory problems was thought to have prevented more serious sequelae. The model for the intervention could be used in various situations of health and illness.

Strategies for Critical Analysis and Application

1. Identify a need for health education in your community, which might be met by a group or community program.

2. Describe how you might involve patients, family members, community leaders, and health care professionals to plan and promote the program.

3. Identify potential costs of offering the program and potential sources of funding.

REFERENCES

Bruce, L. (1989). *Nonlanguage nutrition education: An alternative for a multilingual population in Nutrition Education Opportunities: Strategies to help clients with limited reading skills.* Report of the Second Ross Roundtable on Current Issues in Public Health (pp. 71-75). Columbus, OH: Ross Laboratories.

Calhoun, M. (1985). The Vietnamese women: Health/illness attitudes and behaviors. *Health Care Women International, 6,* 61-72.

Coughlin, R. (1965). Pregnancy and childbirth in Vietnam. In D. Hart, P. Rapidhon, & R. Coughlin (Eds.), *Southeast Asian birth customs: Three studies in human reproduction* (pp. 207-270). New Haven, CT: Human Relations Area Files.

Cowan, A. (1994). Division of adult health promotion and black churches team up to fight cancer. In Health Bulletin. *Raleigh: North Carolina Department of Environment, Health, and Natural Resources, 3*(7), 7-10.

Dickman, F., & Keil, T. (1977). Public television and public health: The case of alcoholism. *Journal of Studies on Alcohol, 38*(3), 584.

Dyson, B., & Dyson, E. (1979). The health team in primal community: A new context for community medicine. *Patient Counseling and Health Education, 1*(3), 122-127.

Gilliss, C. (1983). *Identification of factors contributing to family function following coronary artery bypass surgery.* Unpublished doctoral dissertation, University of California Medical Center Library, San Francisco.

Gilliss, C. (1984). Reducing family stress during and after coronary artery bypass surgery. *Nursing Clinics of North America, 19*(1), 103-112.

Gilliss, C., Gortner, S., & Sparacino, P. (1989). *Improving recovery from cardiac surgery* (2R01-NR1031-03 Final Report). Bethesda, MD: National Center for Nursing Research, National Institutes of Health.

Gilliss, C., & Tack, B. (1990). Nurse-monitored cardiac recovery: A description of the first eight weeks. *Heart and Lung, 19,* 491-499.

Gortner, S., Gilliss, C., & Shinn, J. (1988). Improving recovery following cardiac surgery: A randomized clinical trial. *Journal of Advanced Nursing, 13,* 649-661.

Gortner, S., Gilliss, C., & Sparacino, P. (1986). *Improving recovery from cardiac surgery* (NU 0131-02 Final Report). Bethesda, MD: Division of Nursing, National Institutes of Health.

Gortner, S., Price, M., Rankin, S., (1985). After cardiac surgery: Monitoring recovery by telephone. Abstract No. 339, *Circulation, 72,* III-98.

Green, L. (1980). To educate or not to educate: Is that the question? *American Journal of Public Health, 70*(6), 625-627.

Grosso, C., Barden, M., Henry, C., & Vieau, M. (1981). The Vietnamese American family...and grandma makes three. *MCN; American Journal of Maternal Child Nursing, 6,* 177-180.

Hochbaum, G. (1979). An alternate approach to health education. *Health Values, 3*(4), 197-201.

Hollingsworth, A., Brown, L., & Booten, D. (1980). The refugees and childbearing: What to expect. *RN, 4,* 45-48.

Nguyen, M. (1988). Culture shock—a review of Vietnamese culture and its concepts of health and disease. *Western Journal of Medicine, 142,* 409-412.

Rankin, S. (1988). *Gender, age, and caregiving as mediators of cardiovascular illness and recovery.* Unpublished doctoral dissertation, University of California Medical Center Library, San Francisco.

Rankin, S., & Gilliss, C. (1987). Intervening with middle-aged families recovering from cardiac surgery. In L. Wright & M. Leahey (Eds.), *Families and chronic illness* (pp. 367-380). Springhouse, PA: Springhouse Publishing.

Richman, L., & Urban, D. (1978). Health education through television: Some theoretical applications. *International Journal of Health Education, 21,* 46-52.

Salber, E. (1979). The lay advisor as a community health resource. *Journal of Health Politics, Policy and Law, 3*(4), 469-478.

Scharf, M. (1989). *Eating well without reading well: Designing a guidebook for urban teenagers in nutrition education opportunities: Strategies to help clients with limited reading skills.* Report of the Second Ross Roundtable on Current Issues in Public Health (pp. 33-41). Columbus, OH: Ross Laboratories.

11 Evaluation: Determining and Documenting Patient Learning Outcomes

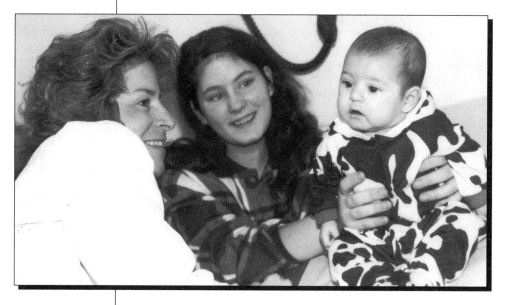

OBJECTIVES FOR CHAPTER 11

After reading this chapter, the nurse or student nurse should be able to:

1 Describe ways in which evaluation and documentation of learning can be integrated in basic nursing care, including medication administration, dressing changes, and bathing.

2 Identify four levels of evaluation and provide examples of patient learning outcomes that can be identified in each level.

3 Discuss how the problem-oriented record (POR) can be used to encourage interdisciplinary collaboration.

4 Describe how evidence of individualized patient care can be shown when "charting by exception."

5 Discuss how evaluation relates to assessment in the nursing process.

Assessing Outcomes of Patient Education

Patient education is an appealing concept. Our visceral reaction is that the instructed patient fares better than the uninstructed one. It is, however, difficult to evaluate concretely the many outcomes of patient education.

Evaluation is an essential component of the nursing process, yet it is one that is often neglected and misunderstood. Why is it that we frequently cannot find time to evaluate patient education or that we fail to document learning? Why does the word evaluation cause us to feel uneasy and uncertain?

To evaluate is "to determine the significance, or worth of by careful appraisal or study."[1] All too often, nurses and patients alike feel threatened by the thought of evaluation. We worry about being personally devalued or judged unworthy. We recall our humiliation when, as children, we failed in a test or a spelling bee, and we do not want to feel that way again. We fear that if we fail to achieve what others expect of us, we will lose love, support, assistance, esteem, and credibility.

The actual intent of evaluation is not to place a value or worth on patients or nurses. Its purposes are to measure the degree to which goals have been met, to define specific outcomes, and to redirect patient care. Evaluation of patient education involves collecting specific and descriptive data related to behaviors targeted as patient learning objectives. Through evaluation, the nurse and the patient determine the value of the nursing interventions in helping the patient to carry out desired behaviors. We must also determine the likelihood that the patient can be safely discharged from our care based on the ability for self-management and what resources are needed for continuing care.

In addition to misunderstanding the meaning of evaluation, many nurses underestimate its importance in patient education. In the past, many nurses thought about patient teaching as simply giving information. Nurses have not always considered patient teaching as a valid nursing intervention for response to specific client needs or problems. As we become aware that the nursing process directs the delivery of patient education, just as it directs other nursing interventions, we recognize that evaluation is a component of the nursing process, deserving of our attention (Fig. 11-1). This chapter offers a better understanding of evaluation, addresses methods of data collection, and discusses how to use the information gained in evaluation to reinforce learning and to plan future learning opportunities for patients. The examples offered in this chapter focus on education of individual patients and their families. Strategies for evaluating organizational approaches and community programs for patient education are discussed in Chapter 2.

Although evaluation is the fourth step in patient education, it is not an end point. As illustrated in Figure 7-1 in Chapter 7, evaluation links us back to assessment, and the nursing process continues. Not only do we determine if the patient met the goal, but we determine why or why not. The barriers that prevented the outcomes we targeted must be confronted as the nurse-patient relationship continues. A staff RN from an outpatient clinic in the Boston area shared this experience:

> There are numerous barriers when educating a client with HIV/AIDS. One of the more pronounced I have encountered in my career is when a goal has been set to change behaviors. A person with HIV/AIDS has a great responsibility to society; that would be to slow the rate of transmission of this virus. The nurse can facilitate education, provide information, and make recommendations for a healthy life-style, but the ultimate responsibility is the client's. The educator is further challenged when the client is an active injection drug user, or when the client has expressed a loss of hope for the future. Instilling that hope and setting individualized goals with clients is the first step in overcoming barriers to patient education and ultimately changing behaviors.

---

[1]By permission. From *Webster's New Collegiate Dictionary* © 1979 by G & C Merriam Company, publishers of the Merriam-Webster Dictionaries.

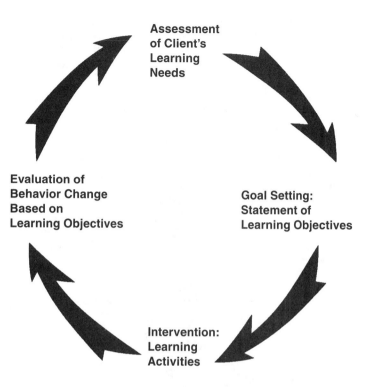

FIGURE 11–1. Evaluation is part of a continuous process in patient education.

Documentation of learning is also addressed in this chapter. The patient's record should reflect what the patient knows, understands, or performs; it emphasizes patient outcomes. Components of nursing documentation systems are reviewed and discussed as they relate to patient education.

Scope of Evaluation

Evaluation is closely related to assessment. Both involve formulating criteria or questions, gathering and categorizing data, and writing a summary statement. These findings are used in patient care planning. *Assessment* usually refers to building a data base that includes nursing diagnoses and outlines the patient's needs or problems. *Evaluation* refers to the *follow-up assessment* that is continuously conducted as nursing interventions are carried out. Therefore, evaluation occurs throughout the learning activities and is used to assess the patient's progress toward meeting learning ob-

jectives. Understanding the information and skills introduced in Chapter 7 is important in preparing for evaluation. We encourage the reader to review that chapter's information about the assessment process.

Evaluation is conducted using the behavioral objectives discussed in Chapter 8. If the patient objectives are clearly defined, evaluation is straightforward. Measurement is based on the stated behaviors. The patient and family should be active participants in evaluating learning. Through self-evaluation, based on his own learning objectives, a patient can define what is expected of him, he can plan and participate in learning activities, and he can seek feedback to direct his performance. Evaluation becomes a learning experience that can increase the patient's self-esteem as he recognizes his own accomplishments and gains positive feedback and support from others.

Evaluation is also a learning opportunity for the teacher. The feedback she receives from the patient's progress or lack of progress helps her to modify her approach and to consider alternate teaching strategies. These may include providing the learner with more review, clarifying learning objectives, and changing teaching or learning methods and media.

Evaluation is thus a continuous process conducted by the teacher and learner throughout patient education. Using the evaluation process, both parties benefit from feedback that reinforces successes and readdresses problems. There are certain times when evaluation is more formally conducted and includes the use of written documentation as well as oral feedback. This documentation usually occurs at the ends of nursing shifts, after classes or skills training, and before the patient's discharge from the hospital or office. Just as the assessment process involves asking questions to gather specific information, so does the evaluation process. The evaluation process should include:

Measuring the extent to which the patient has met the learning objectives: what are the outcomes of patient education?

Indicating when there is a need to clarify, correct, or review information

Noting objectives that are unclear

Pointing out shortcomings in the patient teaching interventions, specifically addressing content, format, activities, and media

Identifying barriers that prevented learning

In patient education, it is the teacher's responsibility to initiate the evaluation, summarize the findings, document findings in the medical record, give constructive feedback to the patient and family, plan future experiences to reinforce learning, and design learning opportunities to foster behaviors that were not initially accomplished.

The teacher must be prepared by knowing what questions to ask and by having a good understanding of each component of the patient education process. In addition to first measuring behavior, the nurse looks critically at nursing care and identifies problems that have prevented learning.

Determination of Patient Learning Outcomes

Evidence of patient learning outcomes has received new emphasis as a result of the guidelines of the Joint Commission on the Accreditation of Healthcare Organizations (JCAHO) that made patient education a special focus survey area beginning in 1993 (JCAHO, 1994). Nurses express concern that with shorter inpatient stays, they are expected to produce unrealistic learning outcomes. Chapter 2 outlines the JCAHO standards, emphasizing that teaching should be appropriate to length of stay and understandable to the patient.

Learning outcomes can be accomplished in any setting, even if the patient is there only a matter of minutes. It is helpful to consider that there are four levels of learning outcomes, addressing different increments of learning (Fig. 11-2). The nurse is able to evaluate a patient's learning in one or more levels.

Level A: Patient's Participation During Interventions

The teacher assesses the level of participation of the learners. Was education provided for this patient? Was the learner present, that is, physical presence at a class or alert presence for individual teaching? Does he ask questions? Does he seem alert and interested? Is he able to comprehend instructions? Is he able and willing to assume responsibility for learning? Are learning experiences relevant to his individual situation? Does he participate in discussion, demonstrations, and problem-solving? Were concepts too basic or did he feel overloaded and overwhelmed by the amount of instruction? Were learning objectives and desired outcomes clear to the learner? (Did he know what he was expected to do?) Did family members participate? Evaluation of readiness should not be overlooked. Counseling patients during the initial shock of an illness or disability, helping them ac-

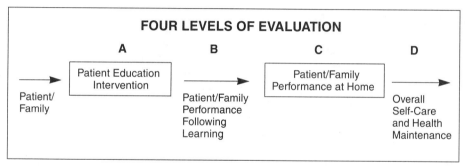

FIGURE 11–2. Levels of evaluation. (Adapted from Brethower, K. S. & Rummler, G.A. [1979]. Evaluating training. *Training and Development Journal, May,* 12–20.)

cept it, and encouraging them to focus on how they will live their lives in the future are some of the greatest challenges facing nurses. Interventions and evaluation related to this counseling and the patient's response are seldom documented.

JCAHO (1994) sees the following outcomes as key:

Patient and family understanding of the current health problem, reason for admission

Patient received informed consent

Patient and family understand the treatment plan and the role they will play

Patient has overview of survival skills needed for safe discharge

Level B: Patient's Performance Immediately After Learning Experience

Was the patient able to meet performance standards (objectives) as a result of the learning experience? To what extent did he meet objectives? Describe the patient's performance rather than what the nurse did. How should future teaching be conducted? Outcomes should reflect knowledge and survival skills to participate in self-care. Individual needs, patient readiness, and patient learning abilities should be assessed. JCAHO is particularly interested in the following areas of teaching:

Safe and effective use of medications
Medical equipment
Potential food-drug interactions
Rehabilitation techniques
Community resources
How to obtain further treatment
Ongoing health care needs

Level C: Patient's Performance at Home

Was the patient given written discharge instructions that were understandable to him? Did patient and family perform the desired behaviors at home? To what extent did they follow the recommended plan? If they had difficulty, was this a result of not remembering, inability to perform the skill, or misunderstanding instructions? Did they change their minds about willingness to perform the behaviors? Did physical limitations or financial barriers prevent them from self-care? Was a continuing care provider identified and given instructions to promote continuity of care?

Step D: Patient's Overall Self-Care and Health Management

Was overall management successful in preventing or controlling health problems? Did physiologic data (blood pressure, blood glucose level, handling emergencies, readmission) reflect successful self-care? What were long-term results?

Which Level of Evaluation Is Best?

Ideally, evidence of learning in each level can be assessed for each patient. However, nurses are limited in evaluation if they are not able to follow the patient's entire course, from admission to home, and possibly to readmission. Nurses must realize that all levels of evaluation provide important evidence. For example, if a patient does not perform a skill at home, we must know whether he was provided and received instruction. Otherwise, it is hard to pinpoint the difficulty and improve the intervention. Valuable time may be lost recreating the assessment of potential barriers to learning. Every nurse who teaches a patient can document an outcome at some level, and learning outcomes can be reflected in documentation in the patient's record on a daily basis.

Frequently we hear, "I'd love to do patient education, but I don't have the time to teach and document it with all the paperwork and other demands placed on me." We feel that many golden opportunities for patient education are lost during the typical day. For instance, bath time can be used for teaching the diabetic about good skin and foot care, the surgical patient about dressing or cast care, the patient with chronic obstructive lung disease about breathing exercises, and so on. Medication time can be used to teach the patient with congestive heart failure how to take his pulse before self-administering medication or to teach the patient with rheumatoid arthritis how he can safely taper off steroids. Any time we enter a patient's room can be an opportunity to do some patient teaching. The astute nurse who does make use of these moments must also remember to document her teaching in the patient's chart.

Evaluation of Patient Education Interventions

This step in evaluation looks at both the teacher and the learner. General principles of assessment and motivation are important. We need to know if the climate was set for the patient to be a colleague and the nurse to be consultant in learning about the self-care regimens. We want to determine if the teaching-learning process was interesting, clear, and stimulating to the learner. We determine the patient's ability and desire to learn by observing both verbal and nonverbal responses. We especially want to know if the patient and family understand the learning objectives and desired outcomes for learning. Data gathered in this step are used to modify the climate or patient education interventions. Data are gathered by interview, questionnaire, and observation.

We suggest that nurses formulate a series of questions to provide direction in the evaluation of the patient education process. We have constructed a checklist with our questions (Fig. 11-3). We have included references to the text to encourage readers to review principles introduced in other chapters.

The nurse should take a critical view of the teaching and learning interventions that were designed to help the patient achieve his goals and gain knowledge, attitudes, and skills. The following questions help in determining which interventions have been effective and in what areas changes might be made to improve nursing care.

Format. Was the patient taught by self-study, individual instruction, or group instruction? Was the format compatible with the learning objectives and with the patient's condition and learning style?

Content. Did the patient receive the necessary facts and training to learn the desired behaviors?

Teaching and learning activities. Was the patient given an opportunity to actively participate, ask questions, and practice? Were the patient's past experiences used as resources for learning? Were the patient's social roles and developmental tasks acknowledged? Was learning practical and problem centered? Was there an opportunity for immediate applica-

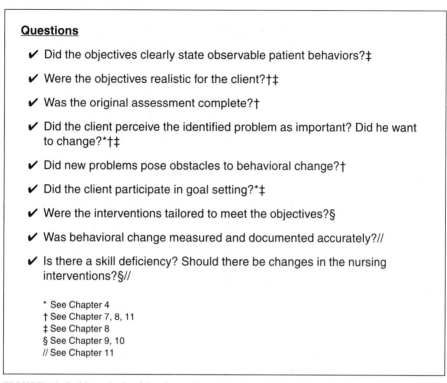

Questions

✔ Did the objectives clearly state observable patient behaviors?‡

✔ Were the objectives realistic for the client?†‡

✔ Was the original assessment complete?†

✔ Did the client perceive the identified problem as important? Did he want to change?*†‡

✔ Did new problems pose obstacles to behavioral change?†

✔ Did the client participate in goal setting?*‡

✔ Were the interventions tailored to meet the objectives?§

✔ Was behavioral change measured and documented accurately?//

✔ Is there a skill deficiency? Should there be changes in the nursing interventions?§//

* See Chapter 4
† See Chapter 7, 8, 11
‡ See Chapter 8
§ See Chapter 9, 10
// See Chapter 11

FIGURE 11–3. Nurse's checklist for evaluation of patient education.

tion by the learner? Were the learning methods and media appropriate for the types of learning objectives?

Media. Were the media able to deliver the message in a manner that the patient and family could understand?

Patient and family satisfaction. Do the patient and the family have suggestions for improving the patient education experience? Which activities did they find most helpful and which seemed least helpful? Did they feel supported in the learning environment? Were their concerns addressed? Did they feel confident of the staff's preparation to teach? Was the content understandable and practical?

Time, cost, and resources involved. Were resources of staff and facilities adequate for teaching? If not, which unmet staff needs posed barriers to patient learning?

Recommendations of the staff. Do nurses and other members of the health care team have suggestions? How do they assess the quality of the patient learning experience? Were the contributions of staff members in teaching the patient and family coordinated? Did they feel prepared to teach? If not, what training should be offered to the staff?

Patient and Family Performance Immediately After Learning

The teacher uses learning objectives as a yardstick to measure the patient's ability to assume self-care. Learning objectives describe the behaviors the patient will perform to show that he has mastered knowledge, attitudes, and skills. They are tailored to the patient's individual goals.

Recall that a learning objective has three components: performance, conditions, and criteria (Mager, 1975). *Performance* states what the learner will do and uses an action verb that describes a measurable activity. In choosing the action verb, the teacher asks: "Can I measure this behavior?" The verb is carefully selected so that the learner and the teacher both have a clear understanding of how the learner will demonstrate competence. *Conditions* state special activities to be included in the learner's performance. Sterile technique used in insulin administration is an example of a condition. *Criteria* state how well or how long the behavior must be performed to show mastery. To summarize, the three characteristics of a learning objective are that it is specific, that it is measurable, and that it is attainable.

To evaluate patient education, the teacher uses performance, conditions, and criteria to measure the patient's progress. The measurements should be collected accurately and should reflect qualitative and quantitative data.

In Chapter 7 the following learning objective was offered as an example: The patient will draw up and administer 22 units of insulin using sterile technique at 7:00 AM on 3 consecutive days.

Qualitative data might include the following statement: "The patient was able to perform sterile technique in preparing the injection but could not accurately measure the units of insulin." Quantitative data might include this statement: "The patient was able to perform sterile technique correctly only once. In the other two efforts, he contaminated the needle by placing it on the table uncapped." Specific data help the nurse and the patient to focus on problem areas and to acknowledge progress that is made toward meeting the objective.

Patient and Family Performance at Home

This area of evaluation is often difficult because in many cases we are not able to provide continuous care. Outpatient follow-up may be difficult because the patient is discharged to a different city, follow-up appointments are infrequent, home health services may not be available, or there is little communication about patient teaching between agencies.

We do need to know how the patient is doing at home. Does the patient feel competent to manage self-care? Does the home environment present any barriers to self-care? Is the regimen flexible enough? Is the patient able to handle problems or temporary relapses constructively? If emergencies have occurred, did the patient or family respond appropriately? Is the patient still assuming responsibility for self-care? Unfortunately, we often don't learn about patient difficulties until a crisis, such as readmission, occurs. Interventions such as telephone follow-up, postcards, home visits by students, and better communication between the hospital and outpatient clinic can improve evaluation of the patient and family performance.

One of the most important things a home health nurse does is to continue patient education. A home health nurse offers the following advice:

> You've got to be a good listener, a teacher, and an observer. They may tell you one thing, and you observe another. You can't assume anything. They have to demonstrate it back to me. Are they living it? You can't force them to change their lifestyle. It's not like the hospital where if you don't want them to have sweets or salt, you simply refuse them. This is the real world where they have a salt shaker on the counter and a daughter who brings in doughnuts. We're there to teach and encourage, not boss and demand. (Bovender, 1994)

Patient Overall Self-Care and Health Maintenance

This method of evaluation takes a broader look at the patient's course before and after the learning of new behaviors. Information is collected about absences from work or school, hospitalizations, episodes of acute complications, and daily management. Research data are usually gathered to measure the long-term value of patient education interventions. In addition, they may be used to substantiate requests for third-party reimbursement of patient teaching and negotiated managed-care contracts.

Methods of Measurement

There are several ways to gather information to evaluate learning. The nurse should remember that adults learn best with immediate application of knowledge, attitudes, and skills. Evaluation becomes a learning experience when it is prompt and when it is an exercise shared with the learner. The feedback reinforces positive behaviors and guides the correction of misunderstandings and performance problems. Because evaluation is a problem-solving process, the learner gains skill in managing problems by working with the teacher.

Seven methods are commonly used by nurses to evaluate patient learning.

Direct Observation

Watching the patient perform a skill or having him role play a situation offers two valuable opportunities. First, accurate, descriptive data can be collected. Second, the learner receives immediate feedback and guidance. We encourage nurses to use direct observation whenever possible, rather than to rely on reports and assumptions. Patients should be encouraged to demonstrate self-care activities and should be given professional guidance to reinforce learning. Examples of opportunities for direct observation are when the patient changes dressings, administers medication, performs breast self-examination, or selects foods according to a prescribed diet plan.

Patient Records

We must often rely on patients to keep records of their performance. Although teaching be-

gins in the company of health care professionals, much of the actual learning occurs in the home when the patient and family assume total responsibility. Although reinforcement of positive behavior is essential to the continuance of learning, it is not easily provided when opportunities for observation are lacking. Asking the patient to keep specific records and to present them to the nurse at a later time reinforces the patient's responsibility, reinforces positive behaviors, helps the patient to evaluate his own progress, and provides the nurse with data for evaluation. This method has worked well in evaluating cooperation with medical regimens, diet modification, stress management, and treatments carried out at home. Whenever it is possible to supplement patient records with direct observation by the nurse, this should be done to increase objectivity.

Reports

Patient and family reports are used as sources of data although their objectivity is often questioned. Reports can be accompanied by measurements such as pill counts, weight, and blood tests. Reporting should be solicited from the patient and family through carefully constructed questions. For example, the nurse will get more specific and descriptive data by asking, "What medications did you take today and at what times did you take them?" than she would by asking, "Are you taking your medication as you were instructed?" Patients can be taught to be good reporters if they are given specific directions about collecting and recording significant information and if they are told how they are expected to contribute to the evaluation process.

Tests

Oral and written tests can be used before learning activities and repeated at intervals following instruction. This method is effective in measuring the patient's progress toward meeting cognitive objectives, and it offers objective data about his ability to retain what he has learned. Tests require the patient to be an active participant in defining learning needs and in recognizing positive change. Tests are often used to teach and evaluate daily management decisions made by patients and their families dealing with chronic illness. As with the tests discussed in Chapters 9 and 10, tests used for evaluation should present problems in a sequence, from simple to complex, and the tool should be appropriate for the patient's literacy level.

Interviews With and Questionnaires Completed by Patients and Family

Patients and their families may be interviewed or given written questionnaires to assess their degrees of confidence in new knowledge and skills. They may evaluate their own progress, define their learning needs, and offer suggestions for future training. We have used questionnaires of this nature in the evaluation of prenatal classes, newborn care instruction, and stress management classes. We emphasize the importance of asking specific questions that do not require long, general responses and of phrasing the questions so that the learner can understand them. Questionnaires are inappropriate for illiterate patients and family members. You may also ask patients to write a letter describing the birth experience or a surgical experience and explaining how prepared they felt for it. They can offer suggestions for how to best prepare others based on their experiences.

Interviews With and Questionnaires Completed by Staff

Staff members contributing to the patient's care can offer important information about his progress. Although one nurse coordinates the patient's care, many health professionals, including those from other disciplines, gather evaluative data. They should be asked to con-

tribute these important measurements. This can be done efficiently with brief, carefully worded questions used in interviews and surveys. The questions should focus on specific, measurable behaviors. Data are also found in their notes in the medical record.

Critical Incidents

Research can be used to follow up patients over a predetermined period of time to look for such incidents as readmission, complications, and mortality.

Length of Stay

Patient education can reduce length of stay by enabling the patient to better participate in his recovery and preparation for discharge. Teaching must be updated and streamlined to accommodate shorter lengths of stay in the hospital. When determining goals for patient teaching, estimated length of stay associated with the diagnosis-related group (DRG) or case type guides the nurse in keeping the teaching plans realistic. The nurse should be familiar with DRGs frequently seen on her unit and the associated length of stay. For example, if the cardiac arrest DRG has a mean stay of 5 days, a cardiac rehabilitation program should be carried out with this discharge goal in mind.

Assessment of Learning: Comparing Four Levels of Evaluation

Data from a combination of evaluation sources should be assimilated and the results should be summarized. This procedure is similar to that of categorization of information and writing a summary statement in assessment.

The first question to be answered is: "To what extent were the learning objectives accomplished?" The answer to this initial question guides us in asking further questions:

If the behavior was successfully performed, how can it be reinforced?

If the behavioral objective was *not* met, was the patient able to perform the behavior in the past?

If he was able to perform it in the past, why has he failed to perform it now?

Evaluation does not simply provide us with one "Yes" or "No" answer. Instead, it becomes another starting point in the continuous nursing process. We gather data and offer feedback about the learning experience from the patient, the family, the health care team, and the institution. We also look to others for return feedback about the quality of our nursing interventions. Feedback is a learning tool that can be powerful in guiding behavior when it is used positively. Tips on giving feedback are offered later in this chapter.

Conclusions drawn from evaluation should be carefully considered. Often data are limited or absent at one level of evaluation. In this case, conclusions at a higher level may be inaccurate.

For example, if information is collected at level D (overall self-care) to reflect that blood pressure has not declined, it is inaccurate to assume that the patient did not know how to follow the regimen (level B) or that he was not following the treatment plan at home (level C) unless evaluation was conducted at all levels. Ideally, evaluation occurs at each level and modifications are made to the teaching plan to build success at each level.

Assessment of Learning: Identifying Needs and Performance Problems

In Chapter 8 we introduced a flow diagram to illustrate the use of behavioral objectives in the learning process (see Fig. 8-1 in Chap. 8). This figure guides the nurse in following the evaluation.

If the desired behavior is accomplished, the nurse provides opportunities for reinforcing the positive behavior. Clinic visits, home visits, telephone calls, and community resources offer such opportunities. The patient and the family can demonstrate the knowledge and skills they have retained and ask for the review or guidance that they need. The health care team should encourage clients to take advantage of these learning resources. When learning behaviors are not accomplished, or are only partially accomplished, the patient educator must reassess and readdress barriers to behavioral change. Mager and Pipe (1970) provide a model for problem-solving to determine client learning needs (Fig. 11-4). We must reconsider whether or not the particular behavior is important and necessary. If so, we ask if a skill deficiency is present. If the patient has never been able to perform the skill, the teacher should provide additional training. If the skill will be used infrequently, feedback and practice should be arranged. For example, insulin injection is often learned with some initial difficulty, but the skill is used so often that it is retained and reinforced. Breast self-examination is performed less often, so this technique and the importance of its performance may need more reinforcement.

If the patient has demonstrated the ability to perform the skill but has not continued to perform it, four additional questions direct the teacher's problem-solving. Mager and Pipe suggest that if performing the skill somehow punishes the patient, we should identify the source of punishment and remove it.

1. Why does the patient feel punished? For example, patients who are on special diets often complain that they are not able to follow their diet while socializing with friends. Locating other sources of support, such as support groups of dieters, may remove the feeling of being different or punished.

2. Does the patient see the performance as unrewarding? If so, the teacher can arrange positive consequences by offering additional support and more frequent follow-up visits and reporting mechanisms, so that the patient will see his improvement more clearly.

**WHEN CLIENTS FAIL TO MEET LEARNING OBJECTIVES:
IS THERE A SKILL DEFICIENCY?**

Yes	No
1. Has the client ever demonstrated the ability to perform the skill? If not, *formal training* is required.	1. Is the performance of the skill punishing? If so, *remove punishment.*
2. Is the skill used often? If not, *arrange practice.* If so, *arrange feedback.*	2. Is nonperformance rewarding? If so, *arrange a positive consequence.*
	3. Does the client feel that it doesn't matter if he performs the behavior? If so, *arrange a consequence.*
	4. Are there obstacles to performing the behavior? If so, *remove obstacles.*

FIGURE 11–4. Assessment of performance problems. (Adapted from Mager, R. F. & Pipe, P. [1970]. *Analyzing performance problems.* Belmont, CA: Fearon-Pitman Publishers.)

3. Does the patient feel that it doesn't matter whether he performs the behavior? If this is the case, as with hypertensive patients who fail to take their medications regularly, more frequent blood pressure checks can reinforce the patient's awareness of the seriousness of omitting the medication.

4. Do obstacles prevent the patient from performing the behavior? If so, the teacher will want to look at these and try to help the patient deal with them. For example, the snack machine at work, which contains only candy and chips, may be less of a temptation if the patient takes a more nutritious snack with him to work in the morning. If a mill worker feels self-conscious about wearing a protective mask on the job, because "nobody else wears one," the company manager and employee health nurse may be able to insist that all employees wear the recommended masks.

The nurse must become a detective to help patients overcome stumbling blocks in the learning process. This requires the skills of making astute observations, using active listening, and approaching individual situations creatively.

The continuous cycle of teaching and learning brings us back to formulating objectives. The nurse, the patient, and the patient's family must once again discuss their mutual goals: where does the patient want to be in terms of his behaviors, and what can the nurse offer to assist him in carrying out these new behaviors? Just as negotiation and the formulation of a learning contract were emphasized in Chapter 8, they are also priorities in evaluation. The original learning contract should be modified according to the oral agreement between the nurse and the patient.

Feedback

Feedback is a communication process that involves a sharing of perceptions. The patient and family can be supported and guided in learning when they are given constructive feedback. They can be directed toward meeting their goals. Nurses often comment that they wish patients, families, and staff would give them more positive feedback about the nursing care they provide. Health care institutions ask for feedback from the public about how they are meeting community health care needs.

Feedback is seen as a valuable commodity. People generally refer to two types of feedback: positive and negative. *Positive feedback* is complimentary of a person's behavior. *Negative feedback* communicates displeasure or disappointment with a person's behavior. Most people describe positive feedback as being of great importance to them. It means more when it comes from someone we respect, from someone who values us, and from someone who understands our situation. Feedback is provided in the home, workplace, and health care settings. In patient learning, patients and their family members expect to receive feedback from nurses and other team members.

Certain guidelines can be offered to increase the likelihood that the feedback given by professionals to clients will be constructive and helpful. Rather than focus on positive versus negative feedback, we consider how we can use the evaluation process to offer a maximum number of opportunities for useful feedback. In Box 11-1, first we describe the characteristics of constructive feedback. Then we offer tips for conveying the message to the patient and family so that it is understood. Suggestions are also provided for the nurse to solicit feedback about her performance from others.

Understanding and Preventing Relapse

The problem of relapse is a challenge faced by all patients and all health care providers. Quite simply, we expect that patients may lapse in performing the health care regimen. We expect it because behavior change is difficult and the patient does not live in a sterile environment. It is the *lapse*, a slip or mistake, that often leads to a more dangerous long-term relapse. Yet seldom does the teacher prepare the patient to handle the lapse and thus prevent the *relapse*. Research in relapse prevention has focused on the addictive disorders of alcoholism, smoking, and obesity. Studies suggest three stages of behavior change: motivation and commitment, initial change, and maintenance. The authors believe that these findings may be

---

BOX 11-1. Guidelines for Obtaining and Giving Constructive Feedback

Characteristics of Constructive Feedback

- It is descriptive rather than judgmental. It offers objective data and suggestions for improvement.

- It is specific rather than general. It does not include absolute words such as *always* or *never*. It is concerned with the here and now.

- It is focused on the person's *behavior* rather than on the person *himself*.

- It is given at the earliest opportunity after the behavior is performed. It is timely.

- It considers the needs of the learner. It is given to help, not to hurt.

- It is directed toward a behavior about which the learner can do something. The person will only become frustrated and discouraged when he is unable to control a situation.

- It involves sharing information and offering guided choices rather than giving advice such as "You should...."

- It considers the amount of information that the learner can handle. It does not overload the person.

Tips for Giving and Soliciting Feedback

- Ask whether feedback is wanted. It is most useful when it is solicited rather than imposed.

- Be prepared to listen.

- Give positive feedback first. Reinforce positive behaviors, then discuss weaknesses.

- Don't argue or push. Present alternatives.

- Check to be sure that your feedback is interpreted correctly.

- When requesting feedback from others, tell them what kinds of specific information you want. Offer them structured questions but encourage them to use open-ended responses.

- When you want feedback from others, be open to it. Observe patients' expressions or comments. Listen for the intended message.

helpful in all behavior modification efforts (Brownell, Marlatt, Lichtenstein, 1986).

Relapse may have positive consequences if it somehow prepares the learner for future success. For example, the patient who experiences a relapse may learn more about his vulnerability under certain conditions and develop better coping behaviors for similar situations in the future. Relapse can be a positive experience if the teacher and learner use it well. This type of learning requires a trusting relationship between teacher and learner.

Nurses learn through experiences in patient education that we can anticipate high-risk situations for relapses and teach patients self-management techniques (coping responses) to get through those situations without experiencing a relapse. These techniques include cognitive, as well as behavioral, acts. In this way, evaluation focus shifts from short term to long term and from compliance to incremental learning. If the nurse and patient fail to recognize this, both may become discouraged and pessimistic about the power of patient education (Marlatt & Gordon, 1985).

More Than Information Alone

Godfrey Hochbaum suggests that the temptation to give more (or more forceful) information to drive home to patients possible dire consequences when they do not exhibit desired behaviors comes from our own assumptions that human behavior is shaped by rationality and sufficient motivation (Hochbaum, 1980). We assume that one or both must be missing if a person does not act as we expect him to.

The learning of information alone does not ensure that behavioral change will follow. To illustrate this point, Hochbaum asks health professionals to compare their own daily behaviors with the behaviors they prescribe for their patients. He reminds us that we tell patients to refrain from smoking, to exercise regularly, to fasten seat belts, to keep their weight within prescribed limits, to floss and brush their teeth every day, to eat a balanced diet, to have periodic dental and medical checkups,

and to follow the physician's instructions accurately. Yet he asks, "How many health professionals comply with all these practices?"

In an attempt to better understand why *patients* do not perform desired health behaviors, Hochbaum asks health professionals to consider why *we* do not practice what we preach. Health professionals are generally more knowledgeable than others about the harmful consequences of not following these practices, and because they see these consequences in their workplace, one would expect them to be "at least as motivated to perform them as the most motivated laypersons" (Hochbaum, 1980).

Identifying Barriers to Behavioral Change

Many factors enter into the choices patients make. The integration of learned facts into everyday life is the key to behavioral change. For example, when a patient agrees with the physician that he should lose 9.1 kg (20 lb), that decision alone does not guarantee that he will lose the weight. We recognize that the initial decision involves making many choices, on a daily basis, that are much more difficult to make than the original decision. These choices involve making sacrifices and overcoming obstacles in day-to-day situations. Patients encounter many strong influences that pose barriers to their maintenance of a medical regimen. Even the most informed and motivated patients have difficult and discouraging experiences where they live, work, and play. Hochbaum suggests that if health professionals can assist patients in identifying these barriers and in finding ways to overcome them, the patients will better cooperate with the medical regimen (Hochbaum, 1980).

Nursing Policies as Barriers to Patient Learning

Patient education skills can be learned, just as we learn to give injections. However, using patient education skills effectively depends on our ability to do things *with* patients rather than *to* them. Especially in the hospital setting, patients are often put in a dependent position, and their choices are made *for* them by well-intentioned nurses. A learning environment should offer the patient an opportunity to try out new behaviors and receive support and instruction from the staff. What often occurs is that the patient is instructed and shown skills, but he remains in a dependent role. He is discharged from the hospital without having had the opportunity to try out new behaviors.

Health care settings make heavy demands on professionals, who often respond to their stressful work by categorizing duties and patients. We formulate teaching protocols to ensure high-quality care for patients with similar problems. We construct standards and adhere to them. We schedule treatments, medications, and meals. All of this is done to provide the best care to patients. If strategies for ensuring high-quality care are implemented so rigidly that they stifle the patient's development in a cooperative learning relationship, they may destroy real patient education.

Documentation of Patient Education

Written documentation of all aspects of patient care, including patient education, is essential. It is important for communication among team members, to provide a legal record in case of a lawsuit, to support quality assurance efforts, to meet JCAHO standards, to promote continuity of care, and to promote reimbursement. Documentation should reflect the following elements of patient care, and all of these elements include patient education:

Initial assessments, reassessments
Nursing diagnoses and patient needs, priorities
Interventions planned
Interventions provided
Patient's response, outcomes of care
Patient and family ability to manage needs after discharge

Nurses view documentation as time consuming, especially in light of increasing patient acuity, complex care, and expanding clinical responsibilities. However, they must find the time for timely, accurate documentation that shows the basis of their clinical judgments and the evidence of nursing interventions provided to the patient (Box 11-2). We believe that nurses should make every effort to improve documentation systems by designing all components to fit together. Documentation can be streamlined to avoid duplication of charting and to accurately reflect the nursing process in which nursing diagnoses are either resolved or referred. To demonstrate quality care, nurses must integrate all clinical data, including those gathered by other members of the health care team. This necessitates a single, integrated, patient-centered data base (Eggland & Heinemann, 1994; Mowry, 1992).

We have witnessed increasing use of computerized documentation systems, with data entry at a bedside terminal. Research on the use of bedside computers shows that automation enhances the amount and accuracy of information documented by nurses (Eggland & Heinemann, 1994).

A documentation system should be concise, organized, and focused on patient outcomes. When charting of patient education is done correctly, the mastery of learning objectives is highlighted, and we get a "snapshot" of what the patient knows and is able to do. Statements in the charts such as "patient teaching done" describe the nurse's behavior

---

BOX 11–2. Documentation

- Initial assessments, reassessment
- Nursing diagnoses and patient needs, priorities
- Interventions planned
- Interventions provided
- Patient's response, outcomes of care
- Patient and family ability to manage needs after discharge

rather than the patient's behavior and in such general terms that evaluation is meaningless.

Although documentation systems look different from one setting to another, and even among units in the same agency, they have common components (Montemuro, 1988; Eggland & Heinemann 1994). Computerized charting systems share these components in a medical record. Katz and Green (1992) argue for an end to former practices of narrative charting and individualized "Kardex" care plans. Certainly, duplication of charting should be avoided and timesaving methods encouraged. Yet, narrative charting can continue to be effective if duplication is avoided and integration of the patient record is promoted. One of the biggest problems with narrative charting has been the quality of data nurses documented and the ability to reflect both the nurse's clinical decision-making and the patient's outcomes.

We are often asked by nurses, "Don't we need a special form for documenting patient education? Wouldn't our documentation improve if we had a better checklist or flow sheet specifically for patient teaching?" We firmly believe that no universal answer to this question is appropriate for every situation and setting. The best advice we can offer is: "Where is patient education currently documented and is it working?" Often staff have no clear understanding or mandate for the use of progress notes and how to chart patient education outcomes as an integral part of care. With the creation of new forms often comes fragmented communication, the perception that patient education is separate from routine care, and the belief that patient teaching requires extra work that is unrealistic. A rule of thumb is: if you create a new form, one or more existing forms should be eliminated.

A review of the common components of a documentation system, listed below, will allow nurses to consider how they can integrate the documentation of patient education into the patient record.

Nursing admission assessment (data base)
Problem list
Care plan

Flow sheets (optional)
Progress notes
Discharge summary

Nursing Admission Assessment

Client profile and history are completed by the RN on admission. Functional assessment is highlighted to aid the formulation of nursing diagnoses. Patient assessment forms are designed to compliment whatever assessment guide is chosen by the nurse. This varies according to setting and patient needs. The assessment is described in Chapter 7 and emphasizes the identification of barriers to learning, such as lack of readiness, culture, language, and physical problems. Assessment forms may be designed strictly for patient teaching purposes to pinpoint potential problems or barriers that high-risk patients may face following medication regimens, for example (Gibson, 1989).

Problem List

A list of actual and potential health problems identified by health care providers, individually or collaboratively, is placed at the front of the chart. Nursing diagnoses are contributed to this list and numbered as they are identified, not necessarily in order of priority or intensity. A date is entered next to each problem as it is identified, and another date is recorded to reflect when the problem is resolved. The problem list is used as an index. Problem numbers are used throughout the record to streamline documentation, whether manual or computerized. Nurses in many agencies use standardized care plans that are generated based on DRGs and nursing diagnoses.

Care Plan

An individualized care plan for each patient is organized by problem. For each nursing diagnosis, patient goals or outcomes (including learning goals) are outlined, interventions or nursing orders (including patient education) are indicated, and actual outcomes are noted. Many different forms can be used to reflect these components. Standardized and computerized care plans, tailored to nursing diagnoses, are increasingly popular. However, these plans must be individualized by the nurse to direct each patient's care.

The care plans used in managed care systems, called care maps, are described in Chapter 13.

Flow Sheets

A systematic way to document routine or repetitious actions can be developed to minimize unnecessary prose and to save time. Flow sheets can be kept at the bedside to record vital signs, medication, positioning, and so forth. Paperless flow sheets can be used at bedside computer terminals. Flow sheets list observations in a clear, concise check-off format to encourage rapid and immediate documentation; abnormal findings or patient responses must be recorded in narrative notes. This method of charting assumes that all abnormal findings, or variances, are charted; this is referred to as *charting by exception* (Eggland & Heinemann, 1994). If flow sheets are used to record patient teaching, they should be organized by patient response, not by "what the nurse did" to teach the patient.

Progress Notes

Narrative notes show the *patient's* progress as viewed by all disciplines. Evaluation of the patient's responses to nursing interventions should be evident. Each problem is referenced with a number corresponding to the problem list.

Patient education is ideally documented in the progress notes section of the medical record. Because patient education is a problem-solving process, documentation includes a clear statement of needs or problems, significant data contributing to these nursing diag-

noses, and the plan for nursing care. The evaluations of the outcomes of care are essential ingredients in the care plan. Narrative notes also encourage the charting of the patient's own words to illustrate outcomes of patient education and evidence of individualized care.

In Chapter 1 we presented comments from health professionals. Many of them addressed documentation concerns or problems. Although many of them stated that progress notes were important to communication and planning, they worried that their contributions to the medical record were ignored.

Dr. Lawrence Weed (1971) developed the problem-oriented record (POR), a systematic tool for communication and problem-solving. All team members (physicians, nurses, physical therapists, dietitians, pharmacists, and social workers) contribute to the one problem list that focuses on *patient* problems rather than on *provider* problems. Team members write narrative and discharge notes using the SOAP format to document subjective and objective data, assessment (or identification) of problems and the planned course of intervention. The SOAP note was later modified to include intervention, evaluation, and revision, and referred to as SOAPIER. This method increases awareness of the contributions of others and encourages the members to function as a team. There are no divisions of nurses' notes, physicians' notes, and so forth. All health care professionals document information on the patient's progress notes. The patient is clearly the center of the team and the focus of care.

We recommend this method, and in our own experiences in patient education, it has increased communication and collaboration. It helps team members to know what has been taught by others and facilitates reinforcement of learned behaviors.

The POR highlights the use of the nursing process, which is based on problem-solving. Narrative notes begin by naming the problem, and they then offer *subjective* and *objective* data, the *assessment*, and the *plan*, as detailed in Box 11-3.

The PIE charting system, developed at Craven Regional Medical Center in New

Bern, North Carolina, incorporates the care plan into the progress note. Problems are identified by number and written in nursing diagnosis form. PIE refers to the components of *Problems, Interventions,* and *Evaluation.* Each problem must be reviewed at least once every 8 hours (per shift), new problems are added, and problems that have been resolved are dropped. Patient teaching is documented along with other interventions on the progress notes (Eggland & Heinemann, 1994; Buckley-Womack & Gidney, 1987).

Focus charting is another format for charting, which directs nurses to address the patient's functional health patterns. It focuses on the patient's response (nursing diagnosis) rather than the medical diagnosis. Narrative charting uses DAR notes, intended to be identified as "patient care notes," rather than "nurses notes" (Lampe, 1985; Eggland, 1988).

> Focus DAR Progress Notes
> Focus: Area of concern
> Data: Data base
> Action: What did the nurse do?
> Result: Patient outcome

We have described three formats that can be used for progress notes. All three create the possibility for interdisciplinary coordination, a focus on the patient's functional health problems, and a record of the patient's learning outcomes as an integral part of documenting care. Regardless of the type of progress note, the nurse should shift the focus of care from the medical diagnosis to the individual patient's response to it (the functional problems). This can be encouraged throughout the course of patient care by asking the following question: "How does this diagnosis *affect this patient?*"

Nurses' responses to this question help us to keep patient care centered on the patient (Box 11-4).

Discharge Summary

Summaries or reports written at the time of discharge or transfer communicate to other health care providers the patient's needs for reinforcement and continued learning. This documentation is important because learning is a process that occurs over time. It is often begun in the hospital, but it must be resumed in the clinic or home. Nurses are encouraged to use written as well as telephone consultations in planning to meet the patient's learning needs. Recalling experiences with patients who have newly diagnosed diabetes, for example, reminds us that much of their learning occurs after they leave the sheltered hospital environment and that most of them need continuous patient teaching to become responsible and capable in managing their daily care. Suggestions for patient-centered one-page discharge instructions are offered in Chapter 9. Many agencies require that discharge instructions be developed in triplicate; the patient and family sign a copy for the patient's record indicating instructions were received, a copy is given to the patient, and a copy is provided to the individual or agency responsible for continuing care.

Patient Contracts

Patient contracts may be also be entered as a permanent part of the patient record. They were first discussed in Chapter 8.

❑ CASE STUDY

Evaluation of Mrs. Dawe's Behavioral Change

After the home visit, this summary of patient learning outcomes was offered by the nursing students. Reassessment of patient needs and modifications to the teaching plan are also noted.

Problem #3: Altered Nutrition

Mrs. Dawe correctly outlined food exchanges for breakfast, lunch, and dinner using her American Diabetes Association (ADA) diet plan. She made up three sample menus for each meal. She included one-half cup of ice cream in one of these meals and substituted accurately. She returned to the clinic for her first weekly visit with 2 days of food intake recorded in her notebook. Both days she had followed her diet plan. She reported that on the last 5 days she "cheated" on her diet and ate several desserts, failing to record what she ate. She stated that she felt guilty not following the diet and proceeded to explain that she knew controlling her weight was important in the management of her diabetes.

Her weight today had not changed from her last clinic visit.

We reviewed her goals and learning objectives. Mrs. Dawe stated that she was still interested in following her diet and wanted a nurse's help in doing so.

We reinforced Mrs. Dawe's knowledge about her diet and her understanding of the importance of weight control in diabetic management. We stressed that she would have to take responsibility for changing her habits but that we would help her to work out strategies to confront problems. She stated that she would like to resume her diet plan today and see us next

week. We agreed and reinforced her 2 days of success with her plan.

Problem #4: Altered Tissue Perfusion

Mrs. Dawe reported that she was taking her medications and showed us the record of medication in her notebook. She reported that she omitted salt in cooking during the week and that she did not use any canned foods except for water-packed fruits. She recalled ten high-sodium foods when asked to do so.

Her blood pressure was 188/96 mm Hg today.

Mrs. Dawe reported that it was less difficult than she thought to avoid high-sodium foods and that Mr. Dawe had encouraged her to do so. In fact, when she was about to use canned tomato sauce in cooking, Mr. Dawe reminded her of its high sodium content. We commended them on their positive behaviors and showed them how the blood pressure measurement also highlighted their success.

Figures 11-5 and 11-6 illustrate SOAP notes written by the nursing students to document Mrs. Dawe's care.

❑ CASE STUDY

Mr. Straminsky's Ambulatory Surgery

Mr. Al Straminsky is 73 years old. His wife, Alice, is 70. They live in the suburbs, 28 miles from the large teaching hospital where Mr. Straminsky is to have his bladder biopsy in ambulatory surgery. He was a patient in the same hospital 3 years before when he had a coronary artery bypass graft.

Nurses in the ambulatory surgery unit recognize that all patients have some degree of anxiety before the procedure. During the preoperative assessment, the nurses ask about concerns the patient and family have. Patients usually come to the ambulatory surgery center 2 to 4 days before surgery. Before beginning patient teaching, the nurse tries to determine the patient's

Knowledge about the expected surgery
Previous surgical experiences or hospitalizations
Other illnesses
Support systems
Occupational or related concerns such as when work or activity can be resumed
Effective ways of coping with pain

3/31/95 HOME VISIT

<u>**Nursing Note**</u>

#3. ALTERED NUTRITION

   S: "I want help with my weight problem. I know I'm too heavy and it's making my diabetes difficult to manage. My diet is too limited. I just can't follow it."

   O: 5'3" tall, weight 170 lb. at last visit. 45 lb. above prescribed weight. Unable to follow ADA diet. Gets little exercise except for housework.

   P: Negotiate weight loss goals. Change diet plan to updated ADA low-fat, high fiber diabetic diet. Outline menus with Mrs. Dawe and make referral to the dietician to build variety into her diet plan. Discuss importance of weight loss in management of diabetes. Refer to diabetic luncheon. Schedule clinic visit for 1 week from now.

#4. ALTERED TISSUE PERFUSION

   S: "I know I need to cut down on salt and lose weight to get my pressure down."

   O: Blood pressure 220/190 today. Reports taking medication.

   A: Blood pressure poorly controlled. Diet recall reveals salt used in cooking and at the table, with canned foods frequently included.

   P: Continue medication as ordered. Patient to keep written records. Follow weight-reduction diet as ordered in No. 1. Omit salt in cooking and avoid canned foods. Mrs. Dawe is in agreement with the plan. We discussed high-sodium foods to be avoided. Return to clinic in 1 week for blood pressure check.

FIGURE 11–5. Nursing entries in the problem-oriented record (POR).

Unfortunately, nurses at the center find that they usually have about 15 minutes to complete the assessment, and often patients do not share their concerns in depth with the nurse. This is particularly true of elderly patients (Kempe, 1987; Leyder & Pieper, 1986).

Patient teaching preoperatively for Mr. Straminsky centered on what to expect in the surgical procedure and instructions for discharge (Connaway & Blackledge, 1986). The patient and his wife seemed to understand the instructions although Mrs. Straminsky made a comment about how they had seen so many doctors, specialists, residents, and medical students, and they were overwhelmed with instructions. They were given a pamphlet explaining the ambulatory surgery unit and told the logistics of arriving the next morning for the surgical procedure.

The nursing diagnoses identified for most patients in this unit were appropriate for Mr. Straminsky:

1. Knowledge Deficit related to the ambulatory surgery unit and the surgical procedure

2. Anxiety related to surgical procedure and discharge from unit

The short teaching session seemed to go well. The patient and his wife asked questions about the procedure and repeated what they should do following discharge. They seemed interested and capable.

When Mr. and Mrs. Straminsky returned for the bladder biopsy, the admissions nurse greeted them. They were asked to report at 6:30 AM, and they arrived early, at about 6:00. Mr. Straminsky was assigned a bed and his wife waited for a few minutes before joining him. Throughout the morning, Mrs. Straminsky seemed to be anxious. Despite the procedure, which by standards of the health care team went well, she seemed distracted and unsettled. She told the nurse assigned to recovery

---

4/7/95 CLINIC VISIT

<u>**Nursing Note**</u>

#3. ALTERED NUTRITION

S: "I followed my diet the first 2 days but cheated after that. I just couldn't pass up desserts when I thought about having them. I didn't keep records of what I ate, because I was embarrassed. I really do want to lose weight and wish you would help me to do it."

O: Weight 170 lb. (unchanged from last visit). The 2 days of recorded meals did follow diet plan.

A: Poor cooperation with diet plan. Understands meal spacing and is able to select menus. Understands importance of weight control but does not perform necessary behavior modifications.

P: Review goals. Stress Mrs. Dawe's responsibility. Offer assistance for problem solving and role playing. Reinforce 2 days of positive behavior. Return visit in 1 week.

#4. ALTERED TISSUE PERFUSION

S: Reports taking medication. Reports omitting salt in cooking.

O: Blood pressure 188/96 today.

A: Blood pressure lower. Good cooperation with reducing sodium intake. Knows name and dosage of medication. Identifies high-sodium foods to avoid.

P: Reinforce progress. Continue weekly blood pressure checks.

FIGURE 11–6. Nursing entries in the problem-oriented record (POR).

that she had not been prepared well for this "ordeal."

The nurse asked Mrs. Straminsky to describe her concerns in writing, reviewing her experience. This evaluation method helps the patient (or in this case the spouse) verbalize her feelings, and it can also be used to better teach other patients. Mrs. Straminsky agreed and began making notes. Three days later, her "surgical experience" was delivered by mail to the nurse.

My Husband's Bladder Biopsy

The various physicians who have sent my husband and me for the many outpatient procedures are intelligent, caring, and extremely busy people. They certainly never indicated that they were sending us to the Ritz, but neither did they prepare us specifically for conditions in a large suburban outpatient facility.

In the preliminary visit, more discussion, or a videocassette, would all have been helpful.

Some of these things could certainly be the responsibility of the hospital.

The first shock to me was the size of the tiny cubicles to which a patient is assigned. The only similar situation I have seen was an emergency room 25 years earlier. My sister had been taken there following an accident. I accepted the lack of privacy because of the need for immediate attention in that case.

This time we were scheduled and asked to report at the usual crack of dawn. One lonely nurse was on duty and she got my husband into bed. I was allowed to sit in a straight chair by his side as many other patients joined us, each in his curtained rectangle, each giving his history, giving blood, giving urine, and surrendering all thought that some items might be personal and private. There was no way to avoid hearing the details of others' dilemmas.

When my husband was finally wheeled away to surgery, it was a relief for both of us. I escaped first to the cafeteria, then to a waiting room near surgery. After the surgeon spoke to me about my husband, I was allowed into a recovery room where he was blessedly alone with a nurse in attendance.

"Good," I thought, "He'll be here in peace and quiet for awhile."

It was a very little while. Responsive but groggy, he was wheeled back to outpatients, now a very busy place. We were informed that as soon as he could urinate on his own, my husband would be discharged. There were many disappointing trips to the lavatory, and often other patients were waiting to use the facility. We waited about 8 hours before he was discharged. I believe it was that time that I inquired about whether it would have been better if he were admitted to the hospital. We were advised that neither Medicare nor our insurance would cover the cost, and the nurse advised against it. Evidently patients do best spending as little time as possible in hospitals!

"You don't want him to be in the hospital; terrible things happen in hospitals," were the exact words from the spouse of another patient. At least in the outpatient facility I could sit with my husband and watch for those terrible things.

The nursing staff was wonderful. Competent, professional nurses stayed aware of all that was going on. I imagine that they too wish for a better environment for themselves and their patients.

This experience (which bothered me much more than it did my spouse) could have been alleviated by some preparation such as the ones suggested at the beginning of this account. In addition, a waiting area adjacent to the patient holding area could be provided with video or slide viewers to help explain what is happening.

The nurse realized that more explanation of the physical layout of the unit was needed in the preadmission program. She also knew that patients and families experience more anxiety than they expect to feel due to the loss of control on the morning of surgery. She decided to convene a group of patients and family members who had surgical procedures on the unit and ask them to share questions or concerns that they each had before, during, or after the procedure.

A 15-minute videotape was added to the preadmission program, showing what the facilities looked like and following a patient through the surgical procedure. It could also be shown the morning of surgery. The videotape featured a spouse who described how she handled such things as waiting, getting information on her husband's status, and so forth. This videotape was shown to groups of patients the day before the surgery, and a nurse was available to answer questions after the film. She found that patients and family members learn from each other and also get support from each other, which may continue through the surgical experience on the unit.

Research indicates that preoperative information alleviates anxiety and aids in postoperative recuperation. However, preoperative instruction for the family has been largely overlooked. Studies have indicated that by alleviating a family member's fear and anxiety, he can be a better source of support for the patient. Fear and anxiety have different characteristics and are subjective experiences. We know through the case study of the Straminskys that sensory experiences of the spouse can be a source of anxiety due to lack of preparation. Particularly with the elderly, nurses should use patient education to decrease anxiety related to the ambulatory surgery environment. Evaluation should continue to be done to see how the patient and family perceive the adequacy of preoperative instruction. Although the results of preoperative patient teaching are well documented, this has not been true for family member teaching. One extensive review of the literature shows a lack of:

> Studies that examine the impact of preoperative instruction on significant family members
> Studies that measure fear and anxiety in family members
> Tools to measure family members' psychological reactions to surgery
> Studies to determine potential positive impact of preoperative teaching interventions with significant family members as well as the patient (Moss, 1986)

❏ CASE STUDY

Ken Horton Enters the Coronary Care Unit

Ken Horton, 67 years old and the owner of a large retail store, was admitted to the coronary cary unit (CCU) with symptoms of coronary artery disease. Like most patients in this situation, he was anxious, depressed, and angry.

The nurses at the medical center CCU were using patient-nurse contracts to help patients regain a feeling of control. They recognized that the routines and sensory experiences of the CCU are depersonalizing and that unit procedures and policies (such as restricting visitors, telephones, and newspapers) made matters worse. They also knew that research studies indicate that stress reduction measures to counteract environmental stressors positively affected patient attitudes and the return of function.

The use of contracting in the CCU is described by Ziemann and Dracup (1989). Patients who were physiologically stable were oriented by audiotape to patient-nurse contracting, and then a nurse worked with each patient to offer choices about visiting privileges, hygiene time, room arrangements, teaching preferences, activity, and other areas of patient concern. Contracts were shared with the nursing staff, who honored the terms of the contract whenever possible. Through this process, patients were taught about how and why to manage aspects of their own care.

The nurses evaluated the effectiveness of this intervention by studying control and experimental group outcomes. They used two questionnaires and a checklist designed to measure anxiety, depression, and hostility. The results of the study were rewarding. Although baseline data indicated no statistical difference between the two groups, significant differences were found when overall scores for both groups continued to change in opposite directions over time. The contract worked as an intervention to decrease anxiety. Ken Horton's anxiety decreased when measured 24 hours following contracting with his primary nurse.

Patients in the experimental groups were most interested in controlling the number and length of family visits, highlighting the support of family as a means to decrease stress. Overall, male patients in both control and experimental groups reported higher levels of stress than did female patients.

The nurse researchers and authors in this study have made an important contribution to patient education efforts in the CCU. We often hear nurses in critical care areas complain of frustration with teaching attempts that are hampered by the patient's anxiety and depression. We encourage critical care nurses to consider contracting as a powerful intervention that gets results.

Summary

Evaluation occurs at different points of the teaching and learning process and uses different methods to gather the types of information needed. The nurse uses evaluation to measure the degree to which patient learning goals have been met and also uses findings to improve or redirect patient care. Documentation of the results of patient education focuses on patient outcomes: knowledge, skill, and health behaviors. Good documentation improves continuity of care, satisfies legal responsibilities for charting patient care, and provides evidence that standards for accreditation are met.

Through evaluation we learn valuable lessons from our patients and their families about priorities for teaching, who needs to be taught, how to share responsibility for learning with the patient and family, and how difficult long-term change can be.

Despite good intentions, new knowledge and skills, and behavior modification strategies, patients may only partially achieve the health outcomes we desire. Obstacles to change are often less tangible than, for example, exposure to party foods or pressure from family and peers. They are closely related to self-esteem—the patient's view of himself as a whole person. The feedback and counseling offered to patients in the health care setting may help them to place greater value on themselves and their health. This often takes time to develop, and many patients have difficulty accepting their own responsibilities in daily health management.

The provider-patient relationship offers an opportunity to help the patient grow in assuming his role as a member of the health care team. It is important to communicate confidence in the patient's ability to choose responsibly. It is also important to offer encouragement and guidance for change. Evaluation is a tool used to strengthen the provider-patient relationship and to continue patient-centered care through the nursing process. Documentation that includes evaluation of patient learning outcomes provides critical evidence of such patient-centered care.

In addition to meeting agency mandates for evaluating and documenting patient learning outcomes, nurses gain important personal and professional rewards by engaging in the process. In acute care settings, teaching can make the critical difference in helping a patient survive through an illness or injury. Nurses on a neurosurgery service described the importance their patient education made during an awake craniotomy. They stated that throughout surgery they showed the patient pictures, answered her questions honestly, provided comfort measures, and cared for her emotionally. "We helped maintain the patient's low anxiety level and received excellent feedback and cooperation" (Fuchs, Porter, & Clark, 1994).

In rehabilitation settings, nurses describe the rewards of patient teaching in different ways. "It makes you feel really good to see your teaching help a patient master self-care activities and to see these regained skills restore self-esteem, a positive outlook on life, and in many cases, independence. Nursing empowers patients to make decisions independently and improve the quality of their life" (McDonald, 1994).

Strategies for Critical Analysis and Application

1. Consider nursing care provided in the following settings. Identify what types of patient learning outcomes are realistic, in which level they belong (A, B, C, or D), and how you would document them in the patient record.

   Preoperative visit in day surgery

   Prenatal visit

   Recovery room

   ICU

   Medical-surgical orthopedic unit

   Pediatric office

   Home health

   Long-term care

   School

   Occupational health

2. How can patients and families become involved in evaluating patient education efforts and offering suggestions?

3. How can members of health care team become more involved in evaluating patient education efforts and offering suggestions?

4. How would you assess whether or not a new form is needed for documenting patient education? What are the pros and cons of creating a new form? Which existing form or forms could be eliminated? How can the health care team provide input in the decision?

REFERENCES

Bovender, N. (1994). Home care: nurses discover the rewards and challenges of this growing frontier. *North Carolina Nursing Matters, 4*(11), 6-7.

Brownell, K., Marlatt G., Lichtenstein, E., (1986). Understanding and preventing relapse. *American Psychologist, 41* (7), 765-782.

Buckley-Womack, C., & Gidney, B. (1987). A new dimension in documentation: The PIE method. *Journal of Neuroscience Nursing, 19*(5), 259.

Connaway, C., & Blackledge, D. (1986). Preoperative testing center. *AORN Journal, 43*(3), 666-670.

Eggland, E. (1988). Charting: How and why to document your care daily and fully. *Nursing, 18*: 83.

Eggland, E., & Heinemann, D. (1994). *Nursing documentation: Charting, recording, and reporting.* Philadelphia: J. B. Lippincott.

Fuchs, K., Porter, M., & Clark, M. (1994). Caring for a patient during an awake craniotomy. *North Carolina Nursing Matters, 4*(8), 5.

Gibson J. (1989). A new approach to better medication compliance. *Nursing, 19*(4) 49-51.

Hochbaum G. (1980). Patient counseling versus patient teaching. Topics in Clinical Nursing, *2*:1-8.

Joint Commission on the Accreditation of Healthcare Organizations (1994). *1995 Comprehensive accreditation manual for hospitals.* Chicago:Author.

Katz, J., & Green E. (1992). *Managing quality: A guide to monitoring and evaluating nursing services.* St Louis: Mosby Year-Book.

Kempe, A. (1987). Patient education for the ambulatory surgery patient. *AORN Journal, 45*(2), 500-507.

Lampe, S. (1985). Focus charting: Streamlining documentation. *Nursing Management, 16*(7), 43-46.

Leyder, B., & Pieper, B. (1986). Identifying discharge concerns. *AORN Journal, 43*(6), 1298-1302.

Mager, R. (1975). *Preparing instructional objectives.* Belmont, CA: Fearon-Pitman Publishers.

Mager R., & Pipe, P (1970). *Analyzing performance problems.* Belmont, CA: Fearon-Pitman Publishers.

Marlatt, G., & Gordon, J. (1985). *Relapse prevention.* New York: Guilford Press.

McDonald, K. (1994). Rehab nursing: Helping patients be all they can be. *North Carolina Nursing Matters, 4*(8), 6-7.

Montemuro, M. (1988). CORE documentation: A complete system for charting nursing care. *Nursing Management, 19*(8), 28-32.

Mowry M. (1992). Computerization and quality. In M. Johnson, ed. The delivery of quality healthcare (pp 153-171). St. Louis: Mosby-yearbook.

Moss, R. (1986). Overcoming fear. *AORN Journal, 43*(5), 1107-1114.

Weed, L. (1971). *Medical record, medical education, and patient care.* Cleveland: Press of Case Western Reserve University.

Ziemann, K., & Dracup, K. (1989). How well do CCU patient-nurse contracts work? *American Journal of Nursing, 89*(5), 691-693.

12 Community Health Promotion: Assessment and Intervention

Ronna E. Krozy

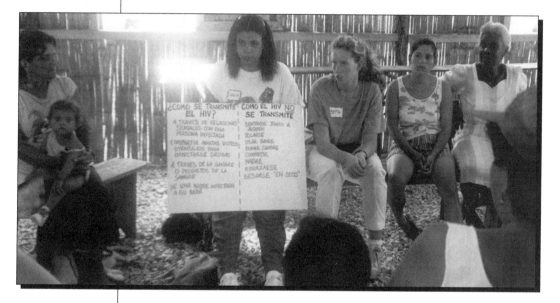

OBJECTIVES FOR CHAPTER 12

After reading this chapter, the nurse or student nurse should be able to:

1 Describe the interrelationship between community assessment and identification of community health education issues.

2 Use several approaches to data collection as the basis for developing a needs assessment.

3 Implement health promotion strategies that effect behavioral change in families, aggregate populations, or community groups.

4 Apply marketing techniques to improve the success of a health education program.

General Considerations About Community Health Promotion

Patient health promotion represents an integral part of the health professional's role. Health promotion addresses activities that prevent the development of risk factors and that facilitate well-being and self-actualization. A major national initiative to improve the health of the nation has been undertaken by the U.S. Public Health Service as evident in its document *Healthy People 2000* (1990). Built on objectives set in 1980, priorities have been established around health promotion, health protection, and preventive services. Examples of areas of concern include smoking, violence, physical fitness, mental health, occupational safety, environmental health, human immunodeficiency virus (HIV) and other sexually transmitted diseases (STDs), cancer, and immunizations. The overall goal is to help people change negative personal behaviors, eliminate unequal access to comprehensive health services, and eradicate many of the chronic conditions that are so costly to treat and are essentially preventable. Ultimately, prevention of disability and suffering also improves quality of life.

Health education comprises an important aspect of health promotion. Community health education differs from patient or family education in that its focus may extend to global, national, state, or local needs. The clients of community health strategies include groups and aggregates that cross all age, socioeconomic, and cultural strata. They may be found in homes, schools, and occupational settings or in shelters and prisons or on the street. Health promotion initiatives may be aimed at an entire country or a small village and the learners may be comprised of people who are homogeneous or extremely dissimilar. Health educators must develop proficiency in group or aggregate teaching because large numbers of participants may be reached more efficiently in less time and with more potential sources of support and sharing.

This chapter discusses factors that must be considered in promoting health in aggregate populations and then describes three health education projects in which the author was involved. In each of these examples, the demographic factors and focus are different, and therefore, the approaches to needs assessment and intervention also vary. Gordon's 11 functional health patterns (1991) are used as the framework to assess the health education needs of a culturally diverse population in a poor Ecuadorian community. The second example demonstrates an assessment and intervention relative to the sex education needs in senior adults. The third example demonstrates the use of force field analysis and behavioral change strategies with staff attending a university health promotion program.

Community Health Promotion and Education

I define health education, a major component of health promotion, as "a helping process using learning theories and teaching techniques that promote the client's knowledge, attitudes, and skill to voluntarily engage in a wellness lifestyle." Part of the educational process requires mobilizing resources and developing supportive relationships with clients. Another aspect is assuming the role of client advocate or political activist for the disenfranchised for whom health education may be a means of empowerment. The health educator must use learning theories and teaching techniques that have been tested, are based on the population's specific needs, and are incorporated into the overall plan. Health education outcomes include learning factual information; developing self-confidence; reexamining or changing values; decreasing fear; and developing competence to make informed decisions and perform desired behaviors autonomously. The overall goals are aimed at enhancing, maintaining, or restoring health and preventing disease.

Poor health habits, chronic illness, and disability pose major challenges and cost communities in terms of lost work and school days, financing of health care and service agencies, and unnecessary suffering; primary prevention is therefore considered the best way to preserve the health of any community. *Primary prevention* is defined as the activities that prevent an illness or negative condition from beginning. Approaches to community health education often focus on the role of individual responsibility, recognizing that many health problems result from such diverse personal habits as smoking, unprotected sexual activity, or overexposure to sun. These habits represent complex behaviors arising from internal and external stimuli; they are not easily amenable to medical intervention or a health professional's advice. Even when actual disease or potential for disease exists, many individuals have difficulty altering their behavior.

Consider for example the number of young people who begin or continue smoking despite multifocused antismoking strategies. A 1994 report by the U.S. Surgeon General notes that most smokers are hooked by age 20 and the tobacco industry spends $4 million on advertising to indoctrinate youngsters to smoke. They do so by making teenagers think that more people smoke than actually do and that it is a means to an enhanced self-image. Smoking is made to look glamorous, with models and cartoon characters conveying independence, healthfulness, and adventure. Cigarette displays, billboards, free samples, and trademarks prominent on clothes and at sporting events provide constant reinforcement of prosmoking messages (U.S. Department of Health and Human Services, 1994). The use of sophisticated marketing strategies poses considerable challenge to public health campaigns where money for outreach is severely limited.

Resistance can result when populations believe a change interferes with perceived quality of life, requires resources that are lacking, or is unimportant. Barriers may also arise from the health system. Health professionals are expected to establish trusting relationships with clients and act as role models. Yet some display negative attitudes or behaviors that prevent individuals from following advice. Health professionals may hold beliefs that certain individuals, especially those from different socioeconomic classes, do not value health, do not want to get well, enjoy their sick role, are too unintelligent to learn new ways, and take up valuable time of professionals. Incongruent or ineffective messages may also be transmitted when a health professional is observed smoking, is overweight, or drives without a seat belt.

Improving the Success of Community Health Programs

Earlier chapters describe specific teaching and learning principles that can be applied to health promotion programs. The following are general questions aimed at increasing the success of any health education campaign.

IDENTIFYING THE NEED. Has a needs assessment been carried out to determine the community's perception of the problem? Specific issues can be identified using such sources as current vital statistics, public opinion polls, discussions with professionals and lay community leaders, focus groups, informal discussions with representatives of the target population, and written surveys (Freudenberg, 1989).

ACCEPTANCE BY THE MAJORITY. Are the health promotion goals and objectives clear? Will the majority of the target community accept the idea or method? Are they able to implement the idea and is it congruent with their lifestyle, needs, and resources? Have barriers and facilitators of behavior change been considered? Are the behavior changes considered practical and realistic? Does the health innovation consider local resources, customs, and environment? Are the positive healthy habits of people capitalized on even if they seem strange?

INVOLVEMENT IN PLANNING. Has the community (or representatives of subgroups) been involved in identifying the health problem or goal or in developing the approach or the evaluation? It is not uncommon to be confronted by many more opponents than proponents. Therefore, opposing views must be considered. Conflict must be seen as a factor requiring discussion and compromise so that energy is not expended negatively but conjointly.

COST BENEFIT AND COST EFFECTIVENESS. Is the expenditure of time, energy, or money in carrying out the action worth the effort, yield, rewards, or inconveniences? Have competing demands that influence learning or behaviors been considered?

COMMUNITY ENHANCEMENT. Will the process enhance the community with regard to job opportunities, environmental protection, and equalizing wealth? Is there enough consumer orientation reflecting the target audience's specific concerns? Consider the resistance that arises from tobacco farmers whose livelihood is the product that causes cancer and heart disease.

SELF-HELP. Are self-help and self-determination the ultimate goals? Will those in greatest need be included and not just those who can take advantage because of sophistication, education, money, maturity, and so forth? Is there a plan for those who are unable to act because of physical, emotional, or social impairments?

USE OF THEORY. Are various theories used that help guide the design, implementation, and evaluation of the health promotion effort (Kreps & Kunimoto, 1994)? Hochbaum and Rosenstock's Health Belief Model, Pender's Health Promotion Model, or Bandura's Self-Efficacy Theory are examples cited in other chapters.

MEDIA EFFECTIVENESS. Are the media used attractive and interesting, understandable, geared to different learning styles and rates, inoffensive and tasteful, personally engaging, and persuasive (Windsor, Baranowski, Clark, & Cutter, 1994)?

Political and Legal Influences on Health Promotion

Political and legal influences refer to formal and informal sources of decision-making and control. Policymakers or special interest groups can influence withholding health promotion programs from segments of society (Freudenberg, 1989). For example, as a result of selection bias, researchers have underrepresented the elderly, the poor, and ethnic minorities in study protocols. These populations need to be included because they respond differently to diseases and interventions (Larson, 1994). Drug companies and manufacturers have withheld information on adverse outcomes to gain a profit. Legislators in tobacco-growing states have supported subsidies to tobacco growers and opposed smoking restriction regulations, despite the evidence of smoking and cancer. Even with the acquired immunodeficiency syndrome (AIDS) epidemic, needle exchange programs have been barred and parents and religious leaders have influenced school committees to vote down comprehensive sex education curricula.

These examples suggest that decision-makers may have vested interests or religious proscriptions. They may be unconcerned or opposed to the issues or approaches needed to prevent certain health problems or they may fear offending others and losing status. They may also be uninformed. The influence of decision-makers can be assessed by asking:

Is health promotion a value?
Who is permitted to learn?
Who controls what is taught?
Who is permitted to teach?
Are sufficient resources allocated?

A needs assessment must be undertaken to answer these questions and to determine whether the allocated budget, human resources, time, space, and materials are sufficient to address the health problem.

Professionals can influence health policy by developing knowledge of political process, establishing a power base, and creating support (Clark, 1992). Health professionals must understand the political structure, how change is effected, and who has the authority to implement change. Political decision-makers need to be apprised of the health needs of the community using both factual data (such as published vital statistics) and personal testimony. The proposed educational intervention must be presented in a persuasive way along with the expected outcomes. Support is garnered through campaigning, lobbying, or establishing a coalition or temporary alliance to work toward a common goal.

Community organization is a similar process that consists of bringing together various segments of the community who act in their own behalf. Their goal is to establish legitimacy, identify and analyze the problem, identify goals and the means to achieve them, select marketing strategies, and establish evaluation criteria (Clark, 1992).

The Influence of Marketing

Marketing is the process of determining a consumer need and meeting the need with a product or service (Tilbury & Fisk, 1989). Through advertising, the product or service is presented in a way that increases usage and loyalty by as many segments of the population as possible. Drexler (1994, p. 18) notes that the alcohol industry is waging an aggressive and successful marketing campaign toward the 21 to 24 year old, using seductive methods (one example is a well-known liquor company hosting parties at numerous local college pubs). In Massachusetts alone, the tobacco industry spends $70 million yearly in cigarette advertising (Cohen, Lederman, Connolly, & Danley, 1991). Unfortunately, unlike the tobacco or alcohol industries that have extensive marketing budgets, sponsors of health education programs frequently have limited finances. Nevertheless, health promoters have been advised to use similar strategies to identify target populations and their needs and to market health behavior accordingly (Frederiksen, Solomon, & Brehony, 1984).

Examples of marketing strategy may be seen in Massachusetts, one of two states (the other is California) to fund a tobacco control program with taxes from tobacco products. Despite a heavily funded counterattack by the tobacco industry, supporters of "Question 1" achieved a 25-cent state excise tax increase on each package of cigarettes, generating $91 million. The Massachusetts Tobacco Control Program (MTCP) is a statewide campaign incorporating advertising and community relations, statewide smoking cessation and education programs, and grants to local boards of health, schools, community agencies, and health advocacy organizations. Their aim is to decrease 50% of the state's tobacco use by 1999 (Massachusetts Tobacco Control Program, 1994a).

With the referendum won, the tobacco industry began buying whole page advertisements, costing close to $30,000 each. Their messages suggest a need for compromise or working the problem out amicably, but they also imply that government control has overstepped its bounds and will ultimately rob the public of freedom. Another tactic is refuting the Environmental Protection Agency's findings on secondhand smoke. The MTCP allocated $14 million to launch the state's single largest advertising campaign (Massachusetts Tobacco Control Program, 1994a). One of their sponsored full-page advertisements cleverly depicts a package of light cigarettes with the message, "Next, the tobacco industry will want us to believe there's such a thing as light cancer" (*Boston Globe*, June 23, 1994, p. 19).

The MTCP campaign slogan is, "It's Time We Made Smoking History." Strategies include support of legislation and ordinances to ban smoking in most public places such as malls, schools, restaurants, and worksites, and extensive exposure in newspapers, public and cable television, and radio that can reach more than 5 million people. Major targets are youth, pregnant women, and persons from culturally diverse communities who may be left out of the education loop and exposed to many more conflicting messages. The MTCP is monitoring statewide changes in sales of cigarettes as well as surveying changes in knowledge and attitudes about smoking. Preliminary findings suggest that for 1993, as many as 7.5% smokers cut down or quit with 37 million fewer packages consumed after the tax went into effect. The media campaign showed 77% of youths, aged 9 to 18, were aware of antismoking ads and over 60% knew the slogan (Massachusetts Tobacco Control Program, 1994b).

The suggestions of Kreps and Kunimoto (1994) for multicultural health communication can be applied to smoking prevention and cessation as well as other areas. Messages of health should appear in all channels of communication, especially those that are popular with the target group (e.g., television shows, soap operas, and age- or gender-oriented magazines). Endorsements from public figures or role models are also helpful. A successful media project in Brazil's antismoking campaign was based on the notion that people are more concerned for social acceptability than health. Five posters were developed by a famous cartoonist depicting the ludicrous and socially inadequate features of smoking. Descriptions of smoking included old-fashioned, tacky, in bad taste, corny, and pathetic. A significant decrease in smoking has been reported since the campaign began in 1986 (da Costa e Silva, 1993).

Community health promotion aims to foster behavior that maximizes wellness and minimizes the development of disease. Health promotion at the community level requires an understanding of the needs and desires of the target population. It is important to consider the behavioral lifestyles and values of the various groups that make up the community and to maximize community involvement. Socioeconomic status, educational level, culture and language, formal and informal power structures, occupation, and marketing forces are some of the important factors that must be considered if a health promotion initiative is to be successful. The influence of these factors is demonstrated in the health promotion programs presented in the following section.

Example 1: The Por Cristo-BCSON Health Project

Despite growing international concern about health promotion and disease prevention, many barriers exist in the aim to promote global health. Among these are overpopulation, social injustice, social disorganization, increasing poverty, and population shifts from rural areas to overcrowded shantytowns where children are born into unsanitary, polluted environments (Kark, Kark, & Abramson, 1993). Future health professionals must be prepared

to make decisions at social, economic, and political levels...to practice in...settings where environmental factors are adversely affecting the population's health...[and to direct practice toward] altering global, national and community environments in order to prevent risks to populations. (Kleffel, 1991, p. 50)

This description aptly applies to the community setting and philosophy for the Por Cristo-BCSON Health Project.

A collaborative venture between Boston College School of Nursing and Por Cristo, a medical missionary group, was initiated in 1991. From a self-supported voluntary health education mission, it has evolved into a credit-granting undergraduate clinical experience in community health nursing. This experience takes place in "Isla Verde", an abjectly poor South American community, where students work with "Father Fred," a British missionary priest who is also an RN.

Students assess and care for families in the home, conduct community assessments, and present community health education programs. Students have set up temporary clinics, diagnosed illnesses, prescribed interventions, counseled, and referred. A simple dispensary now exists and students work with a lay community health worker and part-time physician. Additionally, we have established a relationship with the local university school of nursing. Students have presented classes to their South American peers; in turn, a small group of these students have accompanied us to work in the Isla.

The goals of this experience are to:

- Provide basic health education and service to an underserved population
- Develop creative teaching approaches
- Be immersed in a linguistically and culturally diverse community
- Develop sensitivity and awareness of cultural diversity and universality
- Recognize the dignity of the person irrespective of socioeconomic status
- Help empower the community by enhancing their self-help capabilities
- Observe firsthand the effects of poverty

- Demonstrate the role of the community health nurse

Assessing the Community

An official community assessment and census have not been done in Isla Verde. Although the demographic characteristics appear the same as those in neighboring squatter communities, we realized that an individualized assessment is required to identify specific needs, interests, resources, and community capabilities (Lundeen, 1992; Urrutia-Rojas & Aday, 1991). These data would form the basis for community diagnoses and educational interventions. A descriptive approach to community assessment was planned with the approval of Fr. Fred and community leaders.

Choosing an Assessment Tool

For a number of years, our students have used an assessment tool based on Gordon's 11 functional health patterns (1991) applied to the community (McCarthy, 1994; Box 12-1). Other faculty support this approach as a comprehensive and standardized method of collecting and organizing data (Kriegler & Harton, 1992).

To account for language and life-style differences, the assessment tool required adaptation and a Spanish version was initially developed as a student assignment. This process required back translations and testing to ensure that both nurse and client would exchange exact meanings in their communication (Hatton & Webb, 1993). McDermott and Palchanes (1993) assert that validity in translations must account for colloquialisms, idioms, and other sources of misinterpretation. A bilingual health professional and students (several of whom were bilingual), as well as families, groups, faculty, and students in the host country, took part in the development and testing. Tool refinement is ongoing.

Conducting the Assessment

Students conducted a walking assessment, spoke with community residents and leaders, and toured the institutions in the surrounding city. This allowed the students to observe and record many aspects of the community's life. The following are selected examples of data collected.

Isla Verde is a poor coastal community of squatters living on government-owned property. The community began about 1985 and is divided into cooperatives each run by a council and president. It is quickly expanding and currently about 300,000 people live in the Isla. The community lacks running water, electricity, sanitation services, or fire or police protection; illness is rampant; there is little employment and great educational disadvantage. Many children are malnourished, have multiple parasitic diseases, and frequently die.

The birth rate in the Isla and surrounding areas is high and some deliveries occur at home. Others take place at a local maternity hospital, considered the second or third largest in South America, with 100 births a day and over 500 prenatal visits daily (for problem pregnancies only). One student whose special interest is maternal-child nursing was permitted to return to this hospital for a portion of a day. She observed 16 births within 2 hours with many differences noted in maternity nursing practices. One example was limited use of pain medication.

Many children do not or cannot afford to go to school. They play in the streets, swim or play in polluted waters, urinate and defecate on the ground without handwashing, and run barefoot. Children as young as 5 are left in charge of others much younger while a parent may be at work. A 1-year-old child was observed left in a house alone, unfed and dirty. Many children and adults have lice, fungus, and other skin infections.

Living quarters are frequently one-room shacks built on sand or on stilts over the river's edge, reached by a network of rickety narrow catwalks. Accidental injuries and drownings have resulted from falls into the water. The shacks are constructed of new or salvaged materials such as bamboo, wood, cement block, or cardboard, and frequently

(text continues on page 254)

BOX 12–1. Community Assessment Guide*

I. Health Perception-Health Management Pattern

1. History (community representatives)
   a. In general, what is the health/wellness level of the population on a scale of 1–5, with 5 being the highest level of health/wellness? Any major health problems?
   b. Any strong cultural patterns influencing health practices?
   c. Do people feel they have access to health services?
   d. Is there a demand for any particular health services or prevention programs?
   e. Do people feel fire, police, safety programs are sufficient?
2. Objective data (community records)
   a. Morbidity, mortality, disability rates (by age group, if appropriate)
   b. Accident rates (by district, if appropriate)
   c. Current operating health facilities (types)
   d. Ongoing health promotion/prevention programs; utilization rates
   e. Ratio of health professionals to population
   f. Laws regarding drinking age
   g. Arrest statistics for drugs, drunk driving by age groups

II. Nutritional-Metabolic Pattern

1. History (community representatives)
   a. In general, do most people seem well nourished? Children? Elderly?
   b. Are there food supplement programs? Food stamps: rate of use?
   c. Are foods at a reasonable cost in this area relative to income?
   d. Are stores accessible for most? Meals On Wheels available?
2. Objective data
   a. What is the general appearance of the population (nutritional appearance; teeth; clothing appropriate to climate)? Children? Adults? Elderly?
   b. What food do people purchase (observations of food store check-out counters)?

   c. Are there "junk" food machines in schools, fast food restaurants, etc.?

III. Elimination Pattern

1. History (community representatives)
   a. What are the major kinds of wastes (industrial, sewage, etc)? Are there disposal systems? Recycling programs? Any problems perceived by community?
   b. Is there pest control? Food service inspection (restaurants, street vendors, etc.)?
   c. How is water supplied and what is the quality? Are there testing services? What does water usage cost? Are there drought restrictions?
   d. Is there concern that community growth will exceed good water supply?
   e. Are heating/cooling costs manageable for most? Do help programs exist?
2. Objective data
   a. Communicable disease statistics
   b. Air pollution statistics

IV. Activity-Exercise Pattern

1. History (community representatives)
   a. How do people find the transportation here? To work? To recreation? To health care?
   b. Do people have/use community centers (seniors, others)? Are there recreation facilities for children? Adults? Seniors?
   c. Is housing adequate (availability, cost, size)? Is there public housing?
2. Objective data
   a. Recreation/cultural programs
   b. Aids for the disabled
   c. Residential centers, nursing homes, rehabilitation facilities relative to population needs
   d. External maintenance of homes, yards, apartment houses
   e. General activity level

V. Sleep-Rest Pattern

1. History (community representatives)

(continued)

BOX 12–1. *(Continued)*

a. Is it generally quiet at night in most neighborhoods? If not, why?

b. What are usual business hours? Are there industries operating around-the-clock?

2. Objective data

a. What are the activity-noise levels in business districts? In residential districts?

VI. Cognitive-Perceptual Pattern

1. History (community representatives)

a. Do most groups speak English? Are they bilingual? Other dominant languages?

b. What is the educational level of population?

c. Are schools seen as good/needing improving? Is adult education available/desired? Is vocational training available/desired?

d. What types of problems require community decisions? How are decisions made? What is the best way to get things done/changed here?

2. Objective data

a. Describe the school facilities. What is the drop-out rate?

b. How is the community government structured? Describe the decision-making lines.

VII. Self-Perception–Self-Concept Pattern

1. History (community representatives)

a. Do people feel this is a good community to live in? Is it going up in status, down, about the same?

b. Is this an old community? Fairly new?

c. Does any age group predominate?

d. What are people's moods in general? Do they appear to be enjoying life, stressed, feeling "down"?

e. Do people generally have the kind of abilities needed in this community?

f. Are there community/neighborhood functions?

2. Objective data

a. Racial, ethnic mix (if appropriate)

b. Socioeconomic level

c. General observations of mood

VIII. Role Relationship Pattern

1. History (community representatives)

a. Do people seem to get along well together here? Are there places where people go to socialize?

b. Do people feel they are heard by government? Is there high or low participation in meetings?

c. Are there enough jobs for everyone? Are wages good/fair? Do people like the kind of work available? Do they seem happy in their jobs or appear to have job stress?

d. Are there problems in the neighborhood with riots? Violence? Family violence? Child, spouse, or elder abuse?

e. Does this community get along with adjacent communities? Do they collaborate on any projects?

f. Do neighbors seem to support each other?

g. Are there community get-togethers?

2. Objective data

a. Observation of interactions (generally or at specific meetings)

b. Statistics on interpersonal violence

c. Statistics on employment, income/poverty

d. Divorce rate

IX. Sexuality-Reproductive Pattern

1. History (community representatives)

a. What is the average family size?

b. Do people feel there are any problems with pornography, prostitution? Other?

c. Do people want/support sex education in schools or in the community?

2. Objective data

a. Family size and types of households

b. Male-female ratio

c. Statistics on average maternal age, maternal mortality rate, and infant mortality rate

d. Teen pregnancy rate

e. Abortion rate

(continued)

BOX 12–1. *(Continued)*

    f. Sexual violence statistics
    g. Laws/regulations regarding information on birth control

X. Coping-Stress Pattern

1. History (community representatives)
    a. Are there any groups that seem to be under stress?
    b. What is the need/availability of telephone help lines or support groups (health-related, other)?
2. Objective data
    a. Statistics on delinquency, drug abuse, alcoholism, suicide, psychiatric illness
    b. Unemployment rate by race/ethnicity/sex

XI. Value-Belief Pattern

1. History (community representatives)
    a. Community values: What are the top four issues that people living here see as important in their lives (note health-related values, priorities)?
    b. Do people tend to get involved in causes/local fund raising campaigns?
    c. What religious groups live in the community? What religious institutions are available?
    d. To what extent do people tolerate differences or socially deviant behavior?
2. Objective data
    a. Zoning laws
    b. Scan of public health department reports (goals, priorities)
    c. Health budget relative to total budget

*Adapted with permission from McCarthy, N.C. (1994). The 11 functional health patterns assessment guidelines for communities. Health promotion and the community. In C.L. Edelman & C.L. Mandle (Eds.), *Health promotion throughout the lifespan,* 3rd ed., pp. 209–210. St. Louis, Mosby-Year Book.

do not prevent water or insects from entering. As many as 15 children and adults may live in one room, sleeping on rags on the floor or 6 in one bed. Chickens lived in some homes.

Injuries and deaths from burns are considered a major hazard. They occur frequently because people cook on open flames situated next to bamboo walls; small children pull over pans of hot grease; rubbish is burned in the street, often injuring children playing nearby; and adults get electrical burns and shocks while pirating electricity from main lines.

Without a sanitation system, the people who live on the water have used the tidewaters in place of latrines to carry away human and material waste. Recently, the government has begun to permit people to live in this area. They have filled in parts of the area with tons of sand, permitting housing to be built on a landfill base. The government contends that the sand is the foundation for water pipes to be laid in the future. However, the sand has prevented the natural clearing of waste by tidewater. Groundwater levels have increased particularly after tropical rains and ground waste is accumulating around the homes of families without latrines, increasing the medium for disease transmission.

There is currently no piped-in water system; water is delivered by truck and stored in a covered (or uncovered) barrel outside. It is used for drinking, cooking, bathing, and cleaning. To be potable, water must be boiled for 20 minutes. Where lack of funds precludes buying fuel, water may be boiled for less than the recommended time or not at all. Dysentery, cholera, and typhoid result from ingesting water contaminated with human and animal feces and often cause fatal diarrhea and dehydration. Some families cannot afford even to purchase water.

Extreme poverty makes food purchase and safe storage equally difficult. Food is often eaten with soiled hands or left out uncovered, where flies contaminate it. Many houses have no food visible. One mother admitted to only eating a handful of peanuts the day before. Children are given cola drinks instead of the more costly milk; maternal nutritional deprivation often leads to ineffective breast-feeding; and babies may be given coffee or diluted formula to drink. There is a large outdoor market in the city where vendors sell domestic goods, items in bulk, fresh fruits and vegetables, and meat. Here students observed chickens being freshly killed and then left out without refrigeration. Unfortunately, the market is inaccessible to Isla residents who must find and pay for public transportation to get there. This forces residents to buy goods at small stores in the community where prices and quality of products are problematic.

Health care for the Isla is highly inadequate although it has improved since the recent construction of the small dispensary. Many people cannot afford to pay the equivalent of 50 cents for a visit nor for the resulting prescription. Home remedies, some of which are dangerous, or no treatment at all may be used for a sick individual. Even hospitalized patients may not receive medication, plasma, or bandages until the family prepays.

There are few avenues for rest and recreation in the community. Adults admit they are too poor or tired to do much that can be considered fun. Children have few toys. One day care center was newly established to assist working parents and provide socialization for some children. However, 35 children and infants were tended to by 3 adults. Stress levels are admittedly high and many individuals, particularly men, use alcohol as a relaxant. A number of families attend Sunday religious services or other activities held at the church. The church plays a prominent part in many of the residents' lives. They hold Fr. Fred in great esteem and frequently turn to him for spiritual, emotional, and economic assistance. Fr. Fred has also developed training programs to try to create job skills for interested residents.

Establishing Community Diagnoses

The assessment supported the existence of numerous health hazards in the community, many of which were related to poor hygiene practices and risk-taking behavior. Students were responsible for choosing a functional

health pattern, identifying the associated community diagnoses, prioritizing them according to community need and interest, and planning an intervention based on strengths and weaknesses. Health promotion projects would then be established.

Box 12-2 is a selective list of community diagnoses identified by students. Those starred were given highest priority.

Establishing a Community Health Promotion Intervention

Developing successful health promotion programs for culturally and ethnically diverse populations creates challenges for health educators. Language differences, poverty, prejudice, low literacy, traditional teaching and learning styles, alternative treatment modes and practices, and beliefs about illness are some of the many factors that must be considered if a program is to be effective (DeSantis & Thomas, 1992; El-Katsha & Watts, 1993; Shadick, 1993). The students tried to incorporate the community's needs, interests, values, beliefs, and resources into their health promotion programs while recognizing their own time limitations.

Preparing the Health Promotion Projects

Before arriving in the host country, students arranged themselves in groups and began planning their health promotion projects based on Fr. Fred's feedback and the priority community diagnoses identified by former students. They also incorporated into their teaching activities and materials many of the helpful suggestions found in *Where There Is No Doctor* (Werner, 1992) and *Helping Health Workers Learn* (Werner & Bower, 1982). Spanish versions of these books were also used.

Group 1 chose infant and child care, which included nutrition, immunization, treating diarrhea and dehydration, breast-feeding, hygiene, and accident prevention. Group 2 chose issues of adolescence and women's health, which included understand-

BOX 12–2. Community Diagnoses in Isla Verde

Health Perception-Health Management Pattern

*Health Seeking Behaviors related to (r/t) faithful attendance at classes, active questioning, attentiveness

*Injury: Actual and Potential r/t multiple sources of burns, abuse, drowning, broken glass and syringes on road, bare feet, broken boards in houses on stilts, getting hit by cars, violence (rock throwing, guns, etc.)

Altered Protection r/t wife abuse, child abuse, sexual abuse, lack of police or social protection

Impaired Home Maintenance r/t sense of hopelessness, lack of structural integrity, and inability to purchase repair materials

Infection: Actual and Potential r/t not cleaning wounds, bug bites, using inappropriate remedies for burns (i.e., toothpaste, mud, sputum), multiple sex partners and prostitution, and lack of condom use

Pain r/t lack of medicine, conservative use of analgesics

Nutritional-Metabolic Pattern

Altered Growth and Development r/t altered nutrition and sensory deprivation

Altered Nutrition: Nutritional Deficit r/t inability to purchase food, inability to obtain quality food, knowledge deficit in best use and preparation of local foods, diarrhea

Fatigue r/t nutritional deficit, overworking, etc.

Fluid Volume Deficit r/t diarrhea and knowledge deficit

Elimination Pattern

*Alteration in Elimination: Diarrhea r/t environmental pollution, poor hygiene practices, barriers to implementing prevention strategies

Activity-Exercise Pattern

Diversional Activity Deficit r/t small overcrowded living situations and neighborhoods, deficit of play space or equipment

Ineffective Breathing Pattern r/t environmental dust, untreated asthma

Sleep-Rest Pattern

Sleep Disturbance r/t overcrowding, lack of adequate space, noise

Cognitive-Perceptual Pattern

*Knowledge Deficit r/t AIDS transmission, basic hygiene

Cognitive Impairment: Potential r/t malnourishment before and after birth, child neglect, lack of stimulation

Self-Concept-Self-Perception Pattern

Fear r/t robbery, rape, abandonment, inability to support family units

Powerlessness: Severe r/t lack of education, social control, abuse of women and children

Role Relationship Pattern

*Impaired Social Interaction r/t lack of community cohesiveness, inability to request help despite need

Altered Parenting r/t very young pregnancies, no resources, unemployment, abuse cycles, single female-headed families of many closely spaced children

Violence: Potential for r/t dispiritedness, lack of protection against abuse and injustice, reports of weapons in community

Sexuality-Reproductive Pattern

*Altered Sexuality Patterns r/t lack of sex education, frequent unplanned pregnancies, rape, prostitution, unprotected sex

Coping-Stress Tolerance Pattern

*Family Coping: Potential for Growth r/t observation and report of families supporting and caring for one another and unselfishly sharing all their goods

Anxiety r/t deaths and debilitating diseases

Defensive Coping r/t deplorable living conditions

Value-Belief Pattern

Spiritual Distress r/t lack of basic human needs, human rights abuse, expressions of hopelessness

ing the transmission and prevention of STDs and AIDS and the need for sex education as a preventive approach to adolescent pregnancy. Group 3 chose general health and safety issues. These included burn prevention and treatment, first aid for choking, when to seek medical attention, and principles of nutrition adapted to the customs, income, and available products of the region.

Developing Relationships and Gaining Acceptance

Father Fred helped the students gain acceptance by securing support of community leaders and residents (Michielutte & Beal, 1990). Students are warmly welcomed, however, because of their willingness to "roll up their sleeves and dig in." They have paid for and helped construct latrines, cleaned a poor mother's back yard of broken glass where tiny tots were running around barefoot, and even built a table out of new and used wood for a family who ate on the floor. They have also brought medical supplies, schoolbooks, and many other items that have been distributed to the neediest. The community looks forward to the arrival of students and the numbers of people attending the community 'charlas' or chats run by the students are increasing.

Implementing the Health Promotion Projects

Once in the community, discussion groups were formed to promote community participation, self-select topics, and provide insight on the dimensions of problems (Windsor et al., 1994). The attendees were pleased to have an opportunity to offer suggestions, admitting that few people ever asked for their input. Through their suggestions, students conducted daily 'charlas' or afternoon talks that were publicized by word of mouth and posted notices. Classes were held in either the dispensary or adjoining church and were extremely well attended. Most of the attendees were women, many with children, and it was not unusual to see a standing-room-only crowd.

Teaching Strategies

The students used various approaches, models, and posters in their teaching projects. A large toothbrush and set of teeth were used to demonstrate oral hygiene to children. Each child was then given a toothbrush for return demonstration as well as a sample of toothpaste. A doll of color was used to demonstrate baby care and breast-feeding positions. A realistic model of breasts that could be worn over the chest permitted teaching appropriate positions for breast self-examination. Verbal instructions, posters, and handouts were used to teach how to prevent diarrhea in children and how to prepare and administer oral rehydration therapy. An old donated microscope was used to teach about sources of bacterial contamination and children and adults alike were fascinated to see teeming microbes living in samples taken from an ordinary water barrel. By visualizing the organisms that make people sick, the community could understand the basis for teaching them to cover food and boil water.

Two discussion groups were organized by students: a coeducational adolescent support group to discuss sexual development, prevention of unplanned pregnancy, and rape and a parents support group, which men attended, to discuss community issues such as stress reduction and abuse as well as strategies of empowerment.

One important community-wide project is the burn prevention and treatment program. Nursing students present this program to children, adults, health providers, and teachers, using the clinic, school, church, and day care center for settings. The objectives of this program are for participants to identify sources of burn injuries and deaths, practice preventive strategies, and treat burns appropriately.

Small groups of children are gathered and the nursing students appear with orange gloves, red shirts, or bright yellow tights, simulating fire colors. Participation is encouraged by a question-answer period before and after the program. The children are asked if they know anyone who has been burned. What happened to that person? What caused the burn? What could have been done to prevent it?

The children usually know a burn victim and mention pain and scarring. The causes range from playing with matches to being scalded with hot liquid. Their knowledge of preventive methods is often limited to not playing with matches. They are then asked what they should do if their clothing catches on fire? Some of the students know the correct answer and are complimented. The student teachers then role play with props, actually rolling on the ground or floor while others recite the Spanish version of "Stop, Drop, and Roll." Volunteers from the audience are then selected.

Posters emphasizing burn prevention strategies depict storing matches away from children, turning pot handles inward, observing children when a trash or other type of fire is burning, and securing a metal shield behind a cooking fire.

Proper burn treatment includes understanding how to treat pain, keeping the wound clean, assessing severity, and knowing when to seek medical treatment. Posters depict first, second, and third degree burns. Students emphasize protecting the burn from dirt, excreta, and insects, and using clean cool water on first degree burns and warm salt water as compresses for second degree burns (Werner, 1992). They explain why grease, mud, oil, coffee, feces, urine, or toothpaste should never be used and that severe burns, signs of infection, or extended burns on small children should be treated at the clinic.

An oral quiz is given at the end of each session and questions from the audience are answered. Children are instructed to share what they have learned with their siblings and parents. Teachers are also given materials for reinforcing the lessons.

Outcomes

Evaluation of our various health promotion activities must be ongoing and there are no statistics to demonstrate the outcomes. However, the Por Cristo-BCSON Health Project has helped to create a vehicle for health promotion by establishing support groups for adolescents and adults. Fr. Fred plans to continue these groups and to organize a committee of residents who have volunteered to be group leaders in health promotion activities. As a result of our relationship with the local school of nursing, faculty have expressed an interest in creating an affiliation at Isla Verde for their students and having them continue working on our health projects. In this way, we will promote continuity in health teaching and nursing intervention from within the population. Importantly, teacher and learner satisfaction have been rated as high.

We plan to continue the burn prevention and treatment program and to develop a method for reporting burn data. This will be a challenge in a system where people frequently self-treat except in major crises. However, the community has consistently demonstrated the desire to learn and to promote self-help. They will be asked to help develop a plan for documentation.

The majority of the U.S. population will soon be comprised of people originating from Africa, Latin America, and Asia. An overseas immersion experience provides a milieu for health professionals to develop and incorporate cultural competence and language fluency into their clinical practice. Successful health promotion strategies must be congruent with the health beliefs and practices of the target population, based on fundamental concerns and needs, and aimed at results that are desirable and ultimately achievable (Kreps & Kunimoto, 1994, p. 122). These principles will continue to guide future missions to Isla Verde.

Example 2: A Sex Education Program for Senior Adults

Despite growing efforts to promote positive aging, sexuality has historically been omitted from health education programs for the elderly. In today's era of greater sexual awareness, health professionals must recognize that sexual activity among senior adults can extend throughout a lifetime and does so under favorable conditions. The ability to express oneself sexually remains an important function for many older individuals and sexual health must be viewed as an area of responsibility for health professionals (Krozy, 1984; McCracken, 1988).

Sexual health may be defined as the capacity to express oneself sexually in accordance with one's moral values and choices, free from guilt or anxiety, and in accordance with one's physical capabilities. It includes an understanding of the biologic, psychological, and social determinants of sexual expression. However, myths and stereotypes surrounding sexuality in old age have impeded sexual expression as well as sexual education of older adults.

Sexuality is a legitimate aspect of health promotion; many older adults have questions about sexuality but not the opportunity for frank discussion, and they could benefit from sex education geared to their stage of development (Shomaker, 1980). Many of the barriers to sexual expression, such as suppression of activity, feelings of guilt, and loss of identity as a sexual being (Genevay, 1978), can be mitigated by factual and sensitive sex education. As part of my doctoral research, I developed a sex education program for people 65 and older (Krozy, 1987). Through the years, this material has been presented to various groups of older adults and adapted for health care professionals and lay audiences as a means to eliminate the ageist stereotypes that have a negative impact on the not-yet-old or their caregivers.

Identifying Needs and Interests

A study was undertaken to determine the effect of a sexuality program on older adults' sexual knowledge and attitudes, reasons for attending, the presence of sexual anxiety or guilt (preexisting dissonance), perceived outcomes, topics of interest, and methodologic considerations. Pre- and postprogram questionnaires were developed for data collection. The tools assessed whether older adults perceived a need for sex education, what topics or problems they would want addressed, the materials or methods of presentation they would find appropriate, and their sexual knowledge and attitudes (Box 12-3).

The presence of sexual dissonance was also assessed. *Cognitive dissonance* is the sense of discomfort people feel when what they do differs from what they believe, such as continuing to smoke despite knowing the risks. Neither high nor low dissonance tends to motivate change. However, when the pressure to change is high and the discomfort from the undesired behavior is moderate, individuals may expose themselves to dissonance-producing material as a stimulus to behavior change (Festinger, 1957). The literature suggested that despite potential benefits, some seniors might reject the opportunity to attend a human sexuality program because of discomfort with the topic, fear of experiencing anxiety or frustration, or believing it inappropriate. Others, however, might attend despite discomfort because of a desire to change their sexual knowledge, attitudes, or behavior. Cognitive dissonance theory was therefore used to examine the rationale for voluntary exposure to sex information. Adaptations of Thorne's Sex Inventory (1966) and Janda and O'Grady's Sex Anxiety Inventory (1980) permitted assessing preexisting dissonance.

The pretest showed that many participants were unaware of the following facts.

- Sexual problems can be treated despite having existed for many years.
- Women can learn to become orgasmic at any age.
- People who remain sexually active can prevent a disuse phenomenon.
- Heart attacks do not commonly occur during sexual intercourse.
- Some people can perform sexually after a stroke.
- Few drugs or foods can increase sexual power.
- Elderly men are *not* frequent child molesters.

Many respondents held the following beliefs.

- Men should initiate the sex act.

BOX 12–3. Senior Adult Sexuality Questionnaire

Sexual Knowledge and Attitudes

This section contains various statements about sexuality that participants answered with agree, disagree, or unsure.

1. Most sexual problems are a result of an illness or health condition.
2. There are a number of drugs and foods available which increase sexual power.
3. Menopause (change of life) decreases a woman's desire for sexual activity.
4. It is harder for a single older woman to find a mate than for a single older man.
5. If a couple has had a sexual problem for many years, it is almost impossible to treat it.
6. For most people past 65, sex is just not important.
7. Certain medications decrease a person's sexual ability.
8. Senior adults are unwilling to talk about sex.
9. A common time for heart attacks to occur is during sexual intercourse (making love).
10. After age 60, men cannot father children.
11. People who masturbate (play with their private parts) are generally mentally ill.
12. After a heart attack, a person should not have sex.
13. Most women do not enjoy sex as much as men.
14. The proper way to have intercourse (make love) is with the man on top of the woman.
15. Some women have more sexual interest when they get older.
16. Touching and physical closeness are as satisfying as sexual intercourse.
17. Women can learn to have an orgasm (climax) at any age.
18. Men should initiate the sex act.
19. Oral sex (mouth-genital contact) is something nice people don't do.
20. Most women need stimulation of the clitoris in order to reach orgasm (climax).
21. Women should date or marry men who are older than they are.
22. People have to remain sexually active or they will lose their ability to perform.
23. Living together outside of marriage is sinful.
24. If I didn't have a mate, I would consider having a sexual relationship with someone of my own sex.
25. A person who has had a stroke can no longer perform sexually.
26. The sexual freedom of today's younger generation has produced a society without morals.
27. Child molesters are often elderly men.
28. Dirty movies and magazines (pornography) should be removed from the market.
29. Homosexuals are sinful.
30. Whatever two people decide to do sexually is okay, as long as they both consent.
31. Masturbation is a healthy release of sexual tension.
32. The basic change in older people's ability to perform sexually is that it takes longer.
33. It is more important for a woman to be married to her sexual partner than it is for a man.
34. Most married women stop having intercourse because their husbands are no longer interested.
35. Sex education should be taught in the schools.

Sources of Information

Respondents were asked to indicate whether they had discussed sexual questions or problems, since age 60, with any of the following people:

1. Physician   2. Religious leader   3. Spouse   4. Family member, not spouse

5. Nurse   6. Friend   7. Other _____

Respondents were asked to indicate whether they had learned about sexuality and aging through any of the following sources:

1. Books   2. Magazines   3. Television   4. Newspapers

5. Radio   6. Other _____

- Oral sex was something that nice people didn't engage in.
- Most women didn't enjoy sex as much as men.
- Senior adults are unwilling to talk about sex.
- Today's sexual freedom has produced a society without morals.

These findings supported the basis for the sex education program.

Description of the Learners and Settings

Participants were active, well men and women, aged 65 and older, married and single, without hearing, visual, or mobility deficits that would impede learning. The oldest attendee was 92. They were members of organized groups in religious-sponsored suburban community centers offering health and recreational programs for senior adults. Permission was obtained from administrators and participants. Before each program, written and verbal announcements were given so that there would be clear understanding of the nature of the program.

A group with similar ethnic background and socioreligious affiliation was chosen to reduce population variance, increase learning and lower resistance through perceived commonalities, and increase motivation to attend by perceived moral appropriateness resulting from religious sponsorship (Smith, 1978; Wells, Brown, Horm, Carleton, & Lasater, 1994).

Programs were held in comfortable, well-lighted small rooms with adequate ventilation and temperature, which allowed for general comfort and good visualization of the blackboard and speaker. Table and chair arrangements were flexible to allow for small group discussion, writing, or circular format.

Description of the Program

The program consisted of four 2-hour sessions of didactic information and participatory activities. Box 12-4 presents an outline and sample exercises. The topics selected by

participants in rank order were: the process of aging, research on elderly sexuality, resources for sex information, communicating sexual needs to partner, medications and sexual function, sexual problems and treatment, illness and sexual function, sexual anatomy and physiology, sex and religion, techniques of lovemaking, and sex and cultural beliefs. Homosexuality was not of interest to the majority, but participants ultimately asked a number of questions regarding homosexual practices.

Values clarification exercises (i.e., what did you learn about sex from your parents? religion? school?) helped participants become aware of their own sexual attitudes. Analysis of sexist or ageist humor showed how myths and stereotypes are perpetuated by society. Jokes, comics, and birthday cards served as convenient learning tools (e.g., one card asked, "What does a person your age need to know about sex?" The inside was blank.). The use of humor as a teaching methodology also reduces tension when one can laugh at something that produces anxiety. Sexually explicit films were not used based on participants' written objections. Assertiveness training role play exercises were used to improve communication and protect rights of aging individuals.

Participants found it enlightening to reflect on the influence of their sexuality in most of their experiences throughout the life cycle. For example, discussions and exercises in assertiveness pointed out how women learn submissive behaviors while men learn aggression and their negative outcomes. The pervasiveness of sexual interest, desire, and activity throughout life was also discussed. Each person's sexual expression depends on such factors as needs, beliefs, and opportunities, but sexual appetites differ; thus lack of desire or sexual inactivity are only problematic when so identified.

Outcomes

That older adults are capable of and eager to learn about sexuality was seen in the dra-

BOX 12–4. A Human Sexuality Program for Older Adults

Objectives of the program:

Participants will understand

1. The barriers to sexual fulfillment in old age
2. The effect of illness and medications on sexuality
3. What scientists consider normal sexual behavior
4. How sexual problems can be treated
5. Aging and the sexual response
6. Additional resources for sexual information and treatment

Session I: Overview and Introduction

1. Introduction of teacher and members
   a. Clarify how participants wish to be addressed
2. Establish group norms
   a. Confidentiality
   b. Freedom to refuse to answer or participate
   c. Respect for individuals' ethics, beliefs, values
   d. Sensitive listening and encouragement
      (1). Some issues difficult to discuss
      (2). Appreciate sharing of personal, meaningful information
3. Goals of program
   a. Fact not fiction
   b. Informed decision-making
   c. Self-awareness
   d. Self-confidence
4. Definition of sex versus sexuality
   a. Knowledge (scientific knowledge, self-awareness)
   b. Attitudes (values, beliefs, religion, society)
   c. Behavior (choice, desire, capacity)

Attitudes related to sexuality

1. Sexual behavior learned as a child; male and female roles
   a. From birth
   b. At adolescence (sources of formal/informal sex education)
   c. As an adult (married, single or postmarried)
2. Religious teachings on sexuality
   a. Purpose of sex
   b. Restrictions and sanctions

3. Sex and laws
   a. Purpose of laws
   b. Review of various sexual laws
4. Sex and modern society
   a. Sexual revolution?
      (1). Sexual behavior of today's youth
      (2). Difference between youth and senior adults
      (3). Reason for differences/similarities
   b. Society's attitudes toward senior adults
      (1). Attitudes toward sexuality of senior adults
      (2). Seniors attitudes toward sexuality
         (a). Values clarification: Sex for seniors is....

Summary of session I

Session II: Sexuality, Aging, and Response

1. Warm-up exercise: terminology
   a. Male anatomy and physiology
   b. Female anatomy and physiology
2. Masters and Johnson: human sexual response
3. Comparison of response in younger and older adults
4. Classification of sexual dysfunctions/problems
5. Introduction to sexual problems
   a. Physical causes
   b. Drug causes

Summary of session II

Session III: Sexual Problems and Treatments

1. Warm-up exercise: humor analysis
2. Sexual problems with a psychological basis
   a. Lack of knowledge
   b. Fear
   c. Guilt
   d. Poor self-image
   e. Inability to communicate
   f. Lack of variation
   g. Religious and social taboos
3. Treatment of sexual problems
   a. Education
   b. Counseling
   c. Therapy
4. Modes of sexual expression
   a. Values clarification exercises

(continued)

BOX 12–4. *(Continued)*

Summary of session III

Session IV: General Discussion

1. Warm-up exercise: humor analysis
2. Assertiveness training exercises
3. Review of research on sexuality and aging
4. Course evaluation
5. Termination and refreshments

Sample Analysis of Humor Exercise

Two elderly gentlemen were overheard talking about sex. "Well," said Sam, "I guess I'm not the man I used to be." "Why?" asked his friend. "You see, last night I woke my wife up at 2 AM to make love and she told me that we had made love at midnight. So you see," he said tapping his head, "I'm losing my memory."

Sample Values Clarification Exercises

The beliefs, attitudes, and values that people have are usually a result of lifelong learning. Surprisingly, however, we are not always aware of those values or why we have them. The following exercises ask you to choose what is appropriate or not appropriate, what you agree with or disagree with, your preferences and nonpreferences. In making your choices, you will become aware of your values.

1. Once a person grows old, his or her appearance becomes....
2. You've just learned that your granddaughter is living with a man. You feel....
3. As a child, I learned that masturbation was....
4. What is a man called who "scores" with a lot of women? What is a woman called who "sleeps with" a lot of men? Why the difference?
5. A man should always initiate sexual activity.

Sample Assertiveness Exercises

You are an 80-year-old woman who has spent a great deal of time choosing an outfit for a very special occasion. You overhear a salesperson say, "I don't know why she's being so fussy. Who's going to notice what an old lady wears." How would you react to this remark? What would you do? What would you say?

You are a 66-year-old man who has just recovered from a heart attack. You have been advised that you can resume sexual intercourse but not in the missionary (man on top) position. You would like to ask your wife to change the way you have always made love. What would you do? What would you say?

---

matic postprogram knowledge scores and the less dramatic attitude changes. These results may have been fostered by a climate where confidentiality, sensitivity, and respect were stressed and all questions were encouraged and answered. Participants were able to request clarification and receive positive feedback and reinforcement on their responses.

Neither preexisting dissonance levels nor the desire to reduce dissonance motivated voluntary attendance. More than half the participants attended because they were interested in becoming more comfortable with sexual issues and thought the information would be useful. Others were interested simply in learning new information. Most neither expected nor experienced discomfort, possibly resulting from freely choosing to attend the program. Group discussion of such sensitive subjects as masturbation, the unfounded reasons for its taboos, and its pervasiveness and acceptability into old age may have afforded relief to some individuals. Perhaps, a number of individuals may have found the program uplifting in that the presentation of sexual content gave permission to be sexual and enjoy one's sexuality.

Results of this study suggest that the method of presentation for a human sexuality program was appropriate. Older individuals are interested in diverse aspects about sexuality, willing to discuss sexual issues if sensitively dealt with, neither sexually ignorant, overly conservative nor unchangeable, and able to benefit from sex education.

Implications for Community Health Educators

Sex education for senior adults is an important part of health promotion. Older individuals have questions about sexual response, dating and, in more recent times, risks of STDs and AIDS (Talashel, Tichy, & Epping, 1990; Whipple & Scura, 1989). Discussion groups and forums should be established in community settings such as health centers, nursing homes, or senior housing. Health professionals have a responsibility to learn about the intimacy needs of elders (Rankin, 1989; Roberts, 1989; Rothman & Sebastian, 1990) and to include sexuality in their health promotion programs. This will require that they possess comfort with their own sexuality (Krozy, 1978), awareness of their biases (Quinn-Krach & Van Hoozer, 1988), and the ability to teach creatively, knowledgeably, and appropriately. Once this is accomplished, they will find an eager and interested group of learners from whom they will also learn a great deal.

Example 3: The Challenge— A Worksite Health Promotion Program

Promoting healthy life-styles is both a humanistic and economic concern to employers and those providing occupational health promotion programs. The American Association of Occupational Health Nurses has recommended that by the year 2000, 90% of workplaces will provide their employees with risk reduction and health promotion services (Swanson & Albrecht, 1993). Although not mandated by federal regulation, many companies are taking a proactive approach to health promotion and are offering employees various services promoting wellness.

Successful worksite programs must promote skill in health practices, provide peer support, promote the notion that health is controllable, involve the employee in planning both personal behavior modification as well as change in the work environment, and define health as wellness rather than risk reduction (Pender, Walker, Sechrist, & Frank-Stromberg, 1990). Moreover, Salazar (1991) contends that successful outcomes increase when programs use a theoretical base for planning and development of interventions.

The Challenge is an ongoing health promotion program for university faculty and staff. It occurs during the Spring semester and includes weekly discussions on health, diet, and exercise; organized exercise activities; and establishment of support groups. The model is based on a team approach with points awarded to those who lose weight within a predetermined range, engage in specific exercises, and attend weekly 55-minute presentations on a relevant topic. Each team consists of at least five members, headed by a team captain who tallies individual weight and exercise points weekly. Programs include a nominal registration fee and various prizes and "perks" such as a tee shirt with the program logo.

The School of Nursing faculty and students provide consultation on various aspects of the overall program, conduct height and weight measurement and blood pressure screening at the first and last sessions, and conduct some of the seminars. Topics include principles of behavior modification, choosing the right exercises, understanding one's relationship to food, principles of nutrition, stress management, and maintaining one's health promotion program. Additional nutritional and health counseling and referrals are made available. We incorporated Lewin's force field analysis and various health promotion strategies in teaching participants how to plan and maintain wellness behaviors.

Force Field Analysis

Lewin's force field analysis suggests that first, compliance increases when individuals identify both the stumbling blocks to their own behavior change and the change strategies they would find most acceptable. Second, knowledge of the forces that promote positive behavior change and the strategies that are more likely to effect change will assist the health professional in improving the target population's health outcomes.

Force field analysis, although developed in the 1940s by Lewin and associates, is still considered an important approach to planned change (Lewin, Dembo, Festinger, & Sears, 1944). The behavioral change strategies consist of: *unfreezing* (making one aware of the need for change or increasing the readiness or willingness to change), *moving* (using a variety of cognitive, affective, or regulatory strategies to implement the change), and *refreezing* (that phase of the change when the new behavior is internalized) (Lewin et al., 1944).

Force field analysis refers to a major part of the unfreezing stage. It concerns itself with those forces (factors, determinants) that will assist the change (driving forces) and those that will impede change (restraining forces). Change may be brought about in three ways: adding forces that promote change, reducing forces that impede change, or redirecting forces that support change (Lewin et al., 1944). Forces promoting or impeding change frequently are of unequal strength; for example, resistance to change may be weakened when the behavior is deemed as culturally appropriate, pleasurable, or easy to maintain. When the suggested action is deemed as a loss, painful, culturally incorrect, expensive, beyond the resources of the target population, or without value, resistance will be stronger.

Health Promotion Strategies

A variety of health promotion techniques have been suggested in the literature. Successful interventions often incorporate a variety of approaches because no one technique has been found superior. A combination of strategies that provide factual information, stimulate motivation, help change attitudes and behavior, and promote competence may better address the multifaceted nature of health behavior (Table 12-1).

Helping Identify Personal Barriers, Enhancers, and Change Strategies

The program was introduced with the notion of how challenging it is to advise people to change lifelong habits. Health professionals in looking at stress reduction have often been guilty of simply suggesting changing one's life-style, without assessing the availability of options or resources. It was pointed out, however, that the interest in improving health and fitness shown by so many individuals was a positive sign of motivation. The attitudinal framework for these sessions would therefore be positive thinking and positive reinforcement rather than negative thinking and reinforcement.

It was explained that behavior (what people do) is a result of what people believe or value and the meaning attached to the behavior. The more value (pleasure, reward, satisfaction, or relief of emotional or physical pain) attached to the behavior, the more difficult it is to change the behavior. This leads to habits—both good and bad (e.g., putting on your seat belt every time you get into a car versus reaching for snacks every time you sit in front of a television). Thus, changing our attitudes and customary behaviors requires having knowledge, motivation, resources, and skill.

The purpose of these sessions was to help participants identify their particular strengths and weaknesses, uncover what they valued, examine the bases for their actions, and identify some of the strategies they could use in reaching and maintaining their individual goals. Force field analysis was explained as a method that helps people to identify the forces that promote or prevent their own behavior change. Many of these forces are common to all of us. Participants began to identify barriers to change such as fear of failure and sense of loss.

For The Challenge, forces that promote or impede change were combined into three categories: biologic-physiologic, emotional-cognitive, and social-cultural-economic. Exam-

TABLE 12-1. Behavioral Change Strategies

Informing

Direct learning	Commonly uses a group setting such as the classroom and allows material to be shared and discussed by several individuals.
Audiovisual materials	Include written instructions, videos, tapes, structural models, computerized instruction, or even cartoons where the concepts being taught can be demonstrated.

Motivating

Self-instruction	A popular method but difficult to evaluate. An example of self-instruction is the use of "how to" books.
Bibliotherapy	A promising area of research using a combination of self-instruction and directed reading, evaluation, and group discussion. May involve inspirational story where crisis situation is resolved; reading about health risk information with follow-up counseling (Windsor et al., 1993).
Mass media	Uses persuasion and power of the written word in newspapers, radio, or TV. Influential in changing some behavior (Popham et al., 1993) but readers who experience cognitive dissonance may ignore the message or refute it (Chapman, Wong, & Smith, 1993). Mass media may also have a negative effect because of sensationalist themes of sex and violence and high power advertising.

Skill Building

Demonstration/ return demonstration	Experiential method commonly used for teaching procedures, e.g., how to prepare foods or engage in low-impact aerobics.
Simulation	A representation of a real-life situation to teach new behavioral responses. Practice sessions on responding to emergencies or conducting one's activities of daily living while blindfolded are examples.
Role play	A form of simulation whereby each participant assumes the characteristics of a player in a situation. Through role play, individuals can be taught in a nonthreatening atmosphere how to respond in an effective way (Weston & Cranton, 1986).
Inoculation	Also known as refusal skills training and assertiveness training are methods that prepare people for setbacks and challenges. Individuals role play potential stressful situations or exposure to real-life stress, and rehearse protective responses that will prevent backsliding (Barth, 1993). Assertiveness promotes the ability to say "no" in a comfortable and gracious way (such as upholding the decision to abstain from alcohol or refusing a high-calorie food) while respecting others' rights.
Activism participation	Requires participation in activities such as letter writing or lobbying that create an unfavorable environment for the activity such as smoking. Also stimulates participants to resist or terminate the behavior (Edwards et al., 1992).

Modifying Attitudes and Behavior

Imagery	Creates a mental picture of a habit-free self by focusing on the competing behavior and visualizing the self without the habit. For example, individuals giving up smoking must imagine themselves as nonsmokers; seeing themselves with a cigarette in their hand or mouth must be incongruent with their picture of wholesomeness.
Cueing	A stimulus–response-based approach using human or computer-generated telephone calls, wall charts, or other types of messages to remind an individual to continue an activity. This intervention has been used to enhance medication compliance, immunizations, or appointments (Stehr-Green, Dini, Lindegren, & Patriarca, 1993).

(continued)

TABLE 12-1.   *(Continued)*

Tailoring	Uses compromise as an interim step to change. Valuable when a suggested change is viewed as extremely difficult or impossible (e.g., a stringent dietary restriction of salt or sugar).
Contracting	A verbal or written agreement toward one or more specific actions. Requires feedback to be effective.
Contingency contracting	An "if-then" approach that states a behavioral goal as well as the rewards for its achievement. Each step of change and reward are shared with a health care provider.
Graduated regimens	Implements the desired behavior changes in intermediate steps and goals. Acknowledges each level of success.
Self-monitoring	A method of self-tracking (e.g., one's daily intake or weight) using a journal or diary. Frequently short-lived.
Self-confrontation	Consciously interrupts negative thinking. Person says "stop," claps hands. Works in conjunction with self-reinforcement.
Self reinforcement	Acknowledges positive behavior and verbalizes it frequently out loud.
External reinforcement	Uses social support or continuity of care system to help maintain behavior change.
Self-generated aversive behavioral control	A method of urge control using a negative stimulus such as snapping an elastic band on the wrist or stimulating an acupressure point. Permits time to intervene between urge and acting. Is enhanced by urge replacement/response substitution with another behavioral strategy, such as taking a walk in lieu of smoking.

Other

Hypnosis	A method of behavior modification that requires the individual to be put into a receptive mental state where suggestion influences the behavior.
Acupuncture	Behavioral response believed to be a neurochemical reaction to endorphin production released by stimulating various superficial nerve endings.
Pharmacotherapy	Prescribed therapies often used with drug addictions, e.g., nicotine patches or gum for tobacco addiction, Antabuse for alcoholism, and Methadone for heroin addiction.

ples of biologic-physiologic factors include the effects of genetic makeup (e.g., body type, metabolism), gender, existing disease processes, and age. Emotional-cognitive factors address coping styles, mental status, long- and short-term health goals and knowledge deficits. In the domain entitled social-cultural-economic factors, examples included cultural food patterns, job-related activity patterns (e.g., sedentary work, frequent restaurant dining), and access to health services.

As the beginning step in self-knowledge, participants were instructed to identify a realistic goal and note on an assessment form those positive and negative factors particularly relevant to them (Fig. 12-1). They were then instructed to assign a weight to each factor in accordance with how easy or difficult it

would be to accomplish. This was based on numerous research reports suggesting that self-efficacy, the belief one is capable of carrying out the action, is one of the strongest determinants of successful behavior change (Bandura, 1982; Lawrance & McElroy, 1986; Merritt, 1989). Finally, each participant received a worksheet to list the factors perceived as barriers and the behavioral strategies they felt would be helpful.

Because of the group's diverse makeup, many different issues related to health, diet, and exercise were identified. Participants viewed the university's commitment to health promotion and the availability of excellent resources and supportive fellow staff as external motivators. Written evaluations indicated that this session provided insight

THE CHALLENGE

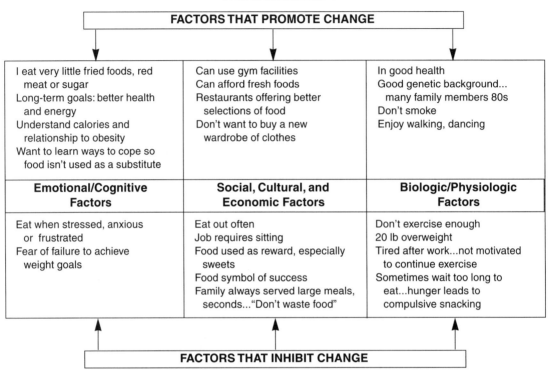

FACTORS THAT PROMOTE CHANGE		
I eat very little fried foods, red meat or sugar Long-term goals: better health and energy Understand calories and relationship to obesity Want to learn ways to cope so food isn't used as a substitute	Can use gym facilities Can afford fresh foods Restaurants offering better selections of food Don't want to buy a new wardrobe of clothes	In good health Good genetic background... many family members 80s Don't smoke Enjoy walking, dancing
Emotional/Cognitive Factors	**Social, Cultural, and Economic Factors**	**Biologic/Physiologic Factors**
Eat when stressed, anxious or frustrated Fear of failure to achieve weight goals	Eat out often Job requires sitting Food used as reward, especially sweets Food symbol of success Family always served large meals, seconds..."Don't waste food"	Don't exercise enough 20 lb overweight Tired after work...not motivated to continue exercise Sometimes wait too long to eat...hunger leads to compulsive snacking
FACTORS THAT INHIBIT CHANGE		

FIGURE 12–1. Behavior change self-assessment, using weight loss as an example.

into behavior patterns that had not been considered.

Given the success of this approach with The Challenge, this method has been taught to students for use with individual or community groups. It remains important that follow-up be done to identify stumbling blocks that may arise and to ascertain that the intervention(s) selected are appropriate, realistic, accessible, and used.

Summary

Health professionals are often responsible for helping clients learn new ways for improving their health and achieving high-level wellness. Earlier chapters provided theoretical models for developing patient education pro-

grams. This chapter presents three health promotion projects that demonstrate how to assess for areas where health education is needed, how to teach people to identify their own behavioral barriers and enhancers to change, and how to promote clients' health through techniques of behavior change. Health promotion occurs in many different settings with diverse population groups. The health educator must therefore develop cultural competence and the ability to act as advocate to promote the community's acquiring necessary resources and successfully achieving health promotion goals. Although personal responsibility for health is recognized, consideration is given to external factors arising from the political climate, the social environment, the economy, and the resources that may or may not be available from the health system.

Strategies for Critical Analysis and Application

1. Compare the differences in planning a health promotion program for an individual, a family, or an entire community. What are the advantages and disadvantages of each approach.

2. You are working in a community comprised of many low-income families and elderly. How would these demographic variables be used in developing a health promotion campaign? What other information would you obtain in prioritizing the community's needs?

3. What are the goals of health promotion programs in accordance with development stage?

4. Discuss how culture and language influence health education programs in a community.

5. Identify the persuasive methods that advertisers use to convince consumers to buy such products as tobacco or alcoholic beverages. How could these same methods be used to foster health-promoting behaviors (e.g., use of seat belts).

6. What strategies are necessary to reach a smoke-free society by the year 2000?

REFERENCES

Bandura, A. (1982). Self-efficacy mechanism in human agency. *American Psychologist, 37,* 122-147.

Barth, R. P. (1993). *Reducing the risks: Building skills to prevent STD & HIV* (2nd ed.). Santa Cruz, CA: ETR Associates.

Chapman, S., Long, W. L., & Smith, W. (1993). Self-exempting beliefs about smoking and health: Differences between smokers and ex-smokers. *American Journal of Public Health, 83,* 215-219.

Clark, M. J. (1992). *Nursing in the community.* East Norwalk, CT: Appleton & Lange.

Cohen, B. B., Lederman, R. I., Connolly, G. N., & Danley, R. A. (1991). *Smoking: Death, disease and dollars.* Boston: Massachusetts Department of Public Health, Chronic Disease Surveillance Program, Bureau of Health Statistics, Research and Evaluation, and Office for Nonsmoking and Health, Bureau of Parent, Child and Adolescent Health.

da Costa e Silva, V. L. (1993). Anti-tobacco posters in Brazil: Fighting smoking with humour, satire, and ridicule. *Tobacco Control, 2,* 189-190.

DeSantis, L., & Thomas, J. T. (1992). Health education and the immigrant Haitian mother: Cultural insights for community health nurses. *Public Health Nursing, 9,* 87-96.

Drexler, M. (1994, October 23). Tapping the youth market. *The Boston Globe Magazine,* 17-24, 30-31.

Edwards, C. C., Elder, J. P., de Moor, C., Wildey, M. B., Mayer, J. A., & Senn, K. L. (1992). Predictors of participation in a school-based anti-tobacco activism program. *Journal of Community Health, 17,* 283-289.

El-Katsha, S., & Watts, S. (1993). A multifaceted approach to health education: A case study from rural Egypt. *International Quarterly of Community Health Education, 13,* 139-149.

Festinger, L. (1957). *A theory of cognitive dissonance.* Stanford, CA: Stanford University Press.

Frederiksen, L. W., Solomon, L. J., & Brehony, K. A. (Eds). (1984). *Marketing health behavior: Principles, techniques, and applications.* New York: Plenum Press.

Freudenberg, N. (1989). *Preventing AIDS: A guide to effective education for the prevention of HIV infection.* Washington, DC: American Public Health Association.

Genevay, B. (1978). Age kills us softly when we deny our sexual identity. In R. L. Solnick (Ed.), *Sexuality and aging* (Rev. ed., pp. 9-25). Ethel Percy Andrus Gerontology Center, University of Southern California Press.

Gordon, M. (1991). *Nursing diagnosis: Process and application* (3rd Ed.). St. Louis: Mosby-Year Book.

Hatton, D. C., & Webb, T. (1993). Information transmission in bilingual, bicultural contexts: A field study of community health nurses and interpreters. *Journal of Community Health Nursing, 10,* 137-147.

Janda, L. H., & O'Grady, K. E. (1980). Development of a sex anxiety inventory. *Journal of Consulting and Clinical Psychology, 48,* 169-175.

Kark, S. L., Kark, E., & Abramson, J. H. (1993). Commentary: In search of innovative approaches to international health. *American Journal of Public Health, 83,* 1533-1536.

Kleffel, D. (1991). Rethinking the environment as a domain of nursing knowledge. *Advances in Nursing Science, 14*(1), 40-51.

Kreps, G. L., & Kunimoto, E. N. (1994). *Effective communication in multicultural health care settings.* Thousand Oaks, CA: Sage.

Kriegler, N. F., & Harton, M. K. (1992). Community health assessment tool: A patterns approach to data collection and diagnosis. *Journal of Community Health Nursing, 9,* 229-234.

Krozy, R. (1978). Becoming comfortable with sexual assessment. *American Journal of Nursing, 78,* 1036-1038.

Krozy, R. E. (1984). Assessment: Sexuality and nursing care. In L. Higgins & J. W. Hawkins (Eds.), *Human sexuality across the life span: Implications for nursing practice* (pp. 108-149). Monterey, CA: Wadsworth.

Krozy, R.E.L. (1987). A human sexuality program for older adults: Effect on sexual knowledge and attitudes, attendance factors and outcomes. *Dissertation Abstracts International 48*(5), 1123-A.

Larson, E. (1994). Exclusion of certain groups from clinical research. *Image - The Journal of Nursing Scholarship, 26*, 185-190.

Lawrance, L., & McElroy, K. (1986). Self-efficacy and health education. *Journal of School Health, 56*, 317-321.

Lewin, K., Dembo, T., Festinger, L., & Sears, P. S. (1944). Level of aspiration. In J. Hunt (Ed.), *Personality and the behavioral disorders: A handbook based on experimental and clinical research* (pp. 333-378). New York: Ronald Press.

Lundeen, S. P. (1992). Health needs of a suburban community: A nursing assessment approach. *Journal of Community Health Nursing, 9*, 235-244.

Massachusetts Tobacco Control Program. (1994a). *Fact sheet.* Boston: Massachusetts Tobacco Control Program, Massachusetts Department of Public Health.

Massachusetts Tobacco Control Program. (1994b). *Preliminary report on the impact of the cigarette tax increase on cigarette consumption in Massachusetts and first wave results of tracking study of the Massachusetts Tobacco Control Media Campaign.* Boston: Massachusetts Tobacco Control Program, Massachusetts Department of Public Health.

McCarthy, N. C. (1994). The 11 functional health patterns assessment guidelines for communities. Health promotion and the community. In C. L. Edelman & C. L. Mandle (Eds.), *Health promotion throughout the lifespan* (3rd ed., pp. 209-210). St. Louis: Mosby-Year Book.

McCracken, A. L. (1988). Sexual practice by elders: The forgotten aspect of functional health. *Journal of Gerontological Nursing, 14*(10), 13-18.

McDermott, M. A. N., & Palchanes, K. (1993). A literature review of the critical elements in translation theory. *Image - The Journal of Nursing Scholarship, 26*, 113-117.

Merritt, S. (1989). Patient self-efficacy: A framework for designing patient education. *Focus on Critical Care, 16*, 68-73.

Michielutte, R., & Beal, P. (1990). Identification of community leadership in the development of public health education programs. *Journal of Community Health, 15*, 59-68.

Pender, N. J., Walker, S. N., Sechrist, K. R., & Frank-Stromberg, M. (1990). Predicting health-promoting lifestyles in the workplace. *Nursing Research, 39*, 326-332.

Popham, W. J., Potter, L. D., Bal, D. G., Johnson, M. D., Duerr, J. M., & Quinn, V. (1993). Do anti-smoking media campaigns help smokers quit? *Public Health Reports, 108*, 510-513.

Quinn-Krach, P., & Van Hoozer, H. (1988). Sexuality of the aged and the attitudes and knowledge of nursing students. *Journal of Nursing Education, 27*, 359-363.

Rankin, D. J. (1989). Intimacy and the elderly. *Nursing Homes, 38*(3), 10-14.

Roberts, A. (1989). Sexuality in later life: Systems of life no. 172: Senior systems—37. *Nursing Times, 85*(24), June 14, 65-68.

Rothman, D., & Sebastian, M. (1990). Intimacy and cognitively impaired elders. *Canadian Nurse, 86*(5), 32, 34.

Salazar, M. K. (1991). Comparison of four behavioral theories: A literature review. *AAOHN Journal, 39*, 128-135.

Shadick, K. M. (1993). Development of a transcultural health education program for the Hmong. *Clinical Nurse Specialist, 7*, 48-53.

Shomaker, D. M. (1980). Integration of physiological and sociocultural factors as a basis for sex education to the elderly. *Journal of Gerontological Nursing, 6*, 311-318

Smith, L. (1978). Sex education in the churches. In H. A. Otto (Ed.), *The new sex education* (pp. 101-116). New York: Association Press.

Stehr-Green, P. A., Dini, E. F., Lindegren, M. L., & Patriarca, P. A. (1993). Evaluation of telephoned computer-generated reminders to improve immunization coverage at inner city clinics. *Public Health Reports, 108*, 426-430.

Swanson, J. M., & Albrecht, M. (1993). *Community health nursing: Promoting the health of aggregates.* Philadelphia: W. B. Saunders.

Talashel, M. L., Tichy, A. M., & Epping, H. (1990). Sexually transmitted diseases in the elderly: Issues and recommendations. *Journal of Gerontological Nursing, 16*(4), 33-42.

Thorne, F. C. (1966). The sex inventory. *Journal of Clinical Psychology, 22*, 367-384.

Tilbury, M., & Fisk, T. (1989). *Marketing and nursing: A contemporary view.* Owings Mills, MD: National Health Publishing.

Urrutia-Rojas, X., & Aday, L. A. (1991). A framework for community assessment: Designing and conducting a survey in a Hispanic immigrant and refugee community. *Public Health Nursing, 8*(1), 20-26.

U.S. Department of Health and Human Services. (1994). *Preventing tobacco use among young people: A report of the Surgeon General.* U.S. Department of Health and Human Services, Public Health Service, Centers for Disease Control and Prevention, National Center for Chronic Disease Prevention and Health Promotion, Office on Smoking and Health.

U.S. Public Health Service, U.S. Department of Health and Human Services (1990). *Healthy people 2000.* (PHS Publication No. (PHS)91-50213). Washington, DC: U.S. Government Printing Office

Wells, B. L., Brown, C. C., Horm, J. W., Carleton, R. A., & Lasater, T. M. (1994). Who participates in cardiovascular disease risk factor screenings? Experience with a religious organization-based program. *American Journal of Public Health, 84*, 113-115.

Werner, D. (1992). *Where there is no doctor: A village health care handbook* (Rev. ed.). Palo Alto, CA: Hesperian Foundation.

Werner, D., & Bower, B. (1982). *Helping health workers learn.* Palo Alto, CA: Hesperian Foundation.

Weston, C., & Cranton, P. A. (1986). Selecting instructional strategies. *Journal of Higher Education, 57,* 263-268.

Whipple, B., & Scura, K. W. (1989). HIV and the older adult: Taking the necessary precautions. *Journal of Gerontological Nursing, 15*(9), 15-17.

Windsor, R., Baranowski, T., Clark, N., & Cutter, G. (1994). *Evaluation of health promotion, health education, and disease prevention programs* (2nd ed.). Mountain View, CA: Mayfield.

Windsor, R. A., Lowe, J. B., Perkins, L. L., Smith-Yoder, D., Artz, L., Crawford, M., Amburgy, K., & Boyd, N. R., Jr. (1993). Health education for pregnant smokers: Its behavioral impact and cost benefit. *American Journal of Public Health, 83,* 201-206.

CHAPTER

13

Case Management, Critical Paths, and Patient Education

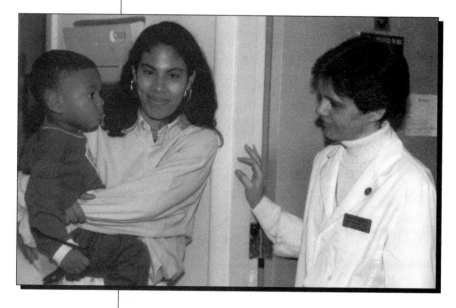

OBJECTIVES FOR CHAPTER 13

After reading this chapter, the nurse or student nurse should be able to:

1 Discuss how the evolution of case management systems can promote interdisciplinary models for patient education.

2 Discuss the concept of "product-line" models for patient education.

3 Describe two ways staff nurses can provide leadership in promoting patient education as an integral part of case management.

4 Identify philosophical differences of traditional and progressive health care providers that can thwart unified patient education efforts.

5 Discuss sources of power that nurses can use to promote patient education and secure needed resources.

Patient Education: Issues, Principles, Practices, Third Edition, by Sally H. Rankin and Karen Duffy Stallings.
Lippincott–Raven Publishers, Philadelphia, © 1996.

Case Management: Controlling Costs and Improving the Quality of Care

Case management has been used for over 20 years as a way to allocate health care resources across a variety of settings to meet individual client needs. The term often described the model used by social workers in welfare settings (Kovner, Hendrikson, Knickman, & Finkler, 1993).

In the last decade, the concept of case management has been adapted to inpatient, acute care settings as well as across a variety of outpatient settings where nurses are recognizing the shift to outcome-oriented and fiscally responsible care. Patient care financing and delivery has shifted from fee-for-service plans to managed care or capitation plans. In response, nurses have developed new professional practice models that incorporate principles of managed care. The models encompass clinical and financial outcomes, nurse as case manager, RN/MD collaborative practice, and increased patient and family participation. Patient education is an integral part of case management because it enables patients and families to participate in care and gain survival skills needed to promote decreased length of stay and safe discharge.

Integrating Patient Education Approaches Into Case Management Models: Product and Process

Nurses provide important leadership in the practice innovations associated with case management models. In doing so, they fulfill various roles and job descriptions. For staff nurses, as well as members of other health care disciplines who provide direct patient care, the need to understand the approaches and tools of case management is essential. The capacity for interdisciplinary collaboration and communication, which has been described throughout the text, and the ability of the health care team to streamline patient education approaches are also critical. To address these issues, the first section of this chapter discusses the *products of case management* and suggestions for designing realistic patient education interventions.

Nurses may assume positions such as managed care coordinator, case manager, clinical specialist, or patient education coordinator. In these positions, nurses fulfill the important roles of manager, consultant, liaison, facilitator, gatekeeper, negotiator, educator, and researcher. They do not directly deliver patient education but are instrumental in the coordination of case management system development. They must also promote innovative, interdisciplinary patient education interventions as part of patient care, design ways of evaluating complex patient needs and responses, and assess nursing staff knowledge and skill to teach patients. These roles increase the nurse's power base to improve patient education, at the same time challenging her to appear neutral in the eyes of the interdisciplinary team and to gain the trust and respect of clinicians as well as administrators. *Process issues*, including assessing and using power, dealing with politics in the organization, and promoting constructive change are key to successfully leading case management efforts (Kortbawi, 1993). The development process for critical paths, one of the tools used in case management, involves nine primary stages, which take place over a period of 2 years for the creation of a single path:

Literature search
Steering group
Targeting diagnoses
Designing paperwork
Gaining consensus
Implementing trial program
Refining program
Full implementation (Hofmann, 1993)

Gaining consensus of many caregivers is the most challenging task of nurses in leadership roles. It is an issue at all stages of group work. The leader must address nurses and other caregivers who do not understand or trust case management and feel it is imposed on them as merely an administrative, money-saving strategy (Hofmann, 1993). Turf battles must also be addressed. The most difficult battles are often waged over how to implement patient education, how to standardize patient education materials, and how to integrate prevention approaches in the acute care setting. As one patient care manager shared: "Accomplishing case management is an issue of process, not product. We must build consensus to develop a plan which can quickly become outdated and need revision. Length of stay is changing before our eyes!"

Addressing process issues, illustrating the use of power and politics, constitutes the second section of this chapter.

Key Elements of Case Management Models: Products

One of the best known and first models of nursing case management was developed by The Center for Nursing Case Management at Boston's New England Medical Center, adapting the concept to the acute care setting with the nurse caregiver as case manager. This model has four essential elements: achievement of clinical outcomes within a prescribed time frame; caregiver as case manager; episode-based RN/MD practices that transcend units; and achievement of patient and family participation in goal setting. Patient education is an essential and integral part of case management efforts (Zander, 1988, 1991, 1992).

Managing care is routinely accomplished by using an overall, standardized plan for a patient, including specific outcomes and time frames, based on their diagnosis-related group (DRG) or case type. The program uses devices called *critical pathways*, one-page summaries of case management plans that plot the course of a patient's hospitalization. *Case type* refers to the medical diagnosis and is used for reimbursement purposes similar to DRGs (Bower, 1988).

The critical path method, an industrial model from the mid-1950s, has been adapted to the delivery of patient care in the follow-ing way. A *critical path* outlines key incidents that typically occur at predictable times during a patient's stay in the hospital according to the patient's case type. A one-page time line accompanies the critical pathway to help nurses and other professionals see with great clarity how key incidents are managed in patient care. The one-page time line describes what is done each day for the particular patient according to the diagnosis and which milestones should be met by the "typical" patient of this case type. If the patient deviates from the goal, the plan is revised. For high-volume case types with predictable care patterns, critical pathways are condensed into "user friendly" documents called *care maps*, which can be used by the nurse to replace the patient care plan. They are shared with the patient in the form of a *patient care map* so the patient can anticipate discharge and track his own progress. Critical pathways are developed collaboratively by nurses, physicians, and other health professionals involved in patient care. The goal is to incorporate an interdisciplinary perspective, identify expectations and events that are critical to achieving a desired length of stay, and implement strategies that improve the quality and cost effectiveness of care. The critical path does not take the place of physician orders. Patient education is one of the key activities sequenced in the care map, along with consultation, diagnostic testing, discharge planning, patient teaching, activity, diet, and medication. Timing and content for effective patient teaching are emphasized. Nursing assessment and documentation reflect the progress or lack of progress made according to the critical pathway.

An example of a patient care map for open heart surgery patients at High Point Regional Hospital in North Carolina is shown in Figures 13-1 and 13-2. It is designed for DRG #106 (CABG with CATH) based on a length of stay of 4 to 5 days. The cardiovascular clinical care coordinator incorporated patient focus groups in the design of the patient care map. Based on patient input, the care coordinator is collaborating with physicians, home health, and
(text continues on page 278)

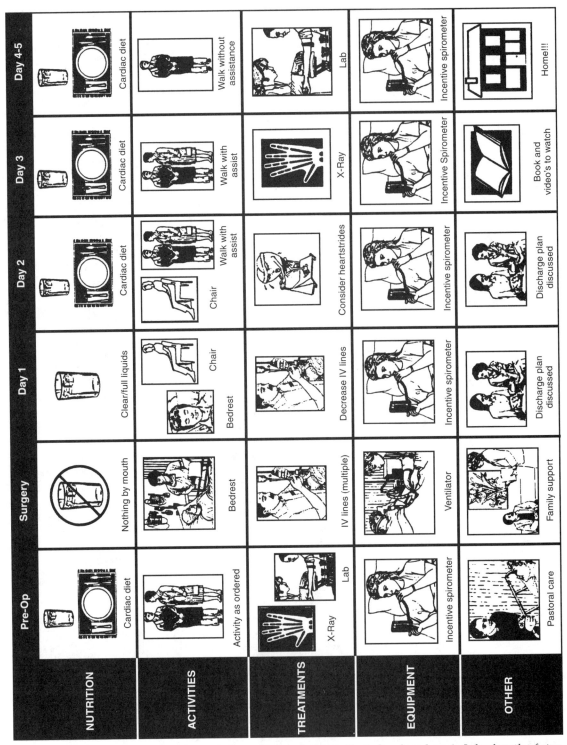

FIGURE 13–1. High Point Regional Hospital open heart surgery patient plan, based on 4- 5-day length of stay, for DRG #106. (Side 1)

276

OPEN HEART SURGERY PLAN

Welcome to High Point Regional Hospital. This plan is to share with you and your family a picture of what to expect during your hospital stay one day at a time. If you have any questions or concerns, please ask your doctor, nurse, or members of our health care team.

Before Surgery: This is a very busy day for you, but you can still enjoy your cardiac diet/food until midnight. You can also do the same activities the doctor has ordered for you until surgery. You will have a chest X-ray and blood and urine tests done. Teaching by your health care team members will also be done today. This will include: coughing, breathing exercises, ankle exercises, the equipment used to watch you during and after surgery, and about the surgery itself. A visit from Pastoral Care is also available.

Surgery: The day of surgery comes early. Medicine will be given to you that makes you sleepy and relaxed. Your only activity will be bedrest. Before surgery, please do not get up after taking your medicine. After surgery, you will wake up in the Surgical Intensive Care Unit (SICU) with a breathing tube in your mouth which is connected to a ventilator (breathing machine). You will not be able to talk until the tube is taken out, but the nurses will ask you yes/no questions so you can let the nurses know what you need. The nurse will explain things to you. Your family may visit you in the SICU at pre-set times, since it is a good idea for them to get some rest, like you, after you return from surgery. The doctors and nurses will also explain to them what is happening and why.

Day One After Surgery: By morning, the breathing tube is usually removed and you can talk again and start taking sips of clear liquid (apple juice, jello). You will wear an oxygen mask and will work on your deep breathing and coughing. An IV will be kept in place, but all the other equipment will be removed, if not needed. Usually you will be transferred to the Cardiac Telemetry Unit (CTU) where you continue your progress towards going home. Your activity will gradually increase during the day and you may get up in the chair. Your emphasis is to stay comfortable and rest.

Day Two After Surgery: Your diet will return to a cardiac diet. Your activity will increase and you will get in the chair several times. Teaching for going home will be continued.

Day Three After Surgery: You will continue with the cardiac diet throughout your stay. Your activities will be increasing each day. You will have an X-ray. You might feel sore, so please take your pain medicine to keep you comfortable. One of the most important activities for you to do is coughing and deep breathing. You and your family or care person will watch videos and learn discharge activities daily to help get you ready to go home. Your discharge plans will be reviewed and finalized.

Day Four or Five After Surgery: You will be walking and doing your coughing and deep breathing exercises by yourself. You will have blood tests. You will be ready to go home.

Remember, each person is special and may progress at a different rate. The plan is adapted to meet the needs of all our patients. It will allow you to set goals for yourself and keep you on course to go home. All your needs are taken into consideration as we work with you to return home. For more information, please read your books: *Going for Heart Surgery, What You Need To Know,* and *Moving Right Along After Open Heart Surgery.*

FIGURE 13–2. High Point Regional Hospital open heart surgery patient plan, based on 4- 5-day length of stay, for DRG #106. (Side 2) (Printed with permission).

cardiac rehabilitation to develop a second care map ("patient plan"), which addresses the patient's course during the first 2 weeks after discharge. The care map is designed as a "picture plan" to aid the teaching of patients with limited reading skills. It also explains in narrative the expected events during the patient's recovery.

Most hospitals have now adopted some form of critical path and care map system to the delivery of patient care. These similar efforts to coordinate and standardize clinical care may be referred to by different names, including clinical paths, practice guidelines, and coordinated care plans. The diagnoses that are often chosen for initial development of critical paths are those that are high volume in the agency as well as predictable in their courses of care, such as vaginal delivery, cesarean section, and open heart surgery. Time lines for critical paths can be by visit (home health), by month (extended care), by week (rehabilitation units), by day (medical-surgical unit), or by minute (emergency department).

The term *patient case management* is often used to describe the close tracking and specialized individual intervention needed to manage high-risk, high-cost patient cases that are vulnerable to patterns of multiple readmissions and an unpredictable course of care.

Variances, which prevent the patient from staying on the expected course, are identified. A *variance* is a deviation from the projected critical path. For example, new nursing diagnoses may be identified, and the plan of care is revised. Quality improvement monitoring involves tracking of variances; if patient outcomes vary from those expected, the nurse or other health care team member documents the variance and its reason. Common reasons for variances may reflect patient, family, and provider outcomes, as detailed in Box 13-1.

Although exceptions are expected as plans are individualized, the targeted length of stay remains unless it can be justified by the variance. It is important to note that variances can lead to a shortened length of stay as well as an extended length of stay because patients may progress more quickly than expected. All variances are noted, with efforts to resolve nega-

---

BOX 13–1. Common Reasons for Variance

- Patient condition, complication
- Patient pain, fatigue
- Patient decision
- Patient's limited mental status
- Medication or treatment not administered
- Additional tests needed
- Care map modified due to admitting diagnosis or preexisting condition
- Family decision or unavailability
- Equipment, medication, referral, transfer bed not available

---

tive variances as priorities in care planning and to examine positive variances that may lead to decreasing lengths of stay.

Documentation that supports case management continues to evolve. The trend toward computerized systems, often entitled "decision support systems," integrates many facets of tracking, communication, and quality improvement. It is also possible to automate the development of critical paths and patient education paths, similar to the development of standardized care plans with which most nurses are familiar. The software programs are capable of developing reports for physicians, nurses, and other staff, which reflect actual length of stay, patient and procedure variances (including those related to patient education outcomes), and actual outcomes of care. A charting by exception format, as described in Chapter 11, is commonly used with bedside computer terminals.

Nursing Leadership in Case Management

This model of case management illustrates the responsibility nurses have assumed in managing patient care, which is goal directed and cost effective.

New England Medical Center nursing staff (Bower, 1988) have identified the following benefits that can be demonstrated with managed care.

1. Patients are more aware of their progress, have more insight into their care, anticipated discharge, and participate more in their care.
2. Nursing assessments are more outcome oriented and address variances that influence length of stay.
3. Length of stay is controlled and in many cases reduced.
4. Staff nurses feel they have more control over the care of patients and feel more satisfied.
5. Orientation of new staff is more effective because they are taught about case types, goals of care, and standards of care.
6. Shift report is more meaningful for each patient on the unit. The nurses share information about estimated length of stay, critical events anticipated for that day, and difficulties in achieving outcomes.
7. Documentation reflects patient progress toward goals.
8. Consultation, collaboration, and continuity of care are increased.

Case management is not restricted to acute care; it can also be practiced in outpatient settings with many of the same successes. For example, nurse case managers have been successfully used to manage care of the elderly who live in the community. In such situations the nurse works as liaison to coordinate services for the elderly client and advocate for the client when he needs additional assistance. A plan of care and goals for rehabilitation are established for the client in a fashion similar to the critical pathways mechanism described above and this plan is shared with the client and family members. For example, as the caseload of acquired immunodeficiency syndrome (AIDS) has grown in the San Francisco Bay Area, the same process has been used to manage care for AIDS clients. Case management goals in the community may differ from those in the acute care setting; however, managed care is still critical for the quality of life of these patients.

Discharge Creep and Issues of Timing: Implications for Patient Education

Patient education is a critical facet of case management. Formal recognition of the periods to initiate patient teaching improves patient learning as well as patient outcomes. The importance of involving the patient throughout the case management process requires a commitment to openness and sharing with the patient and family. The nurse case manager is in a unique position to improve patient outcomes and control health care costs by addressing the need for innovative, product-line approaches to patient education.

As inpatient length of stay decreases, critical paths must be redrawn to reflect a new time line for the delivery of procedures, tests, treatments, and patient teaching. Nurses must acknowledge, and advocate, that 7-day patient education programs cannot be automatically condensed into 4 days with the same patient learning outcomes achieved. Also, all days are not equal; the patient's physical and psychological ability and the need for reinforcement of learning must be considered when allocating teaching responsibilities to the path. Planning integrated patient education approaches that cross service areas is needed to increase patient safety and provide continuity of care. A model of "internal case managers" (specialized in high-risk, high-volume cases) and community-based nursing case managers comprises the system implemented by the Carondelet Health Care System in Tucson, Arizona. The program for heart surgery patients, for example, includes well-managed teaching and care management in preadmission, intensive care unit (ICU), stepdown unit, telephone follow-up, and home visits. By managing the entire service-line care experience rather than only the acute care experience, the Carondelet Nurse Case Management Program documented reduced length of stay by over 30%, reduced costs by over 10%, and reductions in adverse outcomes by 58% (Mahn, 1993).

Patient Input to Streamline Patient Education: Teaching Smarter

Chapters 9, 10, and 11 address a variety of approaches that can be used to streamline teaching in light of the trend for decreased length of inpatient stay. Repeated throughout the text is the advice: Choose no more than three or four critical learning objectives, observe patient performance, and document. Nurses are often stymied at the prospects of teaching less content in favor of survival skills because they worry that patients will be undereducated. The reality of short stays is that teaching too much can mean that the patient learns less, feels overwhelmed and frustrated, and fails to carry out the most essential self-care responsibilities.

One innovative product-line model for educating cardiac rehabilitation patients provides incentive for using patient input to ensure that patient education is streamlined and useful and promotes safety. The model could be applied to other situations in which patients are discharged quickly and cared for across multiple settings, such as obstetrics.

A cardiac rehabilitation coordinator in South Dakota believed that to accomplish effective patient education, nurses must understand the perceived educational needs of cardiac rehabilitation patients and then develop a program that meets both the needs of the patient and the most effective time interval for learning (Hanisch, 1993). Her approach was to study the topics currently taught by the interdisciplinary cardiac team (physician, nurse, physical therapist, social worker, pharmacist, dietitian, and chaplain) during the cardiac rehabilitation period extending 6 weeks to 6 months after hospital discharge. She then constructed a questionnaire that was given to cardiac patients and their spouses. In addition to demographic data, the questionnaire asked patients to rate 30 topics believed by health care practitioners as essential in cardiac patient education.

Respondents were first asked to rate (using a 7-point Likert-type scale) how important learning about the item was, and then to indicate the time interval during which it would have been most helpful. The four choices for time interval were: preoperative, ICU, before discharge (stepdown unit), or posthospitalization.

Over 75% (32 of 41 of respondents) indicated that four items were extremely important during all phases of recovery:

1. Specific instructions on type and amount of activity or restrictions
2. What is normal and to be expected after cardiac event
3. Medication
4. Signs and symptoms of complications that need medical attention

All of these topics could be considered "safety needs."

In addition, patients rated the following items as important during the preoperative period: cardiac risk factors, anatomy and physiology of coronary artery disease, and explanation of the surgical procedure. In the ICU, the priority learning need was about ICU policies and procedures. In the stepdown unit, patient priorities were how to manage incisional pain and receiving written instructions for discharge, including diet. After hospitalization, patients placed priority on a follow-up telephone call, advice on resuming sexual activity, and managing a decreased energy level (Hanisch, 1993). Table 13-1 presents the informational needs of cardiac rehabilitation patients.

Although patients and spouses in this study perceived all 30 items as important, they offered valuable insights to nurses in redesigning and streamlining patient teaching for product-line or critical path models. They singled out the four critical learning objectives targeted for every patient, which could be reinforced in every setting, by every member of the health care team, and reflected in documentation. They also pointed to a limited number of learning needs that were specific to each of the four settings, thus enabling nurses to provide information at a

TABLE 13–1. Informational Needs and Preferred Time to Receive Information for Phase II Cardiac Rehabilitation Patients.

Table 1A								Table 1B			
Likert-type Scale								Time Periods			
(Not Important)						(Very Important)					
1	2	3	4	5	6	7	Informational Item	Pre op	ICU	Post Event	Post Hosp
			3	3	5	30	1. Cardiac Risk factors	23	4	11	2
2	2		3	5	7	21	2. Anatomy-physiology of heart	18	1	12	5
		1	2	6	4	27	3. Atherosclerosis/coronary artery disease	19	2	11	6
			3	1	1	26	4. Explanation of surgical procedure (bypass only)	29		2	
				2	6	25	5. Myocardial infarction	14	7	11	1
	3	2	4	5	4	23	6. ICU/CCU policies & procedures	17	18	4	
1		3	3	3	5	26	7. Effects of cardiac event on body functions	10	5	19	6
4	1		7	4	4	19	8. Effects of cardiac event on sexuality and sexual functioning	8		19	10
1	1		5	5	8	21	9. Possible emotional reactions to cardiac disease/event	11	3	18	8
1		1	2	8	4	24	10. How to communicate special needs to health professionals	13		19	7
	1		1	4	7	27	11. Involvement of partner or family in teaching program	12		13	14
1		1	1	5	10	21	12. How to communicate feelings and concerns to partner/family	8	2	20	9
		2	6	3	8	22	13. Available resources for assistance at home	2		20	18
		1			8	32	14. Specific instructions on type and amount of activity/restrictions	2	1	27	10
1			1	5	11	23	15. Specific time-frame for resuming work and/or leisure activities	2		19	18
2	2		6	10	4	15	16. Suggestions on how to resume sexual activity	2		17	17
					9	32	17. What is normal and to be expected after cardiac event	7	2	21	9
			2	3	8	28	18. Dietary modifications	4		27	9
			2	2	5	32	19. Medications	4	2	28	6
			4	10	6	20	20. Time required for hospitalization and recovery	14	4	17	2
2	1	1	7	7	5	17	21. Follow-up phone call by health professional	2		14	22
	1			5	4	31	22. What will be experienced before, during and after surgery/heart attack	25	5	6	2
				6	2	17	23. Removal of stitches and care of incision (bypass only)	2	5	16	3
			2	5	9	23	24. How to manage incisional pain and/or anginal discomfort	4	6	26	1
	1		2	8	6	24	25. Pulse taking	4	3	23	10

(continued)

TABLE 13–1. *(Continued)*

				Table 1A						Table 1B		
			Likert-type Scale							Time Periods		
(Not Important)				(Very Important)								
1	2	3	4	5	6	7	Informational Item		Pre op	ICU	Post Event	Post Hosp
				2	7	32	26. Signs and symptoms of complications that need medical attention		5	3	23	7
		1	1	2	7	30	27. Common symptoms that occur during recovery		7	5	20	7
	2			8	5	24	28. How to manage decreased energy level		4		18	16
1			1	5	5	27	29. How to care for self after return home		2		19	15
		1	3	4	7	24	30. Written information about cardiac disease		8		15	14

Table 1A shows the rating of information. Table 1B shows preferred time to receive information. The numbers in the columns indicate the number of respondents selecting each informational item and time period. Not all respondents answered every question.

From Hanisch, P. (1993). Informational needs and preferred time to receive information for phase II cardiac rehabilitation patients: what CE instructors need to know, *Journal of Continuing Education in Nursing, 24*(2), 86.

"teachable moment" for the patient, when he is most motivated to learn it. This study should inspire nurses to resist the urge to teach a 30-item list from top to bottom. Rather, patient input helps to streamline the list and the process in ways that promote teaching "smarter" and achieving critical learning outcomes. It would seem that all health care providers, especially nurses, should be eager to abandon outdated patient education approaches and design innovative interdisciplinary models such as the one described.

The remainder of this chapter will address the process issues which, unless skillfully dealt with, can prevent needed innovation.

Philosophical and Power Issues: Implications for Case Management and Patient Education

When care coordinators, case managers, nurse managers, and staff nurses providing leadership in the creation of critical paths are interviewed, they invariably mention issues that can be categorized as philosophical and power or political issues. Confronting these issues is essential if patient education is to be successfully integrated into innovative case management efforts, including the development of critical paths and expert patient teachers. Despite the evidence indicating that patient education improves the quality of care and reduces costs, nurses promoting patient education efforts must compete with other departments in their institutions for budgets and organizational influence (Bartlett, 1986). With the focus of patient education on interdisciplinary planning and coordination involving many providers, and frequently crossing divisional lines in the institution, a political coalition is necessary to support patient education services (Redman & Levine, 1987). In attempting to build coalitions, nurses encounter issues described as philosophical and political.

Philosophical issues concern one's approach to patients and basic beliefs about how patient education should be put into operation. Philosophical issues tend to vary with educational background: nurses or other health care professionals tend to practice patient education in a manner consistent with their own educational preparation. *Power* and *political* issues usually concern control—who teaches what, to whom, and when. Power and political issues produce more tension than any other patient education issue. Most practicing nurses are poorly prepared to deal with power and political issues. This chapter presents skills that will enhance the effectiveness of the practicing nurse who confronts philosophical, power, and political issues in promoting patient education. These skills will also help prepare the student nurse to become an agent for change.

We also explore the impacts different professional roles and institutions exert on the delivery of patient education, criteria to help a practicing nurse determine who has power in a given setting and gain power herself to improve patient education, methods used to bring about planned change, such as change-agentry skills, and, finally, practical suggestions for managing philosophical and political issues.

Traditional Versus Progressive Health Professionals

We have found during our years of nursing practice that, in general, we interact with two different types of health care professionals, those whom we classify as either traditional or progressive. Although we speak of health care professionals as the entire health care team—physicians, nurses, dietitians, pharmacists, social workers, and occupational, physical, and respiratory therapists—the following discussion focuses primarily on the physician and the nurse.

Our image of the traditional health care professional is that of an older man or woman accustomed to a hierarchical approach to medical care, in which the physician is the dominant decision-maker and the focus of patient care activities. Nurses, physicians, and other health care professionals who subscribe to this model view the physician as totally responsible for all aspects of the patient's care and tend to regard the patient as "belonging" to the physician. The physician operates from a position of centralized power. Such traditional models assume that the physician always knows what is best for the patient and that the patient concurs with this attitude. The patient exhibits this concurrence by responding without question to the medical regimen.

Our experience has suggested that physicians who represent this approach generally practice in the areas of surgery, gynecology, and internal medicine and are less frequently found in obstetrics, pediatrics, psychiatry, or family medicine. This impression is supported by a study that examined physicians' opinions of clinical pharmacy. Physicians were found not to favor the expanding role of clinical pharmacy, and those least in favor are older physicians, those in specialties at high risk for malpractice suits, and those who write a large number of prescriptions. Interestingly, physicians with a high risk of malpractice suits tend to be unfavorable toward *any* extraprofessional involvement in physician-patient relationships (Ritchey & Raney, 1981). Physicians practicing in some of the medical and surgery specialty areas are among those with a high risk of medical malpractice suits. This may account for this group's less than enthusiastic acceptance of nurse-sponsored patient education. Implications for nursing are that this group of physicians must be persuaded that patient education can actually reduce litigation. Accurate and concise documentation will establish a channel of communication, keeping the physician aware of all information given to his patients.

Nurses who fall into the category of traditional health care professionals tend to be educated below the baccalaureate level (i.e., either associate degree or diploma graduates) or they may have received their nursing education outside of the United States. Additionally, we recognize that more diploma and associate degree nurses have chosen to return to school, and their nursing education reflects the current emphasis on patient education. The traditional orientation is most likely related to the traditional nurse's educational preparation and the fact that she was educated in an era when nurses were prepared more as the physician's handmaid than as the autonomous health care professional exemplified in nursing education over the past 25 to 30 years. The diploma graduate was also more likely to have been taught according to a "medical model" with physicians as instructors. The current approach to nursing education, which uses the nursing process, has resulted in a more eclectic, holistic appreciation of humankind that is no longer dependent on one particular approach or model. The nurse who is trained to fit into the traditional model will have fewer problems with role inconsistency and role insufficiency than will the nurse educated in the progressive model because traditional role expectations are more likely to be congruent with a "medical model" approach. We have seen more traditional nurses in hospitals than in community, school, and occupational health settings, college and university academic settings, or other outpatient settings.

In contrast to the traditional health care professional, the progressive health care professional may be younger, more accustomed to a team approach with the patient as the focus, and less likely to view the physician as the dominant or only decision-maker. The progressive health care professional eschews centralized power in favor of decentralization, so that all members of the team have authority in their specialty areas.

We emphasize that both traditional and progressive health care approaches are appropriate, and indeed, the traditional approach may be better suited to some situations than the progressive approach. However, as our readers can probably tell, our bias is in favor of the progressive health care professional. We have worked successfully with traditional nurses and physicians, but we feel that the progressive professionals offer better patient education services and greater job satisfaction for all.

Examination of the Issues

Philosophical Issues

Self-Care Approach

A term coined by Dorothea Orem, *self-care* connotes a conceptual basis for nursing practice. Self-care behavior is "the production of actions directed to self or to the environment in order to regulate one's functioning in the interests of one's life, integrated functioning, and well being" (Orem, 1985). The function of the nurse is to assist the client in achieving a level of wellness consistent with the client's own life-style and value system, but not necessarily with the value system maintained by the health care purveyors. Self-care means that the client has control over his medical regimen and makes choices regarding his medical management. The traditional health care system in the United States with its emphasis on acute management leaves the physician little opportunity to assist the client in accomplishing self-care activities.

Patient education is an integral part of self-care practice because most patients lack the requisite knowledge to promote health or to manage problems related to disease. Ideally, patient education is offered to a client to reduce dependency on the health care system, not to increase his need for services. Self-care activities promoted by the nurse attempt to make the system conform to the client's needs. Patient education activities encourage self-care and greater independence from the traditional health care system. Wellness and prevention are also promoted when health care professionals interact with patients and families.

We believe that the traditional health care professional is changing his attitude toward the self-care approach. This is partly a result of consumer desires and pressure and partly because of a changing philosophy in many nursing and medical schools. Also, the standards of the Joint Commission on the Accreditation of Healthcare Organizations (JCAHO) support empowering the patient for self-care and wellness (JCAHO, 1994). The self-care approach is related to the growth of the self-help movement, which will be examined later in the chapter.

Patient Education Model

Progressive and traditional health care professionals adhere to different models of patient education. In our experience, traditional health care professionals tend to approach patient education from the perspective of the medical model: diagnosis, prognosis, and therapy. Teaching is oriented toward imparting knowledge about these three entities. Whereas most medical students receive this type of education, nursing students (especially recent graduates) usually receive instruction in teaching and learning theories, which assert that although information is imparted, there is no guarantee it is learned. Nursing students are required to put teaching and learning theories into practice, and almost all recent nursing graduates can remember being evaluated on a patient education project. But as these theories assert, all students do not learn and practice the precepts as comprehensively as they should. A recently evaluated baccalaureate nursing student in a patient education setting said to the patient, "Since you've had a heart attack before, I know you understand what it's all about. I'll leave you a handout that will give you more information." The student made no effort to assess the patient's level of understanding or his possible misconceptions about the previous myocardial infarction. This student was essentially a product of the medical model approach. (For more information on assessment in patient education settings, see Chap. 7).

The progressive health care professional views patient education as a process with discrete steps, whereas the traditionalist frequently views patient education as the imparting of information. Progressive health care professionals also understand the value of tailoring teaching to individual patient needs and beliefs.

Information Sharing

Another philosophical issue, which also has overtones of issues relating to power and control, is that of sharing information. Progressive health care providers generally tend to be more willing than traditional providers to share information with patients. One nurse related an incident that occurred in a hospital where she worked, in which a number of physicians did not want their patients told about the potential side effects of a particular medication. In another instance, a nursing student was forbidden to make home visits to an oncology patient because the physician did not want the student to tell the patient the possible side effects of chemotherapeutic agents. When a physician forbids a nurse to give information to a patient, issues of power and control are definitely at stake.

Obviously, instances occur when nurses impart incorrect information or choose the wrong time to attempt patient teaching. Many nurses so completely overwhelm their patients with teaching before coronary artery bypass graft surgery that the patients approach surgery with high, unhealthy levels of anxiety. It is the nurse's responsibility to make certain that what she teaches is correct and that she properly assesses the patient's ability to learn. It is the physician's responsibility, in keeping with the patient's right to know, to impart all *pertinent* information to the patient in such a manner that the patient can understand the information.

Holism

The *holistic concept of man* implies that we view the individual as a total, nonfragmented human being, who is a sum of all his parts (Menke, 1985); this concept has an impact on patient education. When we assume the holistic approach, we are interested in the total individual not just the diseased or dysfunctional part. The medical model, which the nursing profession endorsed in the past, separates mind from body from spirit. This model presumes a nonholistic approach—one looks at the child's broken leg, diagnoses it through the use of x-ray films, casts it, and prescribes an analgesic. According to the medical model, the fractured femur is the dysfunctional part, the part that is treated. A holistic approach expands the focus on the child with the broken bone to include assessing the parents' need to be taught childhood safety. When the holistic approach to man is applied to patient education, it is evident that patient education should include more than just teaching about a single dysfunction or problem.

Another example of holism and its effect on patient teaching involves a 44-year-old man with gastric carcinoma. A nursing student who had cared for the patient in the hospital made a home visit to evaluate his status and do any necessary teaching. She found that the patient's family had learned the necessary skills of gastric lavage and jejunostomy tube feedings and that they were doing much better with the physical care than had been expected. However, she noted that the teenage son was exhibiting inappropriate behavior by ignoring his father. During discussions with the mother and son she learned that the son feared a bloody, gruesome death scene. The nursing student was able to clarify the misconceptions and alleviate a great deal of the adolescent's anxiety. Her holistic approach also included a referral to a local hospice group.

In the past, most nursing education paralleled medical education, and nurses were instructed according to the medical model. Some nurses still subscribe to the medical model but, as nursing education has progressed, many nurses have abandoned the old model in favor of a view of man as a unified whole. Note also that many physicians are ascribing to a holistic concept of man, and it is not unrealistic to hope for a unified nursing-medical approach in the future.

Education for the Chronically Ill

Viewpoints about educating chronically ill patients differ between traditional and progressive health care professionals. Most progressive professionals believe that patients with chronic illnesses need more in-depth education than is ordinarily offered by the medical regimen, in other words, more information than indicating on a chart when medications should be taken. Nurses and other progressive health care professionals undertake teaching about chronic illness in

an effort to assist the client in attaining the highest level of wellness possible.

Ruth Wu states in her book *Behavior and Illness* that the chronically ill person maintains a secondary role, the chronic-illness role, on a permanent basis or until he becomes acutely ill, at which point he reverts back to the sick role (Wu, 1973). The chronic-illness role requires greater patient adaptation in most situations than does the more acute-sick role. Social expectations are vague for the patient in the chronic-illness role. He learns that the condition, unlike acute illness (the sick role), is not reversible; this awareness greatly influences the informational needs of the patient. An example will clarify the need for comprehensive patient education. A nurse spent 3 hours with a 12-year-old insulin-dependent diabetic girl and her parents, attempting to educate them about the intricacies of diabetes management. This preadolescent girl and her family not only had to learn about the injection of insulin, diet, exercise, and the signs and symptoms of hypo- and hyperglycemia, but they also had to learn how to work this regimen into the life-style of a 12 year old. At one point they realized that they had to weigh the advantages of less strict control against the possible dangers of later complications and even premature death. Imparting *all* information to the chronically ill patient and his family is especially important. Long-term plans must be made and long-term goals defined by the family and nurse, working together.

The AIDS epidemic and consideration of cancer as a chronic, as well as terminal, illness have resulted in additional efforts to increase the quality of life for these patients through effective patient education (Pollock, 1987). The growth of support groups among the gay community in San Francisco demonstrates the importance of self-help, but also the failure of the established health care community to effectively share information on pharmaceutical agents, treatments, and other issues of utmost importance to the community most at risk for developing AIDS. With prevention and cure of AIDS not expected before the end of this century, the necessity of increasing quality of life for those living with AIDS is imperative. Quality of life can be enhanced through the immediate sharing of information and through hospice agencies that offer emotional and instrumental support.

Quality of life for cancer patients is currently being improved by the research of nurses, which can then be shared and put into practice. Weekes and Savedra (1988), for instance, studied the coping strategies used by adolescents responding to chemotherapy or bone marrow treatments. The implementation of their findings will assist chronically ill adolescent cancer patients to improve their quality of life through patient education.

The nurse educating a patient and the family about chronic illness is responsible for covering the details of the medical regimen. If, however, she does not discuss the regimen in the context of the patient's life-style (including educational background, socioeconomic status, marital and family status, belief system, and occupation), then the teaching is virtually useless.

Power and Political Issues

Compliance

An important topic in any discussion of patient education is compliance. *Compliance* is defined as "the act or process of complying to a desire, demand, or proposal or to coercion" or "a disposition to yield to others."[1] Many traditional health care professionals claim that the goal of patient education is compliance and that patient education is worthless if we cannot prove that it increases compliance.

Our belief is that compliance with a medical regimen is an important goal of patient education, but it is not the only goal. A significant process occurs between education and compliance, in which the client internalizes the teaching and then makes informed choices about applying the teaching to his life. It is the coercive aspect of compliance that relates this issue to power and control. Who has power in

---

[1]From *Webster's Ninth New Collegiate Dictionary*© 1984 by Merriam-Webster, Inc., Springfield, MA.

a patient education situation—the health care provider or the patient? Obviously, the patient should have the control, but too often we try to control the situation for the patient, subtly threatening removal of our support or services if he does not follow our instructions. For too long health care providers, especially physicians, have been viewed as authority figures whose will must be obeyed. As the consumer has begun to require greater accountability of health care professionals, many providers have responded by dropping traditional, paternalistic roles. It is our hope that all health care professionals will eventually put aside their cloaks of authority and view compliance as one small part of the provider-client relationship, instead of as an end in itself.

Responsibility for Teaching

A second power and political issue on which progressive and traditional providers frequently disagree is that of who should teach. Nurses have a legal responsibility to provide health teaching for their patients (see Chap. 5). We have, however, found many physicians who believe that nurses should not perform health teaching. We know of cardiologists in a large medical center who are vehement that nurses not teach their patients who have had myocardial infarctions about management of heart disease. There are also community hospitals whose physicians require nurses to wait for an order before their patients may be shown hospital-approved videos or literature. Although in some instances a physician's order is required to facilitate third-party payment for patient teaching activities, in many situations the requirement of a physician's order for patient education is an issue of power and control.

Physicians' reluctance to allow nurses to perform this as an independent function may be related to incidents they have seen involving nurses who were clinically unprepared to teach. LPNs are not prepared in their educational programs to assess and plan for patient education. This is not to say that there are not many LPN patient educators who carry out effective patient teaching, but it is unrealistic to expect all of them to be as well prepared as the professional RN. Granted, there are some professional RNs who are ineffective as patient teachers because of either personality factors or lack of preparation. A few experiences with these nurses tend to dampen the enthusiasm of even the most strongly patient education-oriented physician. On the other hand, nurses who have been rebuffed in their patient education efforts by physicians are inclined to lose some of their enthusiasm. Patient education must be a team effort and, in our discussion of change-agentry skills, we will further discuss the positive effects of collaboration for patient education.

Most nurses are not interested in appropriating the physician's role in discussing the diagnosis, prognosis, and therapy with the patient. Instead, they interpret their role in patient education as that of making themselves available for clarification and discussion of daily management of the problem. Such a role seems appropriate for the nurse if we accept the goal of nursing as the promotion and maintenance of health in individuals, families, groups, and the community (Weaver, 1985; Roy, 1984; American Nurses Association, 1980). Again, collaboration is a key to effective patient education.

Patient Education Referrals

The third and last political issue is the willingness to refer patients to other patient education resources, especially self-help groups. Frequently, it seems appropriate to refer patients to extramural patient education resources because of various factors (e.g., the need for ongoing support from like-affected individuals and the need for ongoing teaching), as in the case of the education, specialized teaching, and support for Alzheimers disease patients and families, and substance abuse patients.

Too often nurses and physicians are unaware of the existence of groups and online computer resources to which patients could be referred. Ignorance of such resources is undoubtedly partly a result of the proliferation of literature with which health professionals must be familiar. It also represents a lack of concern regarding the development of patients' coping and adaptive resources.

A more disturbing attitude, however, is the paternalism found among traditional health care professionals who refuse to suggest community resources unless they can vouch for their value. The idea of "ownership" of patients by physicians, and occasionally by nurses, is not a viewpoint congruent with the prevailing belief that adults are responsible, autonomous human beings who make their own choices about health care. Thus, when a physician or nurse refuses or neglects to give a patient information about self-help groups, he has single-handedly decided that the patient is unable to judge for himself whether such a self-help group might be useful. We heard one physician who taught in a large medical center affirm his belief that it was unwise to refer patients to community self-help agencies unless the physician could personally verify the integrity of the group. Such an attitude denies the adulthood of patients and effectively places the power for decision-making in the physician's hands instead of in the patient's, where it rightfully belongs.

Considering our mutual interest in patients and their welfare, it behooves all physicians and nurses to acquaint themselves with self-help groups and support groups that may aid patients in the acquisition of an optimal level of health. The health care consumer has already recognized the need for self-help groups and is becoming more aware that the traditional social and medical institutions are not able to provide complete support for the handicapped, the needy, the deviant, or the socially isolated. Recognizing that we, as health professionals, cannot be all things to all people, we must hand over some of our power to self-care and self-help support groups if the client desires it.

Effects of Roles and Settings on Patient Education Approaches

Acute Care Versus Outpatient Settings

In our discussion of philosophical and political issues, we outlined some of the major differences between physicians and nurses in their approaches to patient education. How do differences in roles and settings influence approaches to patient education?

Roles of nurses vary among institutions and even inside institutions. Some institutions employ specially prepared nurses who do all the patient teaching in one area, such as diabetes management or ostomy teaching. These nurses may be referred to as *nurse clinicians* or *clinical nurse specialists.* Staff nurses in these institutions conduct either no patient teaching or only minimal instruction in these areas. Other institutions employ a patient education coordinator, who may or may not be a nurse, and she is responsible for making certain that staff nurses are prepared to teach all aspects of health and illness management with which they come in contact.

Many outpatient settings are placing greater importance on the teaching role of the nurse than are acute care institutions. Thus, community health nurses, school and occupational health nurses, and nurses employed in outpatient clinics are generally spending a greater proportion of their time in patient teaching functions than are nurses working in acute care settings. We believe that this is changing in acute care settings because JCAHO mandates that patient education be documented as an integral part of patient care (JCAHO, 1994). Also, a recent greater emphasis on patient education in nursing schools has produced a young cadre of professional nurses who are aware of the benefits of, and the need for, patient education. Because most of these younger nurses are employed in acute care settings, this has also brought about a change in the emphasis placed on patient education in secondary and tertiary care. The redesign, reengineering, and downsizing of hospitals has also led to trends in role changes of clinical nurse specialists into case management; the primary responsibilities for patient education are now assigned to staff nurses.

Changes in health care reimbursement, which have resulted in shorter hospitalizations, have affected the provision of patient education in the hospital. For example, the average length of stay for coronary artery bypass graft surgery was 7 days in 1986 compared to about 11 days in the 1970s. In 1995, the average length of stay is between 4 and 5 days. Patients being discharged following major surgery are frequently not recovered sufficiently to participate in patient education sessions. Elderly patients are frequently discharged to the home before their mentation is sufficiently lucid to allow for effective patient education. Therefore, the burden of teaching is falling more frequently on the shoulders of home health care nurses, hospice nurses, and other community nurses who are assisting families in caring for increasingly sicker and more disabled patients in the home. Although the home may be a more relaxed setting in which to accomplish effective patient education, issues related to continuity of care and implementation of patient education plans must be carefully addressed if patients are to recover maximally and take responsibility for new medical regimes.

Differences Among Specialists

Our experience with physicians indicates that younger, less specialty oriented, and less traditional physicians tend to stress the importance of patient education. They are more encouraging toward nursing efforts in patient education and are more willing to try various innovative teaching modalities. A group of family medicine residents with whom we worked was extremely enthusiastic about patient education, forming a patient education committee with nursing personnel to enhance and promote patient teaching efforts in the outpatient setting. On the other hand, we have had experiences with pulmonary medicine specialists who refused to let nurses who were working on a respiratory unit initiate teaching of new asthmatics without specific orders. Other unfortunate experiences, such as with internists who have prevented our colleagues from informing patients of the side effects of antihypertensive medications and with obstetricians who refused to let nurses prepare patients psychologically for postpartum depression, have made us believe that the more "medicalized" a physician is, the less likely he is to respond favorably to the prospect of patient education.[2] An additional factor affecting physician attitudes toward patient education is the oversupply of physicians, especially in urban areas and certain specialties, which results in territoriality and fears of "patient stealing." For example, we are aware of settings where physicians practicing internal medicine refuse to refer their patients to a comprehensive diabetes teaching program because they fear that diabetologists will either suggest metabolic management practices, with which they are uncomfortable, or their patients will choose to transfer to the diabetes service.

Lack of Role Definitions

We suspect that one of the reasons patient education is so frequently a battleground for physicians and nurses is the lack of clarification between roles. The nurse-physician relationship was formerly a narrowly prescribed role in which both the nurse and the physician knew what was expected of them. A role transition has occurred in nursing, engendered by nursing education and by new, expanded roles for nurses. *Role transitions* are changes in roles that require new role behaviors and also require role consensus. *Role consensus* is the amount of agreement or disagreement regarding the role expectations of two or more individuals (Burr, Leigh, Day, 1979). As role consensus between physicians and nurses grows, role conflict and the lack of definition of physician-nurse boundaries will subside. Patient education is not the only arena of practice that has been affected by

role conflict. A few of the other areas of conflict are diagnosis, prescription of medications, and midwifery.

Experience with such health professionals as dietitians and pharmacists supports our contention that the more clearly the role boundaries are drawn, the less likely to arise are issues of territoriality and ownership of patients. Dietitians have a long history of involvement in patient education, and nurses and physicians have characteristically called on their expertise in therapeutic dietary teaching. Dietary teaching is a discrete area of patient education, and the need for such teaching can be readily recognized. Likewise, pharmacists occupy a specific role whose boundaries with nursing are easily defined. The pharmacist-nurse relationship is complementary, as is the dietitian-nurse relationship, in that the role functions of each are clear. Pharmacists historically have not been as involved in inpatient teaching as have dietitians and nurses, although this is changing. In outpatient situations, however, pharmacists have been involved in patient education for many years in drugstores and, more recently, in outpatient clinics. We have observed effective medication teaching with lower-income patients in outpatient settings where clinical pharmacists were hired for the express purpose of teaching.

Nursing Staff Skill Mix: Trends in Managed Care

The last issue that should be discussed is the trend toward redesigning nursing staff mix patterns in acute care settings, decreasing the number of RN positions and increasing the use of assistive personnel. The trend for the past 10 years, due to the institution of the Medicare Prospective Payment System (DRGs) and more recent managed care and capitation approaches, is for only acutely ill patients to be hospitalized. Inpatient stays are dramatically shortened, with more care provided in ambulatory or home settings. This means that the hospitalized population is sicker, discharged quicker, with more intensive needs for patient

---

[2]Medicalization is a term coined by Ivan Illich to describe the abrogation by the medical structure of functions that previously were performed societally. A medicalized physician or nurse, then, would buy into this value system and attempt to perpetuate the supremacy of medicine. (Illich, I. [1976]. *Medical nemesis: The expropriation of health.* New York: Pantheon).

education on "survival skills." Managed care incentives to reduce costs have also led to downsizing; fewer nurses are providing care for sicker patients. Many nurses voice concern that care will become fragmented, with nurses spending less time in direct patient care and more time supervising assistive personnel (American Nurses Association, 1994). We believe that nurses must have a strong voice in planning and evaluating staffing patterns to preserve the nurse's role in patient education. Administrators must be knowledgeable about the critical thinking and assessment required for patient education. In addition to adversely affecting patient outcomes, accreditation requirements of JCAHO may be unmet. Nurses must astutely use evaluation data to support their case for adequate professional staffing, citing the cost savings of effective patient education efforts as integral aspects of clinical paths that reduce length of stay. Managerial structures and resources, including nursing staff time and other costs, must be presented to support and justify existing programs (Redman & Levine, 1987).

In summary, we note that patient education practices vary among institutions, as well as among conceptions and implementations of roles. We believe that patient education is undertaken with greater ease and effectiveness when roles are discrete and when respect for various roles and personnel is manifest on a human level.

Power in the Patient Education Setting: Who Has It and How to Get It

We have been referring to power throughout this chapter, assuming that our readers are familiar with our use of the term. Perhaps it is appropriate now to review a few definitions. Stephen Robbins defines power as the influence an individual or group has on the decision-making process (Robbins, 1980). John Wax's definition supplements Robbins'; it is "the control of resources essential to the functioning or survival of individuals and the organization" (Wax, 1971). Traditionally, nurses have been afraid of power, viewing it as "unladylike" or as a magical tool possessed by physicians. More recently, nurses have begun to recognize power as a legitimate function in nursing, and nurse educators have promoted its use. In this section we outline how one recognizes who has power, what the sources of power are, and how to obtain power to implement patient education.

Recognizing Types and Sources of Power

Power is frequently believed to originate from some legendary, mystical source. Many of us believe it is a quality that some of us are fortunate enough to acquire at birth; rather, it is a quality that is developed, over time, with a great deal of hard work. The clues to recognizing power and influence in others are subtle. To implement patient education, first recognize where power resides by asking the questions in Box 13-2.

Because power includes decision-making and control of resources, nurses should learn to answer those questions correctly and approach the power source or sources.

Power emanates from various sources, which in turn strengthen or lessen the power.

BOX 13–2. Questions to Determine Who Has Power Regarding Patient Education in an Institution

- Who decides if this patient is to receive teaching?
- Who assesses the value of a teaching program and mandates its operation in the hospital?
- Whom do I approach for obtaining necessary funding for audiovisual equipment to enhance patient education?
- Who has the "word" on what is really going on in this institution?
- Who seems to be "in control" at meetings on patient education?

The following typology of power outlines its sources, starting with the most influential and ending with the least effective type of power:

1. Expert power
2. Positional power
3. Personality or charismatic power
4. Social power

Expert power is the most effective type of power. The person with expert power knows what she is talking about, and people respect what she has to say. This person may or may not possess positional power. The person who is attempting to coordinate or initiate a patient education program must have expert power if she is to be successful in patient education efforts. Expert power may be a type of formal power, such as that invested in a nurse clinical specialist, or it may be informal power, as exhibited by the staff nurse to whom everyone turns when a diabetic patient needs teaching. Expert power can be developed by formal education or on-the-job training, but expert knowledge must be present to make this person credible. Being an expert on the costs and benefits of patient education efforts, especially financial, are an important source of expert power.

Positional power is always formal power, because it is invested in the individual by an institution or organization. Persons with positional power have the ability to hire and fire, to authorize pay increases, and to set limits of acceptable behavior. Positional power is an obvious asset to the nurse who is trying to initiate a patient education program in the institution. Nurses who have assumed the roles of care coordinator or case manager can learn to use their position and administrative mandates as a source of power.

A third type of power, which is less effective than expert or positional power, is *charismatic power* or *power by personality*. All of us have known individuals with tremendous power because of a dynamism that sets them apart from others. We can readily think of political and religious leaders with charismatic power. There are also people in institutions with power based on their personalities.

We know a physician who began a successful in-house patient education program that was quickly adopted by the medical and nursing staffs because of the power of his personality. Power by personality is more efficacious if it is combined with either expert or positional power. The support of an individual with charismatic power can be a tremendous asset in beginning a patient education program.

The fourth, and least effective, type of power is *social power*. Social power is the power that one has through social relationships and friendships. It is power given by a group to its informal leader. The aspects of social power that make it least useful are its dependence on relationships, its lack of substantiveness, and the underlying premise that something is owed in return for the granting of social power.

Social power, like expert power and charismatic power, can be a type of either formal or informal power. Educators and nurse managers frequently use social power in an attempt to get a staff to accept changes. It is not unusual for chief nurse executive in a large hospital to use charismatic power or expert power; in fact, she is probably more productive if she is able to use these types of power as well as the more formal kinds. A combination of power types is usually effective, but expert power is a necessity for anyone who wants to be recognized as an able leader for patient education.

Developing Power

Once the questions about who has the power have been answered and the type of power has been identified, a number of directions can be taken. An obvious response is to develop expert power. Because this usually takes some time to develop, it may be desirable to gain knowledge from the one with expert power by spending time observing her *modus operandi*. This is also the time to gather as much formal training and education as possible, through reading books and journal articles and attending seminars and classes. One nurse who was hired to develop and assume a job as coordinator for patient education in a community hospital spent the first 6 months in her new position identifying powerful figures among physicians, nurses, and other hospital personnel. She also improved her already formidable knowledge about patient education by attending conferences on patient education, by reading extensively, and by working closely with graduate students in health education to develop a needs assessment for the hospital. She researched innovative patient education models that had been shown to improve patient outcomes and decrease costs. After 6 months she solidified her power, which was previously positional, by displaying her knowledge of patient education needs in the hospital and being recognized as an expert in her field. Positional power continued to undergird her authority, and expert power enhanced and strengthened her power in the hospital.

After assessment of the institutional power structure and establishment of a power base, change may be necessary. The following section addresses the planned change process, and appropriate change-agentry skills are introduced and elaborated.

Planned Change and Change-Agentry Skills

The nature and process of change is still not well understood although many social scientists and some nursing leaders have recently developed theories and models that attempt to explain it (Bennis, Benne & Chin, 1985; Watzlawick, Weakland & Fisch, 1984; Lewin, 1951; Brooten, Hayman, & Naylor, 1978). Planned change entails organizing for change or applying scientific method and problem-solving skills: assessment, planning, implementation, and evaluation (Hall, 1985). Examples of situations in which change-agentry skills (those skills the nurse uses to effect planned change) have been applied to the realm of patient education can illustrate the usefulness of these skills. As Hall states, these "...skills are those which can be employed to facilitate change in client systems and constitute the power arma-

mentarium of the nursing practitioner as a change agent" (Hall, 1985). Five skills listed below greatly enhance the professional image of nurses and help them to develop skills in these power-laden areas where many nurses are somewhat afraid to tread.

1. Coordinating
2. Collaborating
3. Consulting
4. Negotiating and bargaining
5. Confronting

We are introducing two other change-agentry skills we have found useful in diverse patient education settings. We are referring to the first of these as *reframing*, realizing that this term is frequently used in psychotherapy but also appreciating that it is useful in our context. The second skill we are introducing is *coercion*.

Coordinating

Change agentry in patient education involves organizing and bringing together various approaches and health care professionals in such a way that high-quality patient education is delivered. The nurse who uses this type of coordination as a change-agentry skill recognizes the contributions and capabilities of others involved in patient education and arranges patient education programs to meet the needs of varied client groups.

In a community hospital that had hired a nurse with a master's degree to establish a hospital-wide patient education program, the change-agentry skill of coordination was used in the following manner. In committee decision-making situations the coordinator repressed her tendency to want to control and, instead, facilitated the decision-making by *not* asserting her power or authority. She openly recognized the nurses and physicians on the patient education task force as the experts, and she assisted them in designing teaching protocols as part of the critical paths.

Coordination skills were also used to assist the patient education task force in setting goals. The goal was to create a product that would be strongly desired and then to make that product visible. By developing a product, the members of the task force enjoyed an enhanced image, and the entire task force was given increased credibility. Health care professionals were reinforced for doing patient education and perceived payoffs from the patient education program were highlighted.

Collaborating

The process of working in a creative and egalitarian manner can be used to further promote the welfare of the client in the patient education setting. The nurse who integrates such collaboration as a change-agentry skill is respected by physicians, pharmacists, dietitians, and other health professionals because she is willing to share her expertise with others. Collaboration precludes the negative approaches of territoriality and ownership of patients.

In the community hospital discussed above, collaboration was used creatively by the coordinator to set a tone of cooperation. She used *validation* as a strategy to prevent members of the task force from becoming entangled in the decision-making process. Validation consisted of documentation and carefully written minutes that were circulated before every meeting. By validating the process that was taking place, she was able to establish a spirit of mutual cooperation and appreciation of others' contributions.

Another way in which she used collaboration was through her obvious ability to work within the environment of the community hospital and to deal with the constraints imposed by the institution. The fact that she was able to work creatively with administrators, physicians, and the nurse executive immeasurably improved her chances of successfully implementing a hospital-wide patient education program.

Consulting

The relationship between the nurse with proficiency in patient education (e.g., the clinical nurse specialist) and the consultee seeking her skills is reciprocal. The nurse shares her expert knowledge to further the practice of sound patient education concepts. The nurse as consultant has effective communication skills and uses them to assist the consultee in developing patient education resources and programs. Case managers and clinical specialists, by providing consultation for difficult patient situations, can empower staff nurses to teach and provide needed precepting.

In another example, the patient education coordinator assumed her role as consultant by first clarifying her own understanding of her role. She realized that she occupied a staff position and not a line position; thus, there were limits on her authority and ability to discipline, hire and fire, or set policy. Instead, she had been employed for her considerable managerial and organizational skills and to provide the impetus for the establishment of a patient education program.

She avoided a common consultant mistake by refusing to actually practice patient education. She thus did not interject herself into the nurses' work setting. When a patient education coordinator uses consultation to effect change, it is inappropriate for her to assume the actual task of educating patients. Instead, she should teach the nursing staff the principles of teaching and learning theory and other relevant information.

Furthermore, this coordinator took on the role of consultee herself when she sought help from other departments. In addition to increasing her visibility in the hospital, she also managed to secure some valuable contacts for later use. For example, the coordinator consulted the medical records department to determine the most frequent diagnoses on admission. Her ability to move from the consultee to the consultant role provided beneficial role modeling for the nursing staff.

Negotiating and Bargaining

In her role in promoting and providing patient education, the nurse must negotiate agreements. The agreements usually involve the procurement or delivery of patient education to a needy client group. Negotiating is a positive process through which both parties derive satisfaction. In the patient education setting, bargaining may also occur between a nurse and a client with both negotiating for mutually satisfactory and achievable goals.

Bargaining is a splendid change-agentry skill that many of us rarely use. Like all such skills, it must be accomplished in a setting where rationality and calmness prevail. Emotional debates can be avoided by a patient education coordinator; if someone exhibits obnoxious, strident behavior during meetings, it can be ignored and not held against the individual in future meetings.

One coordinator bargained effectively when the goals of certain patient education programs were questioned. Instead of compromising goals, however, she agreed to changes in content and strategy. When bargaining is used as a change-agentry skill, the nurse must remember that negotiating a bargain is a give-and-take proposition and that some important ideas may have to be traded away.

Another nurse who served as associate director of a diabetes teaching center used negotiating as a means to achieve her desired ends regarding establishment of outreach patient education centers for Chinese and Hispanic diabetic persons. The medical director of the center was eager to have the center accredited by the American Diabetes Association, a long and tedious task that he was unwilling to do himself. The nurse informally bargained with the physician, using her willingness to oversee the accreditation process in exchange for the physician's willingness to approve the outreach programs.

Confronting

The various perceptions held by different people in a patient education setting must be clarified and compared. Confrontation involves a face-to-face communicative encounter between the nurse and another health professional or the patient. Reserve the powerful change-agentry tool of confrontation for situations involving a lack of direct, open communication. Use confrontation only after other change-agentry skills have been exhausted.

When using confrontation as a change-agentry skill, be aware of the two levels of response it usually evokes: emotional and intellectual. Recognize and identify the emotional response but do not respond to it. The intellectual response allows room for reasoning. Do not use confrontation in an attempt to impose beliefs on another but to establish an environment that will encourage a new approach to the problem. For example, when a patient education coordinator realized that territoriality was becoming an issue, she turned the decision-making focus toward patient care and patients' rights.

When involved with confrontation, consider the amount of authority and support held by the person being confronted. If he is not powerful, the optimal method of confrontation may be to override him. If he does possess support and authority, summon the committee members to attempt to change his mind. These group members must have equal influence and power for this method of confrontation to work. The term confrontation often has negative overtones. Attempt to remove the emotional "battle lines" aspect of the term.

Reframing

When a situation is viewed in an entirely new light, old ideas and methods can be replaced with new approaches (Clark, 1977). This reframing is different from confronting in that the nurse reworks or restates the situation for the patient or client group. This frequently involves introducing an entirely different perspective into patient education. When old problems are broached in a different light, new avenues can be taken.

This different perspective in patient education may be introduced by the patient or the institution, or it may be the perspective of a particular committee member. An example of reframing occurred when we spoke to the medical staff of an outpatient center, presenting patient education as more than an attempt to gain compliance, but instead as a basic feature of the patient's right to know. One physician who had obviously been pondering this idea said, "I see what you are saying; it's like informed consent."

Coercing

Legal authority can be used to gain an end that is not attainable in any other less forceful fashion. Coercion avoids emotional overtones, focusing instead on institutional and federal regulations. Coercion is better applied to recalcitrant groups of health professionals who are unwilling to institute patient education than it is to individual clients. Coercion is usually a last-resort change-agentry tool; apply it only when all else has failed.

When a patient education coordinator was stymied by one "blocker" physician, she used coercion by having an administrator exert power from above, after showing him that the blocker was obstructing the goals of the organization. This change-agentry skill makes many of us feel uncomfortable; it is not a skill we are taught as nursing students, and women, in general, are not encouraged or taught to use coercion. At times, however, it is the only effective way of achieving the desired goal.

The use of critical incidents, such as a high rate of diabetic readmissions or JCAHO probationary accreditation, can coerce reluctant people or institutions to affect change. When the staff of a community hospital was informed that they did not meet JCAHO criteria for acceptable patient education, they ceased arguing the merits of patient education and began planning better programs.

Other Strategies

Using open-ended questions to probe the attitudes of recalcitrant patient education task force members has led to greater understanding of some unspoken, underlying issues. When opposition to the matter at hand becomes strong, another good tactic can be to

retreat and compromise rather than continue waging war. When using this strategy, however, it is unwise to go back to the beginning of the process because all gains would thus be nullified. A third strategy is to reinforce the base of support and make it stronger. A change agent needs all the help she can get, and she should constantly reinforce her position through the help of others. It is also important to look inward if things are not going well. Perhaps an undesirable response has been provoked by the change agent. Increasing credibility is another strategy to effect change. Showing is better than talking, and it is imperative that other health professionals believe the change agent is an expert in her area. High visibility in an institution does not guarantee credibility.

Summary: Nursing Strategies to Effect Change and Promote Patient Education in Case Management Systems

This chapter has addressed the innovation that is necessary to strengthen patient education as an integral component of case management systems. It is necessary to visibly incorporate patient teaching on the critical pathway and in the process of critical pathway design committees. Patient education should be realistic based on length of stay as reflected by care maps, and variances for patient teaching should be tracked with those for other interventions. Thus, patient education becomes part of total quality programs in the organization and outcomes can be evaluated. Positive outcomes such as safer discharges and cost savings can provide needed support to justify staff time and other resources for patient education programs. Patients and families should also be involved in planning care so that designs are patient centered.

Nurses in all roles can provide needed leadership for the patient education innovations that accompany case management. Staff nurses who are knowledgeable about critical paths, skilled at teaching, and enthusiastic about teamwork with other disciplines can help to make higher quality, lower cost care a reality. Nurses in positions such as case manager, care coordinator, or patient education coordinator advocate for both the patient and the staff nurse not only through their clinical expertise, but also by developing consensus and gaining needed political support. Specifically, they advocate for two of the most needed resources to deliver quality patient education: allocating the time of RNs to teach and providing staff development to promote expertise in practice.

Strategies for Critical Analysis and Application

1. Using Hanisch's model for cardiac rehabilitation teaching described in this chapter, discuss how a product-line patient education model could be developed for prenatal/postpartum patients. Consider the various settings in which care is provided for the patient before, during, and in the first 2 weeks after delivery. Also take into account a discharge of 24 hours after delivery.

2. Continuing the above scenario, describe how the use of patient focus groups could assist nurses in identifying learning priorities and redesigning patient education for the inpatient period.

3. Describe how community-based nursing case management might improve patient education efforts for early discharge postpartum patients and their families.

4. Propose a strategy you could use to gain political support for an innovative new program you developed to replace the exiting, outdated program.

REFERENCES

American Nurses Association (1980). *Nursing and social policy statement.* Kansas City, MO: Author.

American Nurses Association (1994). ANA and SNAs testify on risks of decreasing skill mix. *American Nurse, November/December,* 11,14.

Bartlett, E. (1986). Advocacy skill and strategies for patient education managers. *Patient Education and Counseling, 8,* 397-405.

Bennis, W., Benne, K., & Chin, R. (1985). *The planning of change.* New York: Holt, Rinehart, and Winston.

Bower, K. (1988). Case management: Meeting the challenge: Managed care: controlling costs, guaranteeing outcomes. *Definition, 3*(1), 1-3. Boston: The Center for Nursing Case Management, New England Medical Center Department of Nursing.

Brooten, D., Hayman, L., & Naylor, M. (1978). *Leadership for change: A guide for the frustrated nurse.* Philadelphia: J. B. Lippincott.

Burr, W., Leigh, G., Day, R., Constantine, J. (1979). Symbolic interactionism and the family. In W. Burr, R. Hill, F. Nye, & I. Reiss (Eds.), *Contemporary theories about the family* (Vol. II.). New York: Free Press.

Clark, C. (1977). Reframing. *American Journal of Nursing, 77,* 840-841.

Hall, J. (1985). Nursing as process. In J. Hall & B. Weaver (Eds.), *Distributive nursing practice: A systems approach to community health* (pp. 124-137). Philadelphia: J. B. Lippincott.

Hanisch, P. (1993). Informational needs and preferred time to receive information for phase II cardiac rehabilitation patients: What CE instructors need to know. *Journal of Continuing Education in Nursing, 24*(2), 82-89.

Hofmann, P. (1993). Critical path method: An important tool for coordinating clinical care. *Journal of Quality Improvement, 19*(7), 235-246.

Joint Commission on the Accreditation of Healthcare Organizations. (1994). *Consolidated accreditation manual for hospitals.* Chicago: Author.

Kortbawi, P. (1993). An orientation plan for hospital-based case managers. *Journal of Continuing Education in Nursing, 12*(2), 69-73.

Kovner, C., Hendrikson, G., Knickman, J., & Finkler, S. (1993). Changing the delivery of nursing care: Implementation issues and qualitative findings. *Journal of Nursing Administration, 23*(11), 24-34.

Lewin, K. (1951). *Field theory in social science.* New York: Harper & Row.

Mahn, V. (1993). Clinical nurse case management: A service line approach. *Nursing Management, 24*(9), 48-50.

Menke E. (1985) Conceptual basis for nursing intervention with human systems: Individuals. In J. Hall, & B. Weaver (eds). *Distributive nursing practice: A sysytems approach to community health* (pp 144, 153-157). Philadelphia: JB Lippincott.

Orem, D. (1985). *Nursing: concepts of practice* (p. 31). New York: McGraw-Hill.

Pollock, S. (1987). Adaptation to chronic illness: Analysis of nursing research. *Nursing Clinics of North America, 22*(3), 631-644.

Redman, B., & Levine, D. (1987). Organizational resources in support of patient education programs: Relationship to reported delivery of instruction. *Patient Education and Counseling, 9,* 177-197.

Ritchey, R., & Raney, M. (1981). Medical role-task boundary maintenance: Physicians' opinions on clinical pharmacy. *Medical Care, 19*(1), 90-93.

Robbins, S. (1980). *The administrative process.* Englewood Cliffs, NJ: Prentice-Hall.

Roy, C. (1984). *Introduction to nursing: An adaptation model.* Englewood Cliffs, NJ: Prentice-Hall.

Watzlawick, P., Weakland, J., & Fisch, R. (1974). *Change: Problem formation and problem resolution.* New York: W. W. Norton.

Wax, J. (1971). Power theory and institutional change. *Social Service Review, 45*(3), 284.

Weaver, B. (1985). Distributive nursing practice. In B. Hall & B. Weaver (Eds.), *Distributive nursing practice: A systems approach to community health* (pp. 3-9). Philadelphia: J. B. Lippincott.

Weekes, D., & Savedra, M. (1988). Adolescent cancer: Coping with treatment-related pain, a pilot study. *Journal of Pediatric Nursing, 3*(5), 318-328.

Wu, R. (1973). *Behavior and illness.* Englewood Cliffs, NJ: Prentice-Hall.

Zander, K. (1988). Nursing case management: Strategic management of cost and quality outcomes. *Journal of Nursing Administration, 18*(5), 23-30.

Zander, K. (1991). Care maps: The core of cost/quality care. *The New Definition, 6*(3). Boston: The Center for Nursing Case Management.

Zander, K. (1992). Critical pathways. In M. Melum & M. Sinioris (Eds.), *Total quality management.* Chicago: American Hospital Association Publishing.

CHAPTER

14 | Roundtable: Problems Encountered in Practice Settings

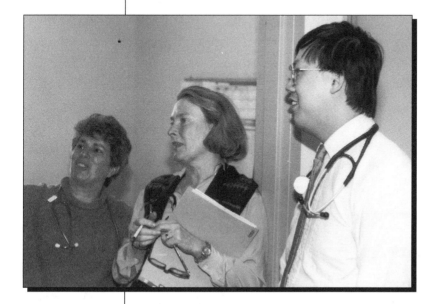

Introduction

This chapter attempts to answer the questions that may have occurred to readers throughout the previous chapters. We try to answer the "yes, but..." questions that probably arose after reading our earlier approaches and suggestions. We have found that many texts propose grand and glorious schemata and frameworks but ignore the daily irritating and confounding problems encountered in practice settings. Therefore, we examine such common problems as how to motivate patients and staff involved in patient education and how to get the health team together. Obtaining publicity and choosing teaching materials are discussed. Delivering patient education to various age groups (pediatric through gerontologic) as well as learners with special needs (learning disabled children) and in special settings (e.g., the dying patient and the psychiatric patient) are also considered.

We begin with a discussion of the differences between patient *teaching* and patient *education*. We have found that these terms are frequently used interchangeably and we feel strongly that they are not synonymous. We present a question-and-answer format to aid in ease of reading.

Patient Education: Issues, Principles, Practices, Third Edition, by Sally H. Rankin and Karen Duffy Stallings. Lippincott–Raven Publishers, Philadelphia, © 1996.

What is the difference between patient education and patient teaching?

Patient education has been defined as "...the process of influencing patient behavior, producing changes in knowledge, attitudes, and skills required to maintain and improve health. The process may begin with the imparting of information, but also includes interpretation and integration of the information in such a manner as to bring about attitudinal or behavioral changes that benefit the person's health status" (Simonds, 1979). This definition states that patient education is a *process* with various components. It considers the patient holistically, with all his needs and concerns, and sets goals with the patient for desired outcomes. The process of patient education also includes an evaluation of the patient's learning, its usefulness to him, and the ease with which he has integrated it into his self-care practices. *Patient teaching* refers to only one component of the patient education process— the actual imparting of information to the patient.

Patient education versus patient teaching is a process versus content issue. The content of the actual teaching is important and, obviously, must be accurate, but the total process of patient education is much more important than the teaching itself. The transfer of knowledge that occurs with patient teaching does not ensure behavioral change. Many research projects give ample evidence of this (Simons-Morton, Mullen, Mains, Tabak, & Green, 1992; Devine, 1992; Brown, 1992; Alexander, Weiss, Helsey, & Papiernik, 1991; Sackett, Haynes, Gibson, Hackett, Taylor, et al., 1975). We believe that it is our ethical obligation to supply patients with information related to their problems. We cannot assume, however, that because we fulfill our responsibility patients will make the desired behavioral changes. If we use the process of patient education, instead of merely imparting the content, we can hope that patients may cooperate more with the regimens. (For more information related to the process of patient education, see Chaps. 6–10).

How can we motivate patients to learn?

Probably the most important factor in motivating patients to respond to patient education with the desired behavioral changes is the recognition of what motivates each individual patient. For one patient, motivation may be assurance that he will be in control of his own life; motivating factors for another patient may be predicated on his desire to please the health care professionals. Some patients are able to state clearly what motivates them, but other patients may not recognize what works as a motivator. Clues to the individual motivation factors can be obtained from the client's life-style, family members, socioeconomic status, and growth and development data. Health care professionals must avoid the assumption that their own motivators apply to their patients.

Frequently motivation is divided into intrinsic and extrinsic factors. *Intrinsic factors* are factors that are internally integrated into the client's personality and *modus operandi*. They include such things as the patient's anxiety level, his success in past educational settings, and his openness to learning. *Extrinsic factors* include the environment for learning, the pleasure of acquiring new knowledge, and the type of interaction in the learning process. Extrinsic motivation factors are factors we, as patient educators, can control. If we establish a climate of mutual trust and safety, the environment for learning can be a positive motivator. Likewise, by injecting fun and some levity into the learning situation, we can make the pleasure of learning become a positive force.

The type of interaction in the learning process is another extrinsic motivating factor that the educator can control. Transactional analysis provides a vocabulary useful to describe the desired interaction. If our interaction with the learner is structured so that the adult learner is programmed as the child in an adult-child or parent-child situation, the interaction will have negative motivational effects on the learner. The adult learner will profit most from an adult-adult type of interaction. An example of an adult-adult type of interaction would be that of group learning experiences for ostomy patients, in which one patient would share with the group his experiences in coping with his ostomy. Another example of an adult-adult type of interaction includes the patient educator who encourages the client to set his own agenda for learning the management of heart disease. Adult-adult interactions require the client to take responsibility for his own learning, an issue that is discussed shortly.

Because motivation also has social mastery and task mastery components, we can use these components to enhance motivation for learning. We know, for example, that adolescents have strong affiliative or belonging needs. The affiliative needs, and related self-esteem and social approval needs, can be used to enhance internal motivating forces when adolescents are engaged in learning how to cease smoking or how to manage contraception. The use of peers who role model desired behaviors is an exceptionally strong motivator for adolescents. One of the most important roles the nurse can play in motivation is that of helping the client to recognize the gap between what his situation is and what he wants it to be. Malcolm Knowles, in his formative text on adult education, describes the gap as a central aspect of motivating patients to learn (1970). For example, a young couple with whom we worked recognized that they did not want to use corporal punishment with their 3-year-old daughter, but they did not know how else to achieve necessary obedience. Once we were able to help them recognize this gap, they eagerly asked for, and then applied, other techniques of discipline. Once patients have recognized the gap, they can be effectively motivated with the use of written contracts. The formulation of such contracts is covered in Chapter 8.

If motivational techniques do not seem to be working, the nurse should consider reviewing the assessment and then reassessing the patient if necessary. Perhaps something has changed in the patient's own situation and previous motivators are no longer effective. For example, a low-to-moderate level of anxiety is an intrinsic motivator and may be used effectively to motivate the patient with coronary artery disease to learn about necessary diet, medication, and life-style changes. However, if this same patient has a successful coronary artery bypass graft operation, he may believe he is "cured" and out of danger; therefore, anxiety may no longer be an effective motivator. The nurse must now reassess the patient and determine other motivators.

There are undoubtedly further questions about motivation, the primary one being, "How much responsibility to learn does the patient have?" When all factors are considered, it is the patient who must ultimately decide whether he is going to accept our attempts to teach him, whether he accepts selectively, or whether he completely ignores us. Nurses and health care professionals are not responsible for patients' behavior. We can try our best to enhance the learning situation and use extrinsic motivation factors, but motivation is essentially an inner drive, and if this drive and a sense of personal responsibility are not operating in our particular clients, there is little we can do to foster these motivators. Ideally, we should be able to teach patients to be their own advocates and to expect patient education services on an inpatient and outpatient basis. Many patients will respond to this approach and, in fact, various books have been written detailing the approach that patients should take when dealing with the medical world (Kleinman, 1988; Cousins, 1979; Illich, 1976). However, we must be cognizant of the few patients who do refuse to take responsibility for their own learning; once we have made every attempt to provide patient education to them, we must finally release our own sense of responsibility for them.

How can we motivate staff to become involved in patient education?

Some of the issues related to motivation of staff in patient education settings are discussed in Chapter 6. Other means of motivating staff to provide high-quality patient education follow.

Nurses and other health professionals frequently complain that they do not understand the process of patient education. One- or 2-day workshops offered to all health professionals are an effective means of imparting teaching and learning principles and securing interest in patient education. The bonus of giving continuing education units may be influential, especially to nurses who work in states with mandatory continuing education requirements. We have offered many of these seminars to nurses, and a basic outline of such a workshop can be found at the end of Chapter 2. We have usually used case studies and role plays in these seminars to enhance the learning process. Sometimes we ask participants to develop their own teaching programs, applying the content learned in the seminar.

Another aspect that can be problematic is the actual disease process or health promotion content that must be conveyed to patients. Many nurses remark that they do not know what to teach. Although we believe that most nurses usually do have the pertinent information stored away, we feel that anxiety can be decreased by *helping the staff to organize* and review the information that patients need. Frequently, staff members become so enthusiastic about teaching after attending such classes that they recognize other areas of need and develop teaching protocols with little assistance from the patient educator. Such seminars and classes satisfy both intrinsic and extrinsic motivational factors for the staff. Negative intrinsic factors such as anxiety about lack of knowledge are modified, and such positive extrinsic factors as gaining continuing education units are resolved.

Nursing rounds oriented toward patient education can be an effective motivating force because they add novelty to the learning situation. In such instances, nurses or other health professionals should be asked to prepare some information about a patient with whom they are familiar. This material may be related to assessment of the client's education needs, to goal setting, to the actual process of teaching skills, or to any number of patient education tasks. During nursing rounds, the nurse performs the chosen tasks with the patient. After rounds the task is critiqued by the observing staff. Nursing rounds can become an excellent means of learning from others and expanding one's own repertoire of patient education behaviors.

Support at the administrative level for patient education is necessary if the programs are to maintain validity and credibility. Such support also is an extrinsic motivator to staff members because they feel that their efforts are being appreciated at the highest levels. Developing and enhancing administrative support is covered in Chapter 2.

Reward and incentive programs for staff who provide patient education can be a strong motivator. Sometimes the reward is the ability to move from night or evening shifts to day shifts. Another possibility is for a staff nurse who has developed special skills to be advanced up a clinical career ladder to a position that may be called clinical teaching nurse. Usually such promotions are accompanied by merit pay raises but have no increase in administrative duties. These promotions keep good nurses at the bedside rather than shift them into administration. Such rewards and incentives also show other staff members that patient education activities are valued in their institution.

Peer support is another important motivating factor for the staff. Staff members who can convene on a formal or informal basis to discuss their problems and their successes in patient education can add a great impetus to the widespread adoption of patient education efforts. As a profession, nursing suffers from a lack of internal validation. Too often we feel we are the only ones on the battle lines, and we refuse to allow ourselves to ask for support when we need it. Greater team efforts and support within nursing would improve patient education efforts and act as a motivator to inexperienced nurses looking for guidance.

We mentioned the benefits that accrue from increased *physician-nurse collegiality* and its resulting improvement in team effort in Chapter 2. Certainly such collegiality can be seen as a motivator for the staff. Nurses who know that physicians approve of their patient education efforts will experience confirmation and validation as motivators. Because collegiality is a two-way proposition, it is important that nurses also validate the patient education efforts of physicians. Collegiality as a motivator can, and should, extend to other health care team members. Another extrinsic motivator is nurses' better sense of their own professional identity in such collegial relationships.

How is the teaching of children and adolescents different from the teaching of adults?

Children are not just small adults, and teaching them demands an ingenuity and an approach different from that of teaching adults. Adolescents' learning needs vary from those of children and from those of adults, and, therefore, are discussed separately.

Teaching and learning principles, when applied to children, should always consider the growth and development level, as well as the cognitive level, of the child. Most research indicates that age is significantly associated with ability to manage distressing situations such as stressful procedures (Fegley, 1988). Table 14-1 is based on Piaget's well-known work regarding the development of perceptual and cognitive processes from infancy through adolescence (Piaget & Garcia, 1974). We purposely chose Piaget instead of Erikson because we feel that an understanding of cognitive processes is of equal importance to an understanding of developmental processes for pediatric patient education. Table 14-1 outlines the cognitive and perceptual stages of development and then suggests an approach to pediatric patient teaching.

Before embarking on pediatric patient education, remember that children have shorter attention spans, have greater needs for support and nurturance, and learn even more easily through active participation than do adults. This means that material must be presented in abbreviated format over short periods of time. Staff members must remember to consistently and persistently show affection and offer praise to their young clients during education sessions. By actively involving children in the learning process, we help them to more readily assimilate the information. It is an old adage that the child's play is his work. In his play he integrates new and unfamiliar information. Play, therefore, becomes a primary vehicle through which he learns about his disease or acute problem, about what will happen, and about how to take care of himself to the best of his ability. Play therapy should also be used to help the child to integrate and understand the painful or frightening experience he has undergone. Follow-up to surgery and procedures is just as important as preparation for these events because most children have many unresolved feelings and questions that need expression.

Although our case study will focus on a school-age child, we note that research is proving the efficacy of early childhood and infant intervention and stimulation (Berrueta-Clement, Schweinhart, Barnett, Epstein, & Weikart, 1984). Parents are being instructed in techniques of infant stimulation by community agencies such as community colleges, public health departments, and voluntary agencies. Certainly pediatric staff nurses should use their knowledge of child development to both initiate and reinforce such infant stimulation techniques with hospitalized infants. Role modeling these techniques is an effective teaching intervention for parents.

This case study illustrates the appropriate teaching for a 10-year-old boy with newly diagnosed idiopathic recurrent seizures.

❑ CASE STUDY

Eric

Eric experienced his first generalized, tonic-clonic (grand mal) seizure during recess at elementary school. He was hospitalized immediately for observation and a diagnostic work-up. Eric's primary nurse initiated patient education 2 days before his planned discharge. Remembering that Eric's stage of cognitive development

TABLE 14-1. Cognitive States and Approaches to Patient Education with Children

COGNITIVE STAGE	APPROACH TO TEACHING
Ages Birth to 2 yrs—Sensorimotor Development	
Begins as completely undifferentiated from environment	Orient all teaching to parents
Eventually learns to repeat actions that have effect on objects	Make infants feel as secure as possible with familiar objects in home environment
Has rudimentary ability to make associations	Give older infants an opportunity to manipulate objects in their environments; especially if long hospitalization is expected
Ages 2–7 yrs—Preoperational Development	
Has cognitive processes that are literal and concrete	Be aware of explanations that the child may interpret literally (e.g., "The doctor is going to make your heart like new" may be interpreted as "He is going to give me a new heart"); allow child to manipulate safe equipment such as stethoscopes, tongue blades, reflex hammers; use simple drawings of the external anatomy because children have limited knowledge of organs' functions
Lacks ability to generalize	Comparisons to other children are not helpful nor is it meaningful to compare one diagnostic test or procedure to another
Has egocentrism predominating	Belief that he causes events to happen may result in guilty thoughts that he caused his own pain, hospitalization, and so forth; reassure child that no one is to blame for his pain or other problems
Has animistic thinking (thinks that all objects possess life or human characteristics of their own)	Anthropomorphize and name equipment that is especially frightening
Ages 7–12 yrs—Concrete Operational Thought Development	
Has concrete, but more realistic and objective, cognitive processes	Use drawings and models; children at this age have vague understandings of internal body processes; use needle play, dolls to explain surgical techniques and facilitate learning
Is able to compare objects and experiences because of increased ability to classify along many different dimensions	Relate his care to other children's experiences so he can learn from them; compare procedures to one another to diminish anxiety
Views world more objectively and is able to understand another's position	Use films and group activities to add to repertoire of useful behaviors and establish role models
Has knowledge of cause and effect that has progressed to deductive logical reasoning	Use child's interest in science to explain logically what has happened and what will happen to him; explain medications simply and straightforwardly (e.g., "This medicine [insulin] unlocks the door to your body's cells just as a key unlocks the door to your house. By unlocking the door to the cell, the insulin can deliver the food and energy in your blood to the cell."

Adapted from Petrillo, M. & Sanger, S. (1980). *Emotional care of hospitalized children* (pp 38–50). Philadelphia: J.B. Lippincott and Kolb, L. C. (1977). *Modern Clinical Psychiatry* (9th ed, pp 90–91). Philadelphia: W.B. Saunders.

had been characterized by Piaget as "concrete operational thought," she began by teaching him the basic pathophysiology of seizure activity (Piaget & Garcia, 1974). Eric was not capable of abstract thought processes, but he did understand the simple drawings the nurse provided of the brain and her explanation that the seizures were caused by too much electrical activity in the brain. The nurse did not stress the term electrical activity; instead, she compared the problem in his brain to an electric toy train that goes so fast that it runs off the track. She completed her analogy by saying that the phenobarbital he was going to take every day would act on his brain as if it were slowing down the speed of the electric train. Eric's nurse remained aware of the fact that at this stage of development in the child's language skills he may not always manage to indicate whether he has fully comprehended her explanation. She therefore used a great deal of repetition and asked Eric many questions.

Children from ages 7 to 12 are generally able to handle many of the aspects of their medical regimen. Eric was made responsible for administering his own medication at the prescribed times. He began preparing and taking the phenobarbital himself while he was still hospitalized.

Children of Eric's age are more socially involved with their peers than are younger children, and it is important not to disrupt their attempts to join groups and participate in team sports. Eric was told that he could continue riding his bike as long as he wore his bike helmet and was accompanied by another child or an adult. He was also informed that he might continue swimming provided there was always someone with him.

Finally, Eric was taught to begin to recognize the signs of his aura. The nurse defined an *aura* as the peculiar sensations Eric would grow to know as a warning sign of a seizure. After determining that Eric had previously experienced nausea and vomiting with the flu, she told him that an aura was the special warning that takes place before a convulsion, just as there was a certain warning that occurred before vomiting. Eric was told that when he began to recognize his aura, which might be a smell, sound, color, or sensation, he should try to lie down immediately.

All the teaching was accomplished with both of Eric's parents present. The parents could later act as reinforcers of the information imparted to Eric and could also offer support to him during the sessions. The nurse presented the material to Eric during three half-hour sessions so that he had an adequate amount of time to assimilate the information and ask questions. She also spent time with Eric's parents alone, giving them more detailed information and answering their questions. Eric was discharged from the hospital, and he and his parents were encouraged to call the nurse or Eric's pediatric nurse practitioner or pediatrician if they had questions or experienced any problems.

Adolescents have a different cognitive style from that of the school-age child. Piaget asserts that around the age of 12 children develop "formal operational thought" (Piaget & Garcia, 1974). During adolescence the ability to think abstractly becomes well developed. Cognitive processes are of an adult type, and the adolescent develops the ability to reason deductively. Therefore, when considering the cognitive style to use during patient teaching, we should be aware that the adolescent can be taught in a fashion similar to the way an adult is taught.

The aspect of the adolescent's development that clearly differentiates him from the adult, however, is his social development and the importance of his peer group. Knowledge of the adolescent's psychosocial task, "identity versus role confusion" as defined by Erik Erikson, is of primary importance to the health care provider working with the adolescent in a patient education setting (Erikson, 1963). The nurse must remember that because the adolescent develops his identity in relation to his peers and in opposition to his parents, teaching should be performed without the parents present.

Use of support groups for families with children with type I diabetes has been found to be an effective strategy in dealing with younger adolescents (11–14 years). One author (Rankin) facilitated a family support group for 3 years, which parents and children attended on a monthly basis. Although parents and children were frequently separated for different activities, many parents stated that the opportunity for their children to be in contact with other diabetic adolescents was a singular experience occurring only during the meetings. On occasion parents and children met together when there were topics of interest to both. For example, representatives from local diabetes summer camps attended the meetings to orient parents and children to camp possibilities. The most popular joint speaker, however, was a diabetic young man who had not been well controlled metabolically during adolescence and who, at the age of 23, was experiencing complications related to retinopathy. This speaker served a twofold purpose. On one level, he allowed children and adolescents an opportunity to see a young adult who had participated successfully in all types of sports and was determined to live as fully as possible, thus modeling a realistic role to adolescents. On another level, the speaker's retinopathy that had resulted from a period of multiple hyperglycemic episodes allowed the parents to understand that parental control would probably be inadequate in terms of protecting their own children from the excesses of adolescence.

Group instruction for parents and children has been successful in significantly decreasing glycosylated hemoglobin levels in diabetic adolescents older than 11 years and in improving knowledge levels in mothers and children (Hackett, Court, Matthews, McCowan, & Parkin, 1989). Group activities, referred to as "structured-fantasy group experiences," that are aimed at decreasing the emotional burden of type I diabetes mellitus in children aged 3 to 15 years have been reported (Basso, 1991). "Structured-fantasy group experiences" involve the use of video to allow children the opportunity to discuss their feelings about diabetes, difficulties in maintaining metabolic control, and stresses involved in peer and family relationships. The intervention entails children who are divided into age-appropriate groups (3–5 years; 6–10 years; and 11–15 years) making a videotape that addresses a topic of choice dealing with diabetes. After the videotape is made, the various age groups use it as a vehicle to discuss their condition (Basso, 1991). Thus, the concept of group teaching and mobilization of groups to deal with children's and adolescents' concerns is believed to be an equally efficacious approach to patient education with children and adolescents.

Frequently, we assume that adolescents have more knowledge about their own anatomy and physiology than they do. This applies to functions of body organs as well as to sexuality. Illustrations are helpful with this age group although they can be more sophisticated than those used with the school-age population.

Honesty with adolescents is extremely important. If a change in body image is expected as a result of surgery or during the course of a disease, the adolescent must be adequately prepared because body image is of paramount importance to this age group. Because of the desire to be "one of the gang" and to look like everyone else, the adolescent who faces a change in appearance will need help from health care professionals in hiding or camouflaging the change.

Developmental readiness for learning should not be equated with biologic growth or maturation. Developmental readiness is instead a combination of maturation, learning, and cognition. These three components must be organized within the individual and be present at the appropriate level to begin teaching. An example is the developmental readiness that must be present for an adolescent to deal successfully with the concept of eating correctly and losing weight. Before the onset of adolescence most children are unable to correctly choose foods that will supply necessary nutrients and also assist in weight loss. However, with increased motivation to gain social acceptance, an increased intellectual ability to understand scientific principles, and a concomitant physical maturation, the adolescent is equipped to build on past learning and prepare and eat foods that are healthy and conducive to weight loss.

How must patient education be modified to meet the needs of children and adolescents with learning disabilities?

Public attention is increasingly focused on learning disabilities in children and adults. The media have recently focused on such disabilities as attention deficit disorder while schools, psychologists, and parents continue to cope with previously recognized disorders such as dyslexia. Greenberg (1991) succinctly outlines the problems encountered by health care providers attempting to perform patient education with learning disabled children. Learning disabled children are not mentally retarded or developmentally delayed in terms of learning abilities; indeed, they are usually of average or higher than average intelligence. However, they may learn better using certain sensory systems—auditory, visual, or tactile—that are different from those used by the nurse or other health care provider. Additionally, certain factors may affect their ability to learn such as problems affecting memory, language, and motor and integrative processing problems (Greenberg, 1991).

Children who are *auditory learners* are thought to have *visual perceptual disabilities*, frequently referred to as dyslexia. Children with visual perceptual disabilities have problems reading and may also have spatial orientation difficulties. Because they learn best through auditory modes, the nurse should not rely on written teaching materials but instead should use auditory-oriented materials such as tapes, records, and verbal instructions. When visual stimuli are used they should be introduced singly, and an opportunity for mastery must be allowed before new visual stimuli are presented. Evaluation of effectiveness of teaching should occur orally so that these children have an opportunity to tell the nurse verbally what they have learned.

Children who are *visual learners* often have an *auditory perceptual disability*. These children often are unable to distinguish subtle differences in sounds and may have problems picking up cues that they are being spoken to, especially when others are speaking in the same room. If instruction needs to take place orally, the nurse should instruct a child who is a visual learner in a quiet room and limit the number of words used. These children usually do well with films, written materials, charts, and other visual learning materials. The child who is a visual learner may not be a good candidate for group instruction.

Tactile learners are children with learning disabilities who are most amenable to learning that includes some type of hands-on, tactile experience. These children may prefer writing and drawing and any other learning process that includes touch and physical exploration (Greenberg, 1991). If these children do not also have other learning disabilities, such as auditory perceptual, they may be good candidates for group games and learning experiences that involve movement.

Integrative processing disabilities usually involve the inability to sequence visual, auditory, or tactile input correctly (Greenberg, 1991). These children may read words backward and be unable to correctly process the word, or they may hear words or sentences improperly and not be able to understand the meaning. The most effective learning strategies with these children involve simple instructions with the opportunity for immediate return demonstration. The use of analogies and jokes is unwise with these children because they may be unable to make the connection between the analogy and the desired learning.

Children with *short- or long-term memory disabilities* have severe deficits remembering information presented to them either recently or in the past. Memory disabilities often accompany other learning disabilities, adding to the problems involved in achieving effective patient education. These children need the opportunity for short and frequent teaching sessions to aid in reinforcement of the material (Greenberg, 1991).

Language disabilities are manifested in children as the inability to answer when some type of response is demanded. The child may be able to spontaneously initiate a question or a topic but when questioned on the same topic may not be able to sufficiently organize his thoughts so that a coherent answer can be given. As Greenberg points out, the most important response of the health care provider is to allow sufficient time for the child to mobilize his thoughts, rather than trying to answer the question for him. These children are not good candidates for learning activities that require quick verbal responses as may occur in a spelling bee format because they will become anxious and increasingly nonverbal.

Motor disabilities can be exhibited in two different ways—gross and fine motor disabilities. Fine motor disabilities are seen in children who are unable to write or draw but may be able to use a computer or paint. Gross motor disabilities result frequently in clumsiness and poor performance in sports activities. In the hospital setting, these children might be recognized by their frequent falls and should be placed in a safe, uncluttered environment when possible (Greenberg, 1991).

Although many children are diagnosed with learning disabilities before their hospitalization or interface with a nurse practitioner in the outpatient setting, it is sometimes the hospital nurse's own assessment skills that detect the child's learning disability and lead to a referral for diagnosis by a specialist. If the child has been previously diagnosed, then the health care provider must pay careful attention to parental suggestions because parents are usually aware of the best learning techniques for their children. Although children with learning disabilities may require more time in a patient education situation, the rewards are great when the appropriate strategy is used. The health care provider should also be aware that the Americans with Disabilities Act provides safeguards to guarantee children and adults with learning disabilities access to necessary equipment, supports, and other devices that may enhance a healthy life-style.

What can we do about physicians who block all our attempts at patient education?

Although we may try our hardest to use change-agentry skills and may try our best to implement a high-quality patient education program, we most likely still will be confronted by physicians who absolutely refuse to allow any of their patients access to patient education offered in the agencies in which they practice. It makes no difference to them that the programs have been approved by the medical staff, and it is usually impossible to tell what is at the root of this intransigence. Fortunately, such physicians are the exception, but they can frustrate the intentions of a conscientious patient educator. If you, as the patient's nurse and advocate, feel that patient education is absolutely necessary for the well-being of the patient, and if you have exhausted every approach including speaking personally with the physician, it may be necessary to have the patient himself request patient teaching and put pressure on the doctor to provide it.

I am documenting all my patient education but no one is reading my notes. What should I do?

This is frequently a problem for nurses who scrupulously document all of their patient teaching in the nurses' notes section of the chart. We feel that all documentation related to a patient should be put in the progress notes section of the chart, so that the entire health care team has easy access to the data. Our experience has been that charting style and format quickly improved when nurses documented in the progress notes, whether this documentation was solely related to patient education or whether it encompassed all of the old nurses' notes data. In many institutions all other health care team professionals (e.g., dietitians, physical and occupational therapists, and social workers) chart in the progress notes section; it seems that someone as important to the team and to the patient as the nurse should also chart there.

Historically, nurses' notes have been poorly written and have conveyed few data. However, as nursing education and nursing's theory base have improved, so has nurses' charting. We believe that problem-oriented charting in the SOAP (subjective, objective, assessment, and plan) format forces everyone to chart pertinent, concise data related to the patient's problems. The SOAP format also lends itself well to charting of the progress of patient education. The nurse who understands and uses problem-oriented charting correctly, with proper grammar, spelling, and punctuation, will find that the charting is read.

How can I get the health care team together to coordinate patient education?

Coordinating patient education can be a difficult job when many disciplines are involved. For example, the patient with newly diagnosed diabetes is usually taught by nurses, dietitians, and, in some settings, pharmacists. The diabetic patient's physician is also involved, and, if some sort of community referral is needed, social workers will frequently join the team. Trying to figure out who is going to do what, and when things will be done, is similar to trying to run a three-ring circus. A general planning meeting can be useful in saving time for everyone and avoiding replication of efforts. If this meeting is set up around the physician's scheduled time on the unit or in the agency, the process will be facilitated. Mutually derived goals should be written at the planning meeting. Notifying the patient's family of a time to be present for planning is also helpful, and, because the focus of the team is the patient, he should also be present. It is also important that the nurse make the patient's family aware of the times when health team members will be teaching the patient, so that they can be present, if this is appropriate.

Continuity of care and logical progression of the teaching plan can be accomplished by having all health care team members use the same problem list and document their teaching in the progress notes section of the chart. The team approach, when applied to patient education, is one of the most effective uses of a group management technique. Communication is rendered coherent and concise, teaching efforts are not replicated, and the entire health care team, especially the patient, benefits.

Some patients seem to be receiving more patient education services than others. What can we do about this inequity?

It is important first to determine why some patients are receiving more patient education

and what underlying circumstances exist. For example, if patients of a certain physician are not receiving diabetes education because the physician refuses to allow the patients to participate, then the patients have to put pressure on the physician. However, if one notes that all the cardiac disease, diabetic, and ostomy patients are being well educated, but that the stroke patients and their families have no services offered, then it becomes necessary to document the need for patient education for the stroke group. In institutions where all patients are assessed a fee for patient education, it behooves the institution to make patient education available to all for whom it is a documented need.

Need can be documented in terms of the numbers of patients hospitalized with certain diseases or health promotion needs, the number of return visits to the agency related to lack of self-care skills, data on local morbidity and mortality, and data obtained from practitioners and national organizations. Once need has been established, agency administrators should be approached with a plan and a request for start-up funding.

When are home visits for patient education purposes efficacious? Which health care professionals should make them?

We are strong advocates of home visits for many purposes, not the least of which is patient education. The different data that discerning health care professionals can gather on home visits far surpass in quality and quantity what they can assess in the hospital. Socioeconomic and educational status, family dynamics, and availability of home and community resources are just a few of the more obvious facts that are evident during home visits.

In addition to home visits enabling us to perform a thorough family assessment, they also help most clients feel more comfortable in patient teaching situations because they are buttressed by familiar objects and family members. We have had successful home teaching sessions with young mothers about basic child health and safety practices, when the mothers were fearful or unwilling to attend teaching sessions in the clinic. Observations from such visits were shared with other members of the team and were often instrumental in making future plans for and with clients.

One of our more unique home visit situations involved introducing two elderly diabetic women to one another, in the home of one, so that they could help one another with management problems. The more experienced patient effectively demonstrated insulin injection and blood glucose testing to the woman whose diabetes was newly diagnosed. This teaching session was facilitated by the nurse but was managed by the patients.

Home visits are expensive in terms of personnel time and driving costs. We are familiar with one outpatient agency that made effective use of senior-year nursing students by using them as liaisons between the clinic and patients' families. The students conducted effective patient education, followed up problems, and assessed the home situations, all of which were course objectives. In this type of situation, it is imperative that communication channels between students and providers be open and that students document their visits. Hospitals can also use students to make home visits following patient discharge; the students can then relay the results of their teaching and other information to the attending physician.

The primary care movement, in nursing and in medicine, has seen a recent emphasis on home visits. Many nurse practitioners make home visits to evaluate the effectiveness of their plan including pharmacologic agents and patient teaching; primary care physicians such as family practice doctors are also making home visits.

How has the implementation of DRGs and shorter hospital stays affected patient education in the hospital and in the community?

The implementation of diagnostic-related groups (DRGs) has resulted in shorter hospi-

talizations for patients of all ages and diagnoses. Indeed, some patients are discharged directly from the intensive care unit. Shortened hospitalizations have resulted in distinctive approaches to patient education. For example, many patients are now receiving their preoperative instructions on an outpatient basis. We are aware of a successful cardiothoracic practice in which patients and family members receive intensive instruction from a clinical nurse specialist before the patient is admitted to the hospital for cardiac surgery. The clinical nurse specialist continues to see the patients during their hospitalization, completes the discharge teaching, and also acts as liaison once the patient has been discharged to the home.

Other approaches to the problem of shortened hospitalizations include teaching only survival skills to patients and family members before discharge. For example, the newly diagnosed diabetic is taught basic skills related to insulin injection and diet and then referred to outpatient teaching centers for more comprehensive instruction.

Although shortened hospitalizations may save health care costs, certain client populations are at risk for poor outcomes related to patient education. For example, many elderly patients are unable to comprehend instructions related to such surgeries as total hip replacements because they are not totally recovered from the effects of anesthesia. Others, such as patients after myocardial infarction, may be too anxious to understand discharge and other educational instructions. Lastly, some patients are discharged from the hospital to the home who, in the past, would have been considered inappropriate for home care. These include patients who need ventilator-assisted breathing, have Hickman or Broviac catheters for the instillation of chemotherapeutic or nutritional agents, are on hemodialysis, or have other high-technology requirements. The staff nurse must be especially skillful in ascertaining individual patient abilities, so that patients who need further instruction, or whose family members need a great deal of instruction, are carefully followed in the community and outpatient setting. Additionally, the nurse should be aware of those groups of high-risk clients for whom follow-up care and teaching are necessitated. These groups include adolescent and primiparous mothers, infants and all other pediatric cases, clients over the age of 65 years, any client who does not have a caregiver available, and any client who has experienced a loss of functional ability. In their excellent text, Malloy and Hartshorn (1989) address the major clinical problems the nurse who is involved in home-based care in the community is likely to encounter. They point out the advantages and disadvantages involved in patient education in the home.

The advantages include the reality of the home setting, decreased anxiety for the patient and family, opportunities for further health teaching after crisis needs are met, and the benefits of being in the client's own environment. The *reality of the home setting* refers to the fact that the nurse is able to readily assess what is available to the client and does not have to set up an artificial practice situation. *Lowered anxiety of the patient and family* means that learning will probably proceed faster in the home than in the hospital. *Opportunities for further teaching after the immediate crisis needs are met* implies that the nurse will have additional opportunities for further health and illness teaching. Lastly, the fact that *teaching occurs in the patient's own environment* contributes to the patient's willingness to take responsibility for his own learning.

The disadvantages of the home setting include time limitations, caregiver burdens, and limited equipment and resources. *Time limitations* can be a problem because most nurses delivering home care have busy daily schedules. It is more difficult to return to the home of a patient to check on his ability to perform ostomy care than to go into a patient's room in the hospital. The *caregiving burden* is undoubtedly greater in the home than in the hospital where the caregiver shares caregiving with the nursing staff. Because many caregivers are performing in other roles in addition to their caregiving role, they are frequently fatigued, and they may be unwilling to engage in lengthy teach-ing sessions. *Limited equipment and resources* refers to the fact that the home care nurse does not have as much equipment and as many supplies available in the home as in the hospital or clinic setting. Therefore, in patient and family education sessions in the home the nurse must be creative and willing to "make do" with what is available.

Is patient education in long-term care settings, such as skilled nursing facilities, realistic?

Because we believe that patient education is an important type of patient empowerment, we advocate its practice in long-term care settings. Family education is especially important in such institutions and can help ameliorate family members' feelings of guilt. As in acute care settings, family members can be taught to assist with bathing and other hygiene tasks and can also be instructed in the best methods of feeding, ambulating, and exercising their relatives.

If there is a realistic potential of discharge from the long-term care facility to the home, then it is especially important for the nurse to teach the patient and family members about managing care on their own. Too often nurses neglect to practice patient education because they believe the patient will never leave the institution or they are overwhelmed with other nursing responsibilities and do not arrange patient and family education.

What types of patient education should I be doing in a day-surgery unit?

Day surgeries are becoming increasingly popular with patients and hospital administrators because they save money for both groups. Nurses working in such units are under greater pressure to perform patient education in shorter periods of time with patients who are frequently groggy and confused.

Patient education in day-surgery units should be oriented toward giving patients and family members survival skills. The nurse should make sure written instructions for follow-up care are given to the patient. For example, therapeutic abortions using the dilatation and curettage method are usually performed as day-surgery procedures. During the recovery period after the abortion, the nurse can prepare the patient for possible mood swings, give instructions about what to do in case of heavy bleeding or signs of infection, and discuss future contraception. Lastly, it is the nurse's responsibility to make sure the patient has a means of getting home and that she knows the date of her follow-up appointment.

What are some of the sources of patient education resources in my own institution?

Frequently, we are vaguely aware that resources for patient education are available in our institutions, but we are not sure what source to tap to find them. The *hospital librarian* is an excellent resource, and we have found that when patient education materials were not available in the library, the librarian always knew where to direct us. Useful audiovisual media are often kept in the library, and, if not, they are at least cataloged so that we know where to find them.

Many patient education resources can be found at the nursing station or somewhere on the nursing unit. One hospital with which we are familiar has excellent *teaching cards* covering diagnostic tests and medications. These are neatly filed at the nurses' station but are rarely used by staff, who either are unaware of their existence or simply do not take the time to deliver them to patients. *Procedure manuals and journals* frequently found at the nurses' station can be valuable teaching resources.

Resources of importance in planning patient education activities include *checklists in the chart* such as the discharge planning checklist, the quality assurance checklist, and patient education flow sheets. In a given institution some or all of these may be found. Occasionally these checklists or flow sheets need revising. They can be useful adjuncts to patient teaching and, if used properly, they make the process more logical and time conserving.

Other resources are *committees* composed of various health care professionals who are planning future patient education programs. Committee members usually have a wealth of knowledge about appropriate resources and are happy to share it. If the committee does not include such professionals as dietitians, pharmacists, social workers, and physical, occupational, and respiratory therapists, do not hesitate to approach such persons; they are valuable resources for nurses seeking help with patient education.

If the hospital is of a moderate to large size, it may have a *patient education coordinator* on the staff. This person is pivotal in the attempts of a hospital to deliver patient education. In an outpatient setting, such as a public health department, the equivalent position is held by a health educator. If there is no health educator, then frequently nursing in-service, staff training and development, or educational services departments have someone who (officially or unofficially) has developed a role in patient education.

Can the idea of "networking" be applied to patient education to increase resources for patients?

Networking is a term currently in vogue that refers to pooling resources to assist a certain cause. For example, a women's network is a group for women with common interests, such as the fact that they are all university faculty members. Networking as a family therapy modality means bringing family, extended family, neighbors, and friends together to help a family resolve a problem and gain needed support.

When we refer to networking in patient education, we mean either bringing together various community services to address a patient's educational needs or developing a bank of resources that we can refer to when we need help. Obtaining referral sources and information from visiting nurse associations, public health nurses, and specialty-oriented nurses is one form of networking. Use of a directory of community resources and the Yellow Pages of the phone book is another method of developing a network.

Another form of networking is sharing the teaching needs of a particular patient with the community nurse who will see the patient after his discharge from the hospital. All too often there is little continuity of care because no one bothers to contact nurses in outpatient settings. If the patient is readmitted to the hospital, then the outpatient agency nurse can give useful information to the inpatient team involved in the patient's care. Information can be shared informally over the telephone. Such reciprocity is unnecessary in many situations, but we are aware of complex patient circumstances in which a great deal of teaching and continuity of care was needed, and in which patients benefited from the extra effort nurses put in to smooth transitions from community to hospital and vice versa. Remember, however, that confidential information regarding patients may not be shared without their permission.

How can I obtain teaching aids without spending a great deal of money?

Patient education has become big business ever since the Joint Commission on the Accreditation of Healthcare Organizations (JCAHO) mandated that hospitals provide it. Many companies already producing learning materials for health care professionals have begun marketing films, filmstrips, videotapes, books, and anatomic models. Some of these products are sophisticated and moderately priced and are able to meet the needs of institutions that are unable to produce their own materials. Other commercial products are expensive and do not meet the needs of most institutions because their content and approach are too general. Audiovisual hardware and software can be expensive, and agencies should carefully consider their needs in this area before purchasing one of the package deals promoted by many of the large companies. Also, research on the effectiveness of such media as closed-circuit television is still not complete, and we may discover that the outcomes do not justify the huge outlay of funds necessary to develop in-house, closed-circuit television, patient education systems.

We have seen agency-developed slide-tape programs, videotape programs, films, brochures, and pamphlets that have met the special needs of the agencies and their patients without being prohibitive in cost. These are often supplemented by commercially printed materials or films. Other sources of free or inexpensive rental audiovisual materials are state health department film libraries and public library systems.

Other resources for free materials are the pharmaceutical, medical supply, and infant formula companies. Sales representatives of these companies are willing to lend films and distribute free literature. We have found that if a given firm does not have the type of brochure we desire for our clients, we can request it and often be supplied with what we need. For example, the brochures produced by the infant formula companies tended to be directed toward Caucasian, upper middle-class families, and we served primarily lower socioeconomic groups of Caucasian and African American clients. We requested a change in format and also inclusion of material in favor of breast-feeding, and we later received these new brochures. One of the authors (Rankin) has effectively used booklets on contraception with female students in a student health service. The booklets were free and were an efficient method of providing information. Obviously, the health care provider needs to screen these resources before giving them to patients because each pharmaceutical or medical supply company is attempting to sell its own products.

The Government Printing Office in Washington, D.C. is also an excellent source of free or low-cost printed materials. They are frequently well illustrated and written simply so that all clients can understand them. There are also numerous patient and provider educational materials available from disease-related associations such as the American Heart Association, American Cancer Society and so on.

My institution plans to buy ready-made teaching materials. How can I best use them?

There are some good ready-made teaching materials that save development time and have the advantage of being pretested for validity and reliability. The most important thing to remember when using these materials is that they must be individualized and tailored for each patient. No teaching materials negate the need for personal instruction. Such materials can supplement instructors but not replace them. Therefore, the patient educator should personally review the materials with the patient, pointing out areas that do not apply and reinforcing others that are more valuable.

Another crucial aspect of using printed materials, or other materials that rely heavily on the written word, is the patient's literacy level. (See Chap. 9 for discussion of the tests for determining literacy level.) We had an unfortunate experience with a patient who had newly diagnosed diabetes that poignantly illustrates the importance of assessing literacy level. The patient was instructed by a dietitian and a nurse about diet, insulin injection, and recognition of signs of hypoglycemia and ketoacidosis. He attended our diabetic teaching luncheon and seemed to be one of our more successfully educated diabetic patients. Three days after discharge he frantically called his physician to report that he had not eaten anything since his discharge because he could not read and did not know what he should eat. None of us had determined his literacy level but, instead, had simply assumed he could read and understand all the written materials we had given him.

What are some examples of quick and easy ways to teach during a busy day?

We feel that many nurses miss golden opportunities to teach because they believe teaching requires long, uninterrupted periods of time. However, often during the care of inpatients and outpatients, the opportunity to teach is readily available. For example, during a dressing change it is easy to talk through the proce-dure with the patient, beginning with the reasons for aseptic technique (explaining why the area is scrubbed with povidone iodine from the inside out). If this patient will have to perform his own dressing changes at home, this talk relieves some of the burden from discharge teaching. When carrying out routine prenatal checks we can say, "I am measuring the height of your fundus (the top of your uterus) to find out how much the baby has grown since your last visit. Usually the fundal height increases about 1 cm a week." When the prenatal patient's urine is tested we can say, "I am checking your urine for sugar and protein. Sometimes pregnant women have a little sugar in their urine, but if you have a lot of sugar, we will want to do some blood tests so that we can make certain you have a healthy baby. We check the protein in your urine because this gives us an idea of your kidney function. During pregnancy more stress is placed on your kidneys. Protein in the urine usually develops with a serious condition called toxemia, and we want to watch you carefully to prevent development of toxemia." Anticipatory guidance and reassurance should always accompany such teaching because some of the information may be upsetting to patients.

Taking blood pressure measurements also presents a good opportunity for teaching. All patients, hypertensive or not, should know the significance of the blood pressure measurement and should know what is normal for them. This is also a good opportunity for health promotion teaching related not only to blood pressure, but also to eating habits and heart disease.

There are literally hundreds of opportunities for brief teaching. By using these opportunities we promote health and self-care practices and also give our patients one more mechanism to reduce their feelings of powerlessness and dependence on us.

What types of things can be done to promote our agency's image as a provider of patient education?

Because the consumer is beginning to expect more patient education services from providers, many hospitals, clinics, and private practice settings are trying to promote an image of themselves as providers of patient education. Such devices as filmstrips, videotapes, and slide-tape programs in waiting rooms help to provide this image and have been used by various agencies (Redman, 1993; Oberst, 1989; Knowlton, 1979).

Less expensive means are posters, either handmade or provided free by organizations such as the American Dairy Association or the March of Dimes. Posters can also be used to advertise seminars or classes open to the public. Many hospitals are promoting their community images by providing free monthly forums on topics of widespread interest such as respiratory disease, prevention of heart disease, and other common health problems. Frequently posters are prominently displayed in hospital lobbies to inform the public of such events.

The hospital admissions brochure may contain information about patient education so that the patient and family are immediately aware of inpatient educational services. Likewise, outpatient offices and clinics can stress their roles in patient education in the brochures that are usually given to new patients.

In the hospital and outpatient units and waiting rooms, information relevant to the unit can be displayed. For example, information related to child safety practices can be exhibited on bulletin boards and waiting room tables. One nurse who taught prenatal classes told us that the free literature on birth control was so popular on the maternity ward that she could not restock it fast enough.

Now that many hospitals and outpatient agencies have begun using computerized billing, it is possible to put a patient education message on the monthly bill. For example, "CPR classes will be held June 1, free of charge for all patients, from noon to 2:00 PM and 7:00 to 9:00 PM" could be programmed to read out on all May bills.

Media coverage of patient education offerings widely extends the image of the agency into the community and can be obtained for free. Public service spots are available on radio and television for community services that are offered without charge to all members of the community. Newspapers will also print notices of such events if they meet this criterion. The University of North Carolina has provided short television broadcasts on safety and emergency techniques such as the Heimlich maneuver. These free public interest teaching spots provided an image of the University of North Carolina's hospital and health professional schools as being concerned about the public.

Another means of making patient education better known in the community is by gaining access to schools and groups such as Parent-Teacher Associations. While employed in a hospital's educational services department, we conducted classes on labor and delivery in a high school's human sexuality classes. These classes were a public service to the high school and were meant to increase the hospital's image as a provider of health education. Obviously such image enhancement is helpful to hospitals worried about use of beds.

Lastly, patient education programs can be initiated in hospitals or outpatient settings by affiliating with franchised, profit-making agencies that have preestablished programs. The benefits of affiliating with the franchised programs are that they have been pretested and the agency offers marketing and recruitment of patients. For example, there are diabetes teaching programs that are branches of hospital supply companies and as such have many resources available to them that smaller community hospitals attempting to establish their own diabetes teaching programs may not have. The disadvantages of affiliation with such groups include the possibility that their programs may be less flexible and less appropriate to disparate sociocultural groups.

What are some of the common mistakes made when attempting patient education?

In our own experience with patient education and in our enthusiasm to try out our ideas, we have made a number of mistakes. We have also noted mistakes made by others and will enumerate them all below.

1. *Assessment mistakes.* Frequently we do not validate our data with the client, a case in point being the diabetic who could not read. Another assessment problem is the failure to reassess the situation and the patient after the passage of time or a change in the experience or life events of the patient.
2. *Refusal to work within the restrictions of the patient's environment.* This mistake is related to assessment and involves the health professional who neglects consideration of such factors as lack of family support, educational level, financial assets of the patient, or cultural or ethnic background. We tend to teach from our own backgrounds and experience and may assume a commonality of background that is not present. For example, in the South it makes more sense to teach the poor rural farmer in need of potassium that greens (e.g., collards, kale, spinach, turnip greens) are a good source rather than to recommend bananas, which are more expensive. In the Los Angeles barrio, it is unrealistic to expect a prenatal patient's husband to be a coach to her during labor and delivery because many Hispanics traditionally do not sanction the presence of men during birth.
3. *Territoriality or "owning" the patient.* Many of us, not just physicians, fall into this trap when we invest much time and effort in teaching our patients. The patient becomes "our" patient, and we are loathe to believe that anyone else can continue the process we started. No one owns patients, and we all need to remember the personal responsibility that the patient has for his own behavior.
4. *Denial or oversight of the patient's right to change his mind.* This is a mistake that frequently occurs when, as above, the health professional has overly invested himself in the patient and his progress. We worked for a long time with an elderly woman who was placed on insulin. We were attempting to teach her self-injection of insulin. We tried many creative approaches because she originally had said she would manage her own injections. However, at some point during this lengthy process she had decided that she did not want to give herself insulin, but rather she wanted her husband and daughter to do it. Because we had a need to make her independent, we refused to recognize her dependency needs or the fact that she had, indeed, changed her mind. The situation became frustrating for all until we finally recognized and respected the interpersonal dynamics of the situation.
5. *Inability to learn from our own mistakes.* Nurses tend to be task oriented and, as such, we often believe that there is only one way to do things. Such an approach is the antithesis of the flexible, open-minded method required with patient education. When conducting the diabetic luncheons, we discovered through an experience with a 12-year-old girl that the luncheon, with its emphasis on food preparation and prevention of long-term complications, was unsuited to any age group other than adult. Later, parents of children and adolescents were invited, but the pediatric patients themselves were seen on a one-on-one basis for teaching.

   We have seen many nurses continue to use medical jargon with patients when all indications suggested the patients did not understand the teaching. Such practices are self-defeating for the staff and frustrating for patients.
6. *Failure to negotiate goals.* Long- and short-term goals should be established at the beginning of any patient education endeavor. It is appropriate for the nurse to have goals in mind, but she also must determine her client's goals so that he can enjoy some sense of progress. Any discrepancy in goals should be acknowledged by both the nurse and the client, with the nurse recognizing that the client's goals supersede hers. For example, the patient with chronic obstructive lung disease may set goals for himself that include administering medications and learning breathing exercises. The nurse

may agree on these goals but also may add a goal of smoking cessation. Obviously, if the patient does not share this goal, he will be unsupportive of, and inattentive to, her efforts, and she will be frustrated.

7. *Lack of awareness of the teaching efforts of other members of the health care team.* Replication of effort is a common and time-consuming problem, but it is easily corrected by good documentation. Well-meaning health professionals frequently repeat teaching in an area that has just been taught by someone else. Although repetition can be a useful teaching device, it should be planned instead of haphazard. Usually patients are not assertive enough to speak up and tell their teacher that they have already heard this lecture before and would like to hear about something else.

   Careful documentation in the appropriate section of the chart (e.g., progress notes, patient education flow sheet) will solve this problem as well as legally document patient education efforts. Also, a good assessment of a patient's areas of knowledge and weakness will prevent this repetition. The planning sessions that we referred to earlier in this chapter will help ameliorate the problem.

8. *Overload of information given to the patient.* In our overzealous attempts to teach patients everything we feel they should know, we run the risk of overloading them with more information than they can absorb. Hospitalized patients have low energy reserves and are not usually amenable to long teaching sessions. Two half-hour sessions are more desirable than one hour-long session. Shorter sessions also allow the patient an opportunity to integrate new information and formulate questions for the next teaching session; this opportunity would be unavailable if everything is taught in one hour-long session.

   Even the outpatient, whose physical status may be better than that of the inpatient, benefits from shorter sessions. Shorter sessions are also more workable in terms of staff time.

   Signs that a patient has been saturated

and cannot handle any more material include inability to answer questions regarding the material, fidgeting, yawning, and staring, glazed eyes. When these signs occur, tell the patient to prepare questions for the next session and, if appropriate, leave some pertinent literature.

9. *Poor timing and inattentiveness to patient stress levels.* This problem is related to the previous mistake and is usually caused by a focus on the needs of the nurse rather than on the needs of the patient. There are advantageous times for teaching and there are some that are poor. A patient who has just received upsetting or unexpected news should not be burdened by a nurse who wants to teach. Likewise, the time periods immediately before or after diagnostic procedures, surgery, or painful episodes are not propitious for teaching.

   A patient under great stress, such as a new mother with a Down syndrome child, is not a good candidate for teaching. Other patients who are not amenable to teaching are patients in denial. For example, a young woman whose acute leukemia had just been diagnosed was in such a strong state of denial that it was impossible to teach her anything about the planned chemotherapy, the importance of diet, or the prevention of infection. Instead, we focused our teaching on her mother and other family members, telling them that we would work with the patient when she came in for chemotherapy on an outpatient basis.

   Sometimes the length of inpatient stay does not allow for adequate teaching, in which case either the patient must return to the hospital or plans must be made for outpatient teaching through the visiting nurse association or public health department nursing service. It is important for someone to take charge of the situation so that the patient does not lose the services he needs.

10. *Failure to arrange for feedback and evaluation.* As nursing instructors, we see this mistake made more frequently than any other by students, and we suspect that it is also one

of the most common errors committed by health professionals. Most of us spend time familiarizing ourselves with the material to be taught and then get so involved in our teaching that we forget to evaluate and gather feedback on the patient's comprehension of what we have taught. Patients tend to want to appease and please the nurse or other health care professional who is teaching them and usually act as if they understand more than they really do. When we do ask for a return demonstration or verbal feedback, we are frequently appalled by how little we have managed to make comprehensible.

Another facet of this problem is our failure to provide time for patients to ask questions. Typically we teach an instructional unit at a rapid pace, quickly ask for questions, and then leave the room satisfied that the patient has understood our teaching because he did not ask any questions. In reality the patient probably either understood so little that he was unable to formulate questions or felt that the nurse did not have time to answer him.

Skill building is an important aspect of the teaching and learning process and must also be considered as an important item when planning time requirements. Any type of skill requiring physical manipulation must be practiced by the patient alone and in the presence of the instructor to ensure its integration into the necessary self-care behaviors. Lack of time for building skills frequently accounts for patients who do not want to be discharged when the physician says it is time. Good communication among members of the health care team will alleviate this common problem.

All of this discussion emphasizes the importance of completing the total process of patient education: assessment, goal setting, teaching, and evaluating (see Chaps. 7–11).

11. *Using materials that have not been reviewed or using media exclusively.* The development and popularity of patient education has been followed by the emergence of so-phisticated patient teaching media. We have used media to great advantage with groups and single patients, but we believe in the importance of carefully reviewing the media and evaluating their applicability for the intended audience. This point was delineated clearly to us on one occasion when we made the mistake of showing a film on breast-feeding that we had not previewed. The film had been produced by one of the breast-feeding advocacy groups and not so subtly suggested that adequate mothering and bonding could only be achieved through breast-feeding. We were dealing with a group of women who had received little family or social group support for breast-feeding and, unfortunately, the film had the effect of polarizing or frustrating our prenatal patients.

Total reliance on media is obviously an inadequate approach to patient education. Such an approach makes it impossible to individualize patient teaching, to allow the patient to ask questions, or to gather feedback from the patient. Mail campaigns and large mass media health education projects use this scheme with the assumption that some information is better than none. Some data indicate that this assumption is untrue. For example, mass media are believed to be efficacious in informing the better-educated segments of society, but most of the public believes mass media are part of a ploy to sell something (Chaisson, 1980). In any case, individualized patient education for clients who must learn skills or information for managing self-care practices is essential and cannot be managed by reliance on media.

What does the nurse practitioner bring to patient education?

Nurse practitioners are RNs with additional education and training in various primary care specialty areas (e.g., family primary care, pediatric and adult primary care, and women's health primary care). The nurse practitioner movement began in the 1960s, but not until the late 1980s did a tremendous surge occur in applications to these programs. Nurses are attracted to the nurse practitioner role because of its emphasis on primary prevention and health maintenance; additionally, the nurse practitioner role is accompanied by greater autonomy than is available to nurses in most other roles.

The expert nurse practitioner is one of the best examples of excellent patient education. She performs many of the same functions as a primary care physician (e.g., health physicals, management of common acute conditions and some chronic conditions) but brings to the role an expertise in patient teaching and counseling gained over many years of practice. Studies indicate overwhelming satisfaction with nurse practitioners as judged by their patients; other research demonstrates that the quality of primary care provided by nurse practitioners is equivalent to that by physicians (Mundinger, 1994). Patients are particularly pleased with the health education nurse practitioners provide.

An example of the attention given to patient education by nurse practitioners is the following SOAP note pertaining to a 9-year-old Hispanic girl, a fourth grader, who was seen by a family nurse practitioner in a clinic with a translator. The child's chief complaint was a sore throat.

S: *History of present illness*—sent home from school on 11/18/94 with fever (102° p.o.), plus complaint of headache and sore throat; Tylenol brings relief

Pertinent past medical history—no known allergies to medications or food

Has had four documented strep throats in the past 3 years; last one 1/94

History of gastroesophageal reflux disorder

Family history—not applicable

Review of systems-

Skin—no complaints of rashes

HEENT—dull headache; sore throat; denies nasal or eye discharge; denies difficulty swallowing

Respiratory—denies productive cough; occasional dry cough; no dyspnea

Gastrointestinal—no vomiting or diarrhea; taking fluids and minimal food; no abdominal pain

O: Temp = 100° p.o.; pulse = 84; respirations = 20; BP = 90/60; weight = 30 kg (66 lb)

Skin—no rash; moist mucous membranes

HEENT—normocephalic; conjunctivae clear; PERL; no mastoid tenderness; tympanic membranes dull, mobile and with a positive light reflex, landmarks visible, no erythema; nares patent; no sinus tenderness; petechiae on soft palate; pharynx erythematous, tonsils enlarged at 4+ and touching, hemorrhagic, cryptic, no exudate; uvula retracted toward left tonsil

Lymph—enlarged, nontender anterior cervical nodes

Chest—breath sounds clear anteriorly and posteriorly; no adventitious sounds; no retractions

Heart—S1, S2, no murmurs, rate regular

A: Probable streptococcal pharyngitis

P: *Diagnostic*—throat culture

Therapeutic—Pen VK 250 mg p.o. t.i.d. X 10 days

Motrin (100 mg/tsp) 1.5 tsp p.o. q6–8h PRN pain

Tylenol elixir (160 mg/tsp) 2.5 tsp po q4–6h PRN fever

Patient education—take all of Pen VK even after symptoms resolve

Push fluids

Monitor temperature

If difficulty with breathing occurs return to clinic immediately

May return to school 11/28/94

Follow-up—return to clinic if condition worsens and for follow-up check on 11/30/94

The concerted effort to chart patient education results in patient teaching being incorporated into practice. Charting of patient education also allows for later evaluation of patient care as well as legal protection.

What is the role of the student nurse in patient education?

We believe that providing for patient education is an integral function of nursing practice. Because nursing students are learning to be practitioners, they should deliver patient education as part of nursing care. Patient education is not something that should be excluded from nursing school curricula in the belief that it will be learned on the job. It is a function basic to all good nursing care and, therefore, must be emphasized in nursing school while the theoretical framework for nursing is being presented. As students progress through the program, the faculty should stress the importance of applying teaching and learning concepts, as well as appropriate content, to patient education situations in clinical settings. Clinical evaluation tools should be designed to evaluate student competency in patient education.

Most nursing students are not involved in formulating agency needs assessments or planning large-scale programs while in nursing school, but they should be familiar with the issues involved so that they can buttress their array of skills for future use.

Many times the most creative teaching of patients is completed by students. Nursing students frequently have recent knowledge about patient education and enthusiasm for attempting innovative approaches. Staff members can learn a lot from students if they drop their defensive attitudes and approach students with a greater sense of collegiality. Students, in turn, can learn a great deal from the staff by observing the techniques staff members have found useful in teaching patients.

We have found it useful to accompany students on home visits that have been planned for patient education purposes. Another means of evaluating students' skills in patient education is for the instructor to arrange for students to conduct discharge teaching, diagnostic test teaching, or perioperative teaching and to then accompany the students when they instruct the patients. The instructor must first ascertain, however, that the students know the material because unfamiliarity with the content embarrasses the students and confuses the patients.

In our desire to encourage varied clinical experiences, instructors frequently push students into situations in which they do not feel comfortable. Sexuality is an area with which the younger student, and perhaps even older students or practicing nurses, may feel uneasy in teaching situations. Until students express an ease with material related to human sexuality, we believe they should not approach this sensitive area. We remember one nursing student who had professed a desire to teach the prenatal class unit on contraception. When she did so, however, she remained suffused with a deep blush and was obviously ill at ease. Patients greeted her teaching with nervous laughter, and we suspect little was learned that evening about contraception.

How do physical limitations of the patient and the environment affect my patient education?

Physical limitations that may impinge on effective patient education include poor eyesight, poor hearing, and lack of small muscle control that affects coordination. All of these physical limitations influence our media selection, goal setting, and implementation of patient education.

The client who is unable to successfully perform tube and dialysate bag changes because of arthritis is not a good candidate for continuous ambulatory peritoneal dialysis teaching. This form of peritoneal dialysis requires the client's unremitting participation in manual skills. To set goals for patients with disabilities that prevent learning and acquisition of management skills is not only unrealistic but also frustrating and cruel.

Physical limitations in the environment of the client must also be assessed. For example, a patient in chronic renal failure was considered for home hemodialysis until the nursing staff discovered that the client lived in rural poverty with no electricity or running water. If goals are mutually derived, there are fewer chances that physical limitations will hamper patient teaching.

How can I conduct effective patient education in extreme conditions such as situations involving homelessness?

Situations involving homeless clients with health problems are some of the most difficult in which to intervene. Consider the case of a homeless type I diabetic client living on the street during the day and in a shelter at night. Neuropathies make this client more likely to develop skin breakdown and foot sores, and because of constant walking during the day in poorly fitting shoes, major foot ulcers are more likely to develop than in nonhomeless persons with diabetes. Additionally, self-monitoring of blood glucose is almost impossible to accomplish because of the amount of equipment involved and the cost of the blood glucose strips. Added to this are problems related to syringes, which on the streets are frequently shared or stolen for use in injecting intravenous drugs, thus increasing the diabetic client's risk of hepatitis B and human immunodeficiency virus infection. Standard teaching regarding diabetes management for type I patients is not realistic for these clients. Indeed, at best, the client should be encouraged to come to a health clinic in a shelter on a daily basis for insulin injection and occasional blood glucose monitoring.

Other problems related to patient education in situations involving extreme conditions such as homelessness include the psychosocial problems that arise. For example, one nurse practitioner working in a homeless shelter told us that because homeless people must spend their days on the streets since shelters are closed, and then line up for meals at various agencies who feed the homeless, circadian rhythms and sense of time quickly become confused. Those who are newly homeless need constant reorientation to time and place and frequently state that they feel like they are "losing it" and "going crazy." In this type of situation nurses are unlikely to be able to provide the same type of patient education to which they aspire. Instead, health care providers try to provide some stability for the homeless client and attempt to solve some of the underlying problems related to homelessness such as unemployment, alcohol and drug abuse, and mental illness.

What are the effects of pain, illness, or fatigue on patient education?

The effects of pain, illness, and fatigue should be manifest to nurses. However, because we become somewhat inured to these behaviors over time we forget to assess for them and their effects on planned health teaching.

Pain can be an all-encompassing experience. If the client is experiencing severe pain, our only intervention should be alleviation of pain either through medications or nonpharmacologic techniques. Once pain has been lessened, relaxation and breathing techniques can be taught for use in the future. Alleviation of pain also ensures that necessary skills can be taught. For example, we may realize the patient needs to learn how to use crutches or cough, turn, and deep breathe, but until the patient enjoys a modicum of comfort, these skills cannot be taught because the patient will not attend to us.

Illness and fatigue can deplete the client's resources to such an extent that he has no energy left for learning. If the client is not listening or focusing on the patient education session or is unable to retain simple information, it is preferable to plan teaching either when he is more rested or when family members are present.

What is the relationship between anxiety and learning?

Research indicates that mild or moderate anxiety may be helpful to learning. Janis (1958), a psychologist, found that patients who had mild or moderate levels of anxiety preoperatively actively sought information to help them build up adequate defenses. Postoperatively, these patients exhibited less anxiety than patients who had no preoperative anxiety. Patients who had high levels of anxiety preoperatively also had high levels postoperatively. Some practitioners believe that the implications from this study are that if we can determine that our patients do not have appropriate levels of anxiety, either mild or moderate, it may be helpful to raise anxiety so that adequate learning can occur. For the severe levels of anxiety, we obviously need to decrease anxiety to a moderate level so that learning can take place. Additionally, results of other classic studies by nurse researchers indicate that preoperative teaching and support will lessen postoperative anxiety (Lindeman & Stetzer, 1973; Lindeman & Van Aernam, 1971) Experientially many of us would support these findings from our own practice.

How can patient education principles be applied in the psychiatric setting?

Traditionally we conceive of the application of patient education to pediatric and adult medical-surgical settings. This is most likely a remnant of our medical model approach and not representative of a holistic model of man in which we consider the total individual. Psychiatric patients have the same basic patient education needs as have medical-surgical patients (i.e., to function to the best of their ability on the wellness-illness continuum and in a manner consistent with their expressed needs and desires).

Benfer (1980) recognizes patient education as one of the functions of the psychiatric nurse on an interdisciplinary health team. The psychiatric nurse should perform the traditional function of teaching necessary information about medications and health. In addition, she should also teach the patient how to relate to the environment of the psychiatric agency, how to use unstructured time, and how to establish necessary structure in daily life.

It is the nurse's responsibility to orient patients to the psychiatric environment, whether inpatient or outpatient. This orientation can be crucial to the patient's adjustment to the therapeutic milieu. Hamer's study of psychiatric inpatients demonstrated that patients felt their learning needs soon after hospitalization involved reestablishment of homeostasis, that is, learning how to achieve a balance between sleep, activity, and food consumption

needs (Hamer, 1991). They also recognized their need to learn how to manage anger. Patients who had been hospitalized for long periods reported needing education in the area of involvement in the community, especially through support groups. Thus, learning needs of psychiatric inpatients change over time just as the learning needs of patients with other chronic illnesses shift.

Many psychiatric patients have had problems structuring their time to meet the demands of daily existence. Therefore, the nurse's role in facilitating the patient's ability to order his time in a meaningful manner is pivotal to his ability to function in the community. Lancaster (1979) recognizes this need to help patients structure their time and feels that patients can be taught to develop leisure-time skills through group therapy. Planned recreational activities, such as exercise, volleyball, crafts, and cooking classes, are other means of helping psychiatric patients gather tools to structure their time. These activities can be taught in inpatient or outpatient settings. We observed senior nursing students teaching a successful cooking course to clients attending sessions at an outpatient mental health center.

Inpatient psychiatric clients with long histories of institutionalization have problems adapting to the communities into which they are discharged. On admission these patients already have been recognized as having difficulties with social interaction and problem-solving skills. If reintegration into the community is to be successful, it is imperative that coping skills are taught both before and after discharge. Social interaction and problem-solving skills are frequently learned in group therapy contexts. Other skills, such as the ability to perform the basic activities of daily living, can be taught by nurses in a combination of didactic and practical approaches. In many instances patients must be taught such basic activities as personal hygiene or how to use a stove, or they must be oriented to a technology that has overtaken them, such as the use of microwave ovens, automatic bank tellers, or fax machines. Stanley (1984) suggests the use of goal attainment scaling to evaluate the psychiatric patient's achievement of treatment goals. The patient decides on the goals he wishes to achieve and weights the goals in terms of importance. When the patient and nurse review achievement of the goals, a goal attainment score is calculated that gives the patient and nurse an indication of the progress made. Such ongoing evaluation reinforces patient education with the psychiatric patient.

Lastly, patient teaching of families, always an important aspect of patient education, may be even more important with the care-giving family members of psychiatric patients. Family members need assistance in decreasing stigma or guilt and in learning how to explain behaviors of their family member to friends, other relatives, and the public. Other aspects of family education include involvement of the family in the treatment plan if indicated, preparation for hospital discharge to the home, and realistic long-term planning. Patient teaching with psychiatric patients and their families requires creativity and patience, but the rewards can be great.

What are some of the special aspects and needs related to teaching the gerontologic patient?

Many health professionals, recognizing that the gerontologic patient is different from the younger or middle-aged adult patient, approach him as if he were a child. Although there are some qualities of the two age groups that are held in common, it is both insulting to the patient and demonstrative of the health professional's lack of sensitivity and knowledge to take this approach.

We know that as people grow old, their cognitive efficiency declines. Older people have been found to have increasing difficulty understanding complex sentences, to be less proficient in drawing inferences, to demonstrate problems with perceptual motor tasks, and to have more difficulty in determining the point of a story (Eliopoulos, 1987, 1990; Feier & Leight, 1981). Institutionalized elderly persons do even more poorly on tests of cognitive ability than do their counterparts living in the community. The presence of such illnesses as Parkinson's disease and Alzheimer's disease should be considered when teaching is attempted. Research comparing Parkinson's disease, Alzheimer's disease, and normal age-matched controls found that although the Parkinsonian patients performed significantly better than Alzheimer patients in terms of learning ability, when compared to normal age-matched controls their learning ability was significantly worse (El-Awar, Becker, Hammond, Nebes, & Boller, 1987). Despite these sobering facts, many creative programs have been implemented. These emphasize conversation and problem-solving skills. They result in improved cognitive abilities and help to prevent deterioration of existing abilities.

In patient education situations with the elderly, the following points (Carnevali & Patrick, 1993; Eliopoulos, 1987; 1990; Fielo & Rizzolo, 1988; Burnside, Ebersole, & Monea, 1979) should be remembered.

Present information at a much slower rate than usual.

Speak in a low tone of voice because elderly persons hear low tones better than high-pitched sounds.

Allow plenty of time for the assimilation and integration of conceptual material; emphasize concrete rather than abstract material.

Reduce environmental distracters.

Keep in mind that any or all of the following causes may be related to the elderly client's reduced capacity to learn: cerebral changes, psychosocial issues, and changes in self-concept with probable loss of self-esteem.

Be aware that group experiences can improve the elderly client's problem-solving ability.

Remember that aged clients are cautious and do not make changes easily.

The implications for patient education are that we must take more time in teaching and that we should deliver the educational material in small increments so that the material can be integrated. Research examining educational strategies to improve knowledge about medications as well as improving compliance support the previous statement. Ascione and Shimp (1984) found that teaching interventions that provided the least amount of information about drugs were more successful than those that provided the most amount of information when drug knowledge was the outcome measure. Increased compliance to medications was related to interventions that focused on compliance such as oral instructions with a reminder calendar than those that focused on oral instruction with or without written instructions (Ascione & Shimp, 1984).

A more recent study that examined medication compliance in the elderly found that patients were taking 80% or less or 120% or more of essential medications than had been prescribed (Hawe & Higgins, 1990). When this group was assigned to a variety of teaching interventions to increase compliance, no program effects in terms of medication compliance were detected 1 and 3 months after the teaching programs (Hawe & Higgins, 1990). These findings support the need for continued teaching emphasis on the importance of taking prescribed drugs in the recommended dosages.

Health professionals should be aware of the causes of the elderly individual's reduced capacity to learn so that they can intervene and perhaps change such modifiable causes as psychosocial losses and low self-esteem. Other modifiable causes include problems related to multiple medications or medications that are incorrectly used. Additionally, physiologic causes pertaining to reduced ability to learn include such conditions as hypoglycemia secondary to diabetes mellitus and hypoxia secondary to congestive heart failure.

Many skills involving social interaction can be successfully taught in a group setting. Examples would be helping the elderly to acquire assertiveness skills to secure better housing or more neighborhood police protection. In deference to the cautiousness and reluctance to make changes that older people display, the health professional should avoid making changes in the medical regimen, whenever possible, and should attempt to maintain a constant environment and schedule for the elderly patient. The reader is referred to Chapter 4 for a discussion of lifespan development and some of the factors that may influence the context of patient education for the elderly client.

What should the health care professional remember when working with persons with AIDS?

Obviously patient education services are appropriate for persons with acquired immunodeficiency syndrome (AIDS), especially during the period when decisions regarding treatment must be made. Although persons with AIDS are living longer now that the treatment armamentarium has been increased, a diagnosis of AIDS portends certain death. The gay community has successfully pushed the medical community to offer as many treatment options as possible. Indeed, the gay community often informs health care providers of the latest treatment strategies. Thus, the nurse attempting patient education with an informed person with AIDS should persevere in attempts to maintain the most up-to-date information about pharmacologic and nonpharmacologic interventions and be open to suggestions from patients. Because many health care providers are unfamiliar with the lifeways of the gay community, the health care professional should admit this to the person with AIDS and maintain an open, caring, and professional relationship. As Scaffa and Davis (1990) point out, moral debates regarding sexual behavior and gay life choices have no place in the health care arena. If health care professionals are unable to care for persons with AIDS in a nonjudgmental manner then they should not be working in this area of health care.

The terminally ill gay person with AIDS may be faced not only with mortality but also with the need to tell his family of impending death and his life-style choices. The informed nurse can be exceptionally helpful to family members in terms of giving them information, offering support, and allowing for needed privacy. The definition of family should be redefined to include the lover and other gay friends who have become part of the family of the AIDS patient.

Intravenous drug abusers (IVDAs) are the fastest growing group of persons with AIDS in the United States. They may be of any cultural, ethnic, or racial group and they may be men or women, or the female partners of male IVDAs. Sharing of syringes is responsible for the huge surge of cases in this population. The IVDAs are a challenging group with which to work. Because chemical dependency is often associated with denial, pharmacologic treatment may be more difficult to maintain. Patient education is difficult with this group until abstinence from alcohol and intravenous drugs has been achieved. Therefore, referral to Alcoholics Anonymous and Narcotics Anonymous support groups is essential. Self-destructive behavior is common and the health care provider should be alert to signs of impending suicide (Scaffa & Davis, 1990). The health care professional should be aware that this group of persons with AIDS is one of the most stigmatized groups in American society and thus a vulnerable population. Patient education should always be accompanied by caring concern.

Are patient education services appropriate for the terminally ill patient?

One might logically assume that once a patient's illness status has changed from chronic to terminal, patient education would no longer be involved. However, as long as a patient has options open and choices to make, patient education should be available. Patient teaching is a form of offering hope to our dying clients because it is a way of telling them that they can make choices about their futures.

Examples of patient education for terminally ill clients include delineating the choice between going home and staying in the hospital. If a patient wishes to go home to die, he and his family will have questions about control of pain; ability to manage baths, hygiene, and meals; and the impact on the remainder of the family. Sometimes we can tell the dying patient about the services of a local hospice organization, and this may offer the necessary support he needs in making his decision to go home. The dying patient must be given the opportunity to revoke his decisions in the same way as any other patient. The offering of choices allows a sense of control that must be respected until the end.

The emotional support aspects of patient education, which are always an important thread, become even more paramount with the dying patient. We may decide to teach the patient's family members or friends how to use reminiscence as a therapeutic treatment modality, allowing the client an opportunity to view his life in retrospect with a sense of unity and completion. Emotional support is also given by the nurse who offers her physical presence and shows family members how they can make the patient more comfortable.

In which situations should one-on-one teaching be used? When should group teaching be used?

We feel that there are distinct advantages inherent in both one-on-one and group teaching. It is difficult to generalize and say when one is more effective than the other because of the individual characteristics of patients.

We have determined individual patient teaching to be more effective than group teaching (whether with a family group or a large, unrelated group) in the following situations.

- When the health professional has little knowledge of the patient and an assessment of the patient for education purposes has not been completed, then teaching will proceed more effectively on an individual basis. Trying to assess individual knowledge in a group situation is difficult and usually impossible because most clients do not want to reveal their knowledge deficits to a group.
- When family members or friends try to co-opt teaching sessions, individual teaching is

more effective. Some family members have been noted to use teaching sessions to make the patient feel guilty for not following a medical regimen or to attract attention to themselves and their roles as caregivers.

- When the information to be taught provokes a great deal of anxiety (such as teaching related to cardiac surgery) or is considered to be in the realm of topics not generally discussed in public (such as sexual function, reproduction, or bowel function), then one-on-one teaching is preferable. When a patient does seem to be a good prospect for a group learning experience, he should first be assessed individually.

We have found group teaching to be useful both as a helpful adjunct to one-on-one teaching and also as the primary format for patient education. Group teaching sessions lessen the feelings of alienation and being different that many people experience with acute and chronic conditions. Patients frequently remark after attending group teaching that it was helpful to hear that others share the same problems and feelings. Groups in which patients are encouraged to formulate their own agenda and conduct the group session seem to be even more successful in terms of compliance than instructor-led groups. Nessman, Carnahan, and Nugent (1980) studied a large group of noncompliant hypertensive patients who were divided into an experimental patient-operated group and a control group of traditional one-on-one nurse management. The patient-operated group was supervised by a nurse and a psychologist, but the emphasis was on the patients' feelings of control and group self-help; the patients concentrated on learning to take their own blood pressure and choosing an appropriate antihypertensive drug. At the end of 6 months, both groups demonstrated reductions in diastolic blood pressure levels, but the experimental group had a significantly greater reduction. In addition, groups have been shown to potentiate behavior modification techniques aimed at weight loss (Glanz, 1985).

Such groups as the patient-operated one mentioned above, self-help groups, and the groups at our diabetic teaching luncheons also offer a second benefit: they encourage sharing among patients of coping techniques and useful hints. We believe, for example, that it is difficult for health professionals who have never had to struggle with an ileostomy or asthma to understand or be aware of the many problems of daily existence involved with those problems. The sharing and social support that occur in such groups can be augmented by technical assistance from health professionals, as long as they do not attempt to co-opt the group.

Another reason to use group teaching formats is to save the costs in time and money of using health professionals. If it takes 12 hours, as estimated by some dietitians, to teach a diabetic the fundamentals of diet, then obviously a group teaching session is going to save manpower and money. Hassell and Medved (1975) found that when they used simple overhead transparencies in conjunction with instructor-led group sessions on diet, this experimental group performed significantly better on posttest scores than did patients in a control group, who were instructed in the traditional fashion with bedside training.

Another benefit of group teaching that accrues to family members is the support they gain from health professionals and other patients and their families. Even if the group teaching session includes only the patients' family members, insight, knowledge, and support can be gained from the group teaching session. The fact that families gain support from one another is especially evident in pediatric settings and is one of the reasons for the success of the Ronald McDonald Houses for parents of critically ill children. This mechanism seems to transfer to more structured settings, such as group teaching classes, so that we see one spouse of a heart disease patient sharing recipes with another. The feeling that "we're all in this together" is especially gratifying to family members, who are frequently more overwhelmed than the patient with the magnitude of the problem.

All of the data are not yet in on the advantages and disadvantages of group versus individual teaching, and we would like to see more evaluation research conducted in this area. Whether to use one or the other or a combination of the two is at the discretion of the health professional, who must constantly remember the individual needs of the patients.

What is the state of the art in international approaches to patient education?

Although nurses and other health care professionals from the United States tend to view the U.S. health care system in a rather provincial manner as the premier example of excellent health care, most western European countries as well as Canada and Australia have equally good medical care that is frequently more efficient and less expensive. These similarities extend to patient education, which in international comparisons demonstrate efficacious and intelligent uses of health education strategies in different countries. For example, the Netherlands instituted a system of patient education coordinators in the late 1970s following governmental policy support for public health measures to assist the public in taking responsibility for their health. With governmental support, a strong consumer movement, and a populace accustomed to autonomy in health care, the Dutch were able to provide patient education coordinators in 60% of their hospitals by 1990 (Fahrenfort, 1990).

In 1990, only 37% of all Canadian hospitals reported having health promotion policies or activities (Bartlett & Jonkers, 1990). However, the federal/provincial-mandated and funded, single-payer health care system is already a more efficient system than the fragmented system in the United States. Although the hospitals may be slow to formalize patient education resources, the problems related to who is going to pay for patient education, that is, the consumer in terms of out-of-pocket expenses or third-party payers, are nonexistent in Canada.

A national survey of patient education in Australia revealed that most hospitals conducted some form of patient education with most being conducted in teaching (95%) and metropolitan (88%) hospitals (Degeling, Salkeld, Dowsett, & Fahey, 1990). Programs tended to be directed toward management of some type of chronic disease problem, such as diabetes (80% of all hospitals offering programs), heart disease (52%), and cancer (36%). Degeling and her colleagues (1990) noted that many of the hospitals did not have planned programs, that is, programs designed for a specific patient group with goals and objectives and that programs tended to reflect the resourcefulness and diligence of individual hospital personnel. They report that there is no formal governmental, legislative, or regulatory support for patient education. Australia, like Canada, has a national health care system that allows Australians to seek no-cost health care at public hospitals. One of the textbook authors (Rankin) noted better developed and more comprehensive patient education programs for type I diabetic children and their families than any in the United States.

Summary

Patient education services seem to be more generous and less of a personal burden in countries with some type of national health care. Provision of patient education is linked, as Bartlett and Jonkers (1990) point out, to "...those countries which have paid most attention to individual rights and freedoms and which have achieved greater economic development.." (p. 99). However, the current health care environment in the United States may circumvent attempts to continually improve patient education. This climate is one in which the attitude "if you can't fix it don't get involved with it" prevails. This attitude results in hospitals that are unwilling to become involved in family burdens resulting from illness because they cannot correct or improve the problem and in third-party payers refusing to pay for diabetes education and home blood glucose monitors for type II diabetic patients. Indeed, the lack of health care reform in the United States during the 1990s does not bode well for patient education efforts in the hospital setting. With poorly coordinated attempts to cut the costs of health care by offering less in terms of health promotion and disease prevention, nurses and other health care providers must maintain a commitment to patient education if the gains made in the 1970s and 1980s are to flourish in the next century.

REFERENCES

Alexander, G. R., Weiss, J., Mulsey, T. C., & Papiernik, E. (1991) Preterm birth prevention: An evaluation of programs in the United States. *Birth: Issues-Perinatal Care and Education, 18,* 160-169.

Ascione, F. M., & Shimp, L. A. (1984). The effectiveness of four education strategies in the elderly. *Drug Intelligence and Clinical Pharmacy, 18,* 926-931.

Bartlett, E. E., & Jonkers, R. (1990). Patient education: An international comparison. *Patient Education and Counseling, 15,* 99-100.

Benfer, B. (1980). Defining the role and function of the psychiatric nurse as a member of the team. *Perspectives in Psychiatric Care, 18,* 166-177.

Berrueta-Clement, J. R., Schweinhart, L. J., Barnett, W. S., Epstein, A. S., & Weikart, D. P. (1984). *Changed lives: The effects of the Perry preschool program on youths through age 19.* Ypsilanti, MI: High/Scope Press.

Basso, R. (1991). A structured-fantasy group experience in a children's diabetic education program. *Patient Education and Counseling, 18,* 243-251.

Brawn, S.A. (1992). Meta-analysis of diabetes patient education research: Variations in intervention effects across studies. *Research in Nursing and Health, 15,* 409-419.

Burnside, I. M., Ebersole, E., & Monea, H. E. (1979). *Psychosocial caring throughout the age span* (p. 478). New York: McGraw-Hill.

Carnevali, D. L., & Patrick, M. (1993). *Nursing Management for the Elderly* (3rd. ed.). Philadelphia: JB Lippincott.

Chaisson, G. N. (1980). Patient education: Whose responsibility is it and who should be doing it? *Nursing Administration Quarterly, 4*(1), 1-11.

Cousins, N. (1979). *Anatomy of an illness.* New York: W. W. Norton.

Degeling, D., Salkeld, G., Dowsett, J. & Fahey, P. (1990). *Patient Education and Counseling, 15,* 127-138.

Devine, E. C. (1992). Effects of psycoeducational care for adult surgical patients: A meta-analysis of 191 studies. *Patient Education and Counseling, 19,* 129-142.

El-Awar, M., Becker, J. T., Hammond, K. M., Nebes, R. D., & Boller, F. (1987). Learning deficit in Parkinson's disease: Comparison with Alzheimer's disease and normal aging. *Archives of Neurology, 44,* 180-184.

Eliopoulos, C. (1987). *Gerontological nursing.* Philadelphia: J. B. Lippincott.

Eliopoulos, C. (1990). *Caring for the elderly in diverse care settings.* Philadelphia: J. B. Lippincott.

Erikson, E. H. (1963). *Childhood and society* (2nd ed., pp. 261-263). New York: W. W. Norton.

Fahrenfort, M. (1990). Patient education in Dutch hospitals: The fruits of a decade of endeavors. *Patient Education and Counseling, 15,* 139-150.

Fegley, B. J. (1988). Preparing children for radiologic procedures: Contingent versus noncontingent instructions. *Research in Nursing and Health, 11,* 3-9.

Feier, C. D., & Leight, G. (1981). A communication-cognition program for elderly nursing home residents. *The Gerontologist, 21*(4), 408-416.

Fielo, S. B., & Rizzolo, M. A. (1988). Handle with caring: Meeting elderly clients' special learning needs. *Nursing and Health Care, 9*(4), 192-195.

Glanz, K. (1985). Nutrition education for risk factor reduction and patient education: A review. *Preventive Medicine, 14,* 721-752.

Greenberg, L. A. (1991). Teaching children who are learning disabled about illness and hospitalization. *American Journal of Maternal Child Nursing, 16,* 260-263.

Hackett, A. F., Court, S., Matthews, J. N. S., McCowen, C., & Parkin, J. M. (1989). Do education groups help diabetics and their parents? *Archives of Disease in Childhood, 64,* 997-1003.

Hamer, B. A. (1991). Health teaching needs of psychiatric inpatients. *Canadian Journal of Nursing Administration, 4,* 6-10.

Hassell, J. & Medved, E. (1975). Group/audiovisual instruction for patients with diabetes. *Journal of the American Dietetic Association, 66,* 465-470.

Hawe, P., & Higgins, G. (1990). Can medication education improve the drug compliance of the elderly? Evaluation of an in hospital program. *Patient Education and Counseling, 16,* 151-160.

Illich, I. (1976). *Medical nemesis: The expropriation of health.* New York: Pantheon.

Janis, I. L. (1958). *Psychological stress: Psychoanalytic and behavioral studies of surgical patients.* New York: John Wiley & Sons.

Kleinman, A. (1988). *The illness narratives: Suffering, healing and the human condition.* New York: Basic Books.

Knowles, M. S. (1970). *The modern practice of adult education: Andragogy versus pedagogy.* New York: Association Press.

Knowlton, C. (1979). How our audiovisual system upgrades and simplifies communication with patients. *Pharmacy Times, 45*(2), 60-62.

Lancaster, J. (1979). Community treatment for mental health's forgotten population. *Journal of Psychiatric Nursing, 17*(20), 20-27.

Lindeman, C., & Stetzer, R. (1973). Effect of preoperative visits by operating room nurses. *Nursing Research, 22,* 416.

Lindeman, C., & Van Aernam, B. (1971). Nursing intervention with the presurgical patient—the effects of structured and unstructured preoperative teaching. *Nursing Research, 20,* 319-332.

Malloy, C., & Hartshorn, J. (1989). *Acute care nursing in the home.* Philadelphia: J. B. Lippincott.

Mundinger, M. (1994). Sounding board. Advanced-practice nursing—Good medicine for physicians? *New England Journal of Medicine, 330*(3), 211-213.

Nessman, D. G., Carnahan, J. E., & Nugent, C. A. (1980). Increasing compliance: Patient-operated hypertension groups. *Archives of Internal Medicine, 140*(11), 1427-1430.

Oberst, M. T. (1989). Perspectives on research in patient teaching. *Nursing Clinics of North America, 24,* 621-628.

Piaget, J., & Garcia, M. (1974). *Understanding causality.* (D. Miles & M. Miles, Trans.). New York: W. W. Norton,

Redman, B. K. (1993). Patient education at 25 years: Where we have been and where we are going. *Journal of Advanced Nursing, 18,* 725-730.

Sackett D. L., Haynes, R. B., Gibson, E. S., Hackett, B. C., Taylor, D. W., Roberts, R. S., & Johnson, A. L. (1975). Randomized clinical trials of strategies for improving medication compliance in primary hypertension. *Lancet, 1,* 1205.

Scaffa, M. E., & Davis, D. A. (1990). Cultural considerations in the treatment of persons with AIDS. *Occupational Therapy and Health Care, 7,* 69-85.

Simonds, S. (1979). *National task force on training family physicians in patient education: A handbook for teachers* (p. 3). Kansas City, MO: The Society of Teachers of Family Medicine.

Simons-Morton, D. G., Mullen, P. D., Mains, D. A., Tabak, E. R., & Green, L. W. (1992). Characteristics of controlled studies of patient education and counseling for preventive health behaviors. *Patient Education and Counseling, 19,* 175-204.

Stanley, B. (1984). Evaluation of treatment goals: The use of goal attainment scaling. *Journal of Advanced Nursing, 9,* 351-356.

15 Research and Patient Education: What It Can Tell Us and How We Can Do It

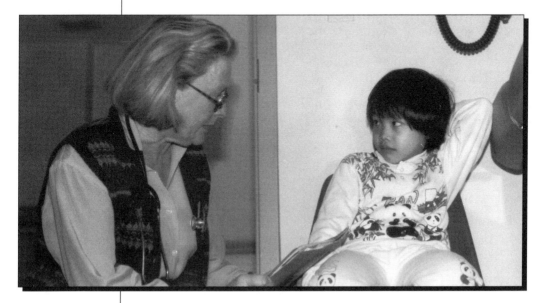

OBJECTIVES FOR CHAPTER 15

After reading this chapter, the nurse or student nurse should be able to:

1 List three problems with patient education research.

2 Compare the progress of patient education research in three major chronic illness areas: diabetes mellitus, cancer, and heart disease.

3 Write two specific aims for a proposed study to test the efficacy of patient education in the area of prevention of sexually transmitted diseases in adolescents.

Overview

Nursing is a practice discipline and, in a manner similar to other disciplines, uses research as a basis for its science and its practice (Gortner, 1983; Kim, 1993). Research, a tool of science, facilitates the development of a knowledge base for practice. Nursing research endeavors to describe, explain, and predict outcomes of nursing interventions with one of the most important interventions being the practice of patient education. This chapter describes the state of the art in terms of research in patient education, examining primarily nursing research, but also appreciating the contributions made by other nonnursing health professionals. The research examined does not represent an exhaustive review of all research in patient education. Instead, we attempt to reflect the state of the art in patient education research so that research can be summarized and made useful for practitioners. Current trends in patient education research are highlighted, and implications for practice and future research directions are suggested. The chapter suggests methods of designing patient education research projects using concrete examples from the authors' own research.

Patient Education Research: The State of the Art

A number of factors have enhanced nursing research over the last two decades. Among the contributions to a greater sophistication in nursing research have the been the widespread growth of graduate programs in nursing, both master's and doctoral, greater sophistication in research methods, and the availability, through technology such as the personal computer, of sophisticated statistical procedures. Early research in patient education was usually pretest-posttest in design, and statistical procedures were generally univariate. Many reports of patient education programs were basically anecdotal in nature with no outcome measures reported. Although many of the earlier studies, particularly those by Lindeman and others in the 1970s (Lindeman & Stetzer, 1973; Lindeman & Van Aernam, 1971), were excellent studies and are still cited as models, later patient education research has demonstrated the importance of considering multiple independent variables and their impact on patient teaching outcomes.

Patient education, a primary cornerstone of health promotion and disease prevention, received a boost with the publication of *Healthy People 2000* (U.S. Department of Health and Human Services, 1990) because patient education objectives are now reflected in this important public health document. The objectives were developed from a participatory process in which 298 objectives were developed in the area of contemporary public health and preventive medicine. Twenty of the objectives focus explicitly on patient education and many more assume patient education as a means of achieving the desired outcomes (Tolsma, 1993). Fortunately, part of the mandate of *Healthy People 2000* was to conduct research in important areas: quality of life, efficacy and utilization of clinical preventive services, and the impact of different forms of reimbursement on the provision of clinical preventive services (Tolsma, 1993). As Tolsma points out, attainment of the patient education objectives entails all of the research areas. For example, objective 17.14 deals with diabetes and chronic disabling conditions; the patient education portion states that patient education must be provided for chronic and disabling conditions. Obviously, patient teaching oriented toward reduction of diabetes complications and better management of blood sugar levels will result in better quality of life for diabetic individuals. Implications for the other areas of research are also clear using diabetes and other disabling conditions as examples. As the objectives of *Healthy People 2000* are incorporated into preventive care and health promotion, research in the area of patient education should receive additional attention. Nursing has been prompt in its embrace of *Healthy People 2000*; one hopes that all health care professionals will join this important health promotion strategy and use it as a means to enhance patient education research.

Problems With Patient Education Research

Although patient education has become more formalized and institutionalized since the first edition of this book in 1983, confusion still exists about the goals of patient education and how to best measure outcomes (Oberst, 1989; Redman, 1993). Oberst (1989) points out that the educational outcomes of most importance in patient education research, and in practice, are knowledge, attitudes, and compliance. In earlier attempts to determine the effectiveness of patient teaching, knowledge was often the only outcome measured. However, as a better understanding of behavioral change has emerged, research scientists realized that knowledge is not always linked with behavior change. Indeed, Oberst states that even knowledge is not well evaluated because *norm-referenced measures* rather than *criterion-referenced measures* are usually used (Oberst, 1989). Norm-referenced measures are used to determine cognitive performance as measured against a norm, such as the performance of others; criterion-referenced measures evaluate how the individual performs in reference to certain predetermined criteria (Waltz, Strickland, & Lenz, 1993). Whether a patient demonstrates an understanding of the biochemical regulation involved in hypertension is not as important as if he knows that hypertension is a chronic problem that requires constant, continuing medication and monitoring. Thus, a criterion-referenced test would enable the health care provider to determine the patient's ability to manage his hypertension 100% of the time, whereas a norm-referenced test would only give us an indication of his cognitive abilities in relationship to others, or perhaps to his past scores on a knowledge test.

A second educational outcome that can be problematic in terms of goals for patient education and measurement of the attainment of the goal is attitude change (Oberst, 1989; Redman, 1993). Changes in attitudes toward a particular health problem or belief are more difficult to effect than changes in knowledge. For example, attitudes related to cessation of cigarette smoking in adolescents are notoriously difficult to change, even with massive dosages of health education, because adolescents typically do not experience any noxious symptoms when they smoke, view themselves as essentially invulnerable, and find smoking pleasurable. On the other hand, adults resistant to exercise may change their attitudes once they discover that exercise promotes increased feelings of well-being as well as desired cardiovascular benefits. Therefore, measuring attitude change is complicated by issues related to the appropriate time of measurement, that is, after the new behavior has been inculcated, and the appropriateness of the attitude measure.

Thirdly, compliance to the treatment regimen, although an important educational outcome, is also difficult to measure because of its multidimensional nature (Oberst, 1989). Oberst suggests that compliance as an outcome has three levels: *feasibility*, *adherence*, and *health status*. *Feasibility* is the extent to which the patient has not only the needed information to act but also is able to master and apply the skills so that compliance can be achieved. An example of problems achieving feasibility, so that appropriate outcomes can be achieved, is the case of older women after myocardial infarction (MI) who are referred by their cardiologists for phase II cardiac rehabilitation programs. Although older women may have the knowledge regarding the importance of engaging in cardiac rehabilitation, they may not have either the financial resources or the willingness to engage in behaviors that have not been part of their previous repertoire. If the nurse researcher were evaluating the program effectiveness of cardiac rehabilitation for women, she might note the lack of feasibility in terms of traditional cardiac rehabilitation to meet women's needs.

The second level of compliance noted by Oberst (1989) is *adherence*, which refers to the necessary behavior change that accompanies compliance. Behavior change is an elusive variable because we cannot always assume that patient teaching was responsible for the behavior change. Additionally, because evaluation of behavior change usually hinges on the patient's self-report, the data may be unreliable. Adherence is measured more easily in some disease processes such as diabetes because nearly all type I and most type II diabetic patients use home blood glucose monitoring devices today. Many of these devices store the blood glucose levels with the date and time the reading was obtained. When the devices are downloaded, or hooked up to a computer, it is possible to ascertain blood glucose readings for 30 days. The blood glucose monitor, therefore, not only allows the health care provider to obtain an indication of adherence to the medical regimen, but it also reveals whether the patient has been monitoring the blood glucose level as recommended. Thus, such devices are not only useful as data collection tools but they also are an intervention that may induce desired behavior change.

The third level of compliance that Oberst suggests should be considered in patient education research is *health status indicators*. Again, diabetes mellitus is a good example of a disease with a rather straightforward health status indicator, that is, glycosylated hemoglobin blood tests. These blood tests give the health care provider an indicator of the degree to which the patient has engaged in behavior change to achieve euglycemia (appropriate blood sugar levels) over the past 60 to 90 days. However, anyone who has worked extensively with diabetic clients is aware that other variables influence blood sugar control and that some of the most compliant patients have the worst blood sugars, whereas some of the least compliant can have glycosylated hemoglobin readings within desired limits. Such is the case with other disease processes that may not have such reliable indicators of health status. Thus, patients who attend smoking cessation programs and stop smoking may lead the program directors to believe that smoking cessation was a result of the patient education when in fact it was due to some other unrelated event.

In addition to problems measuring educational outcomes achieved as a result of patient education, other problems related to research methods have been identified (Holloway, Spivey, Zismer, & Withington, 1988; Oberst, 1989; Redman, 1993). For example, the teaching interventions themselves are usually incompletely described so that replication of both the intervention and the study are impossible. Because many programs have developed outstanding curricula that could be used throughout North America, it seems important that reporting of patient teaching interventions be carefully delineated. Such reporting would give greater support to the comparisons and meta-analyses that are frequently done assessing the efficacy of patient education.

Oberst (1989) points out that in some programs there is no testable relationship between the program's objectives and the interventions. As standards of practice are developed, this problem is being solved. The American Diabetes Association (ADA) has developed standards of practice as guidance for educational programs that desire certification from ADA. The ADA requires that objectives be developed in 15 different areas that are considered crucial to diabetes education. The program must demonstrate where, and when, achievement of the objectives is implemented and how they are evaluated.

Other problems involve the failure to include a control, or comparison, group and to account for intervening or mediating variables (Holloway et al., 1988; Oberst, 1989). The nature of the teaching intervention for control groups is usually poorly described or simply referred to as "standard care." Thus, the reader of the research has a limited understanding as to what the experimental intervention is being compared.

Mediating variables include such factors as age, gender, socioeconomic status, and educational level. As Holloway and colleagues (1988) point out, they also include personality and aptitude factors that may interact in such a manner as to influence the effectiveness of the teaching intervention. Holloway's group notes that studies should be planned that have sufficient sample size so that a range of learner characteristics such as previous knowledge, personality factors, and attitudinal or predispositional attributes can be measured. It should be noted here, however, that to search for such interactions mandates a large sample size and random selection.

Age, gender, socioeconomic status, and educational level are powerful mediating variables that should always be considered in research on patient education. As Chapter 4 pointed out, it is important to consider age not only from the vantage point of maturation but also from the viewpoint of contextual factors such as historical and cohort effects that influence attitudes toward patient education. Gender effects intersect with age across the life span and these interactions require even larger sample sizes to determine their influence on patient educational outcomes. Socioeconomic status and education are also entwined and are frequently found to be the most powerful predictors of patient educational outcomes with higher education predictive of better outcomes.

Important intervening variables that should be considered in any patient education research are patient illness factors and characteristics of the health care educator (Oberst, 1989). Most patient education occurs in the hospital setting; however, shortened hospital stays frequently mean that patients are no longer amenable to in-depth patient teaching while hospitalized because their physical condition mitigates against it. Surgical patients who are still experiencing the effects of anesthesia and medical patients whose cardiac function has been impaired by an MI may be discharged to a long-term care facility or home before they are capable of understanding any but the most basic patient teaching. Therefore, the effects of the in-hospital patient teaching program are likely to be minimal and measurement of educational outcomes appear poor when the intervening variable, patient condition, is not considered.

Another important intervening variable is the characteristics of the patient educator (Oberst, 1989; Redman, 1993). If patient education research is supposed to test the efficacy of the intervention, then the individuals conducting the intervention should not vary. However, as all of us know, nurses and other health care providers vary in their ability to teach, their enthusiasm for teaching, and their commitment to patient education. If possible, differences between educators should be examined by group so that we can say with certainty that outcomes are a result of the entire program and not merely dependent on a particularly charismatic patient educator.

Characteristics of Patient Education Research

Carol Lindeman is a noted nurse researcher and educator who conducted some of the seminal research on patient education (Lindeman & Van Aernam, 1971; Lindeman & Stetzer, 1973). Her 1988 review of nursing research on patient education published in the *Annual Review of Nursing Research* is the last, systematic integrated review of nursing research in patient education. She examined five variables influencing human learning. These research variables are characterized as: patient characteristics, nurse characteristics, nurse-patient interaction in teaching situations, health- and disease-specific characteristics, and health care setting characteristics (Lindeman, 1988).

Lindeman summarized the findings for each of the five variables affecting patient education outcomes. The following generalizations were made for those studies that were primarily examining *patient characteristics*. First, psychological factors alone are not strong predictors of outcomes, but when used in interaction models with specific teaching strategies, psychological factors are predictive of patient education outcomes. Second, socioeconomic status and educational levels are positively related to patient education outcomes. A third generalization involved the timing of patient teaching. Lindeman's review indicated that the timing of teaching did not seem to be important. The fourth finding was related to family involvement, and research indications are that inclusion of the family enhances patient outcomes. More and more, research by nurses and other health care providers documents the family stress caused by illness (Rankin & Monahan, 1991); however, it is not always easy to support the effectiveness of family education (Reeber, 1992). Some research conducted since Lindeman's review has substantiated the importance of including spouses and other family members in patient education (Gilden, Hendryx, Casia, & Singh, 1989).

Only two studies focused on *characteristics of the nurse as teacher*, and, as Lindeman remarks, it is difficult to generalize from only two studies. One study cited by Lindeman, however, supported the authors' contention that higher levels of nursing education are related to better patient education outcomes.

The third and fourth variables in patient education research that Lindeman reviewed were *health- and disease-specific patient populations* and *nurse-patient interaction* in terms of instructional strategies developed for each. The greatest number of studies (n = 92) reviewed by Lindeman were in this group. The specific patient populations included in this review were: maternal-child, surgical, cardiovascular, chronic illness, psychiatric-mental health, and diagnostic procedures. The first generalization involved the efficacy of patient teaching. Lindeman reports that although patients do indeed reflect knowledge and skill improvement after patient teaching, that other more complex patient education outcomes, such as compliance, are affected by multiple independent variables in addition to exposure to patient education. A second generalization involved the effectiveness of various types of teaching strategies, and Lindeman states that most strategies are effective. She qualified this statement, however, by noting that it is impossible to determine if the teaching strategies themselves are effective or if findings are related instead to the nature of the research designs. Third, group teaching is reported to be just as effective as individual teaching, and, fourth, all patient groups showed some favorable outcomes as a result of patient teaching.

The fifth variable examined by Lindeman was the *health care setting characteristics*. Generalizations based on the nursing research reviewed indicated that the organizational structure of the health care setting was less important than the value attached to the delivery of patient education by staff and administration. Studies indicated that patients viewed education as important, and quality assurance programs are an effective vehicle for evaluating the effectiveness of patient education programs.

Lindeman's review reflected nursing research on patient education published from 1965 through 1986. Although some of the 120 studies were conducted with scientific rigor, others were limited in their generalizability by their small sample size, lack of randomization, and design and methodology problems. As the following review of patient education research in major illnesses reveals, however, these problems are certainly not limited to nursing research.

The next section reviews research conducted by nurses and other health care professionals to determine what we presently know about patient education. Most of the research reviewed is based on meta-analyses or literature reviews and includes important work in the areas of diabetes, coronary heart disease, and cancer.

Patient Education Research in Disease- and Condition-Specific Areas

Although nursing's contribution to patient education research has been substantial, other disciplines and professions have participated in equally important ways. Important patient education research has been conducted for specific target populations by other health professionals. A review of patient education research follows; this review is in the area of three chronic illnesses—diabetes, cancer, and coronary heart disease—illnesses that are especially amenable to patient education as well as being among the greatest causes of morbidity and mortality in North America and western Europe.

Diabetes

The efficacy of patient education in accomplishing desired outcomes in terms of diabetes management, metabolic control, and prevention of complications has been an area of controversy for some time. Although the evidence seems to support diabetes teaching and treatment programs (DTTP), the methods of best accomplishing the desired outcomes still require clarification (Assal, Muhlhauser, Pernet et al., 1985; Brown, 1992; Brown, 1990; Delamater, Bubb, Davis, et al., 1990; Gilden et al., 1989; Miller & Goldstein, 1972; Moffitt, Fowler, & Eather, 1979).

The emergence of laboratory tests, such as the glycosylated hemoglobin A_{1c} (HgA_{1c}) and of home blood glucose monitoring devices, has made possible more accurate evaluation of metabolic control. Brown's meta-analysis of diabetes research revealed that younger patients had better knowledge outcomes but that patients of all ages demonstrated improved glycosylated hemoglobin levels between 1 and 6 months after the teaching intervention, but then declined to the 1-month level (Brown, 1992). Muhlhauser and others documented long-term improvement in HgA_{1c} values up to 22 months for type I diabetics who attended DTTPs in West Germany (Muhlhauser, Jorgens, Berger, 1983). Assal and colleagues reported an incidence rate of 0.19 severe hypoglycemic reactions in 434 patients attending DTTPs (Assal et al., 1985). Muhlhauser and others compared this rate to 0.54 episodes per patient for the general diabetes population (Muhlhauser, Berger, Sonnenberg, 1985).

Prevention of complications, such as peripheral vascular problems, gangrene, and amputations, has also been viewed as an important outcome of diabetes patient education. Assal and associates found a decrease of 85% in below-knee amputations in a group of patients at the University Hospital of Geneva following specific foot care teaching (Assal et al., 1985). They asserted that the surgical savings are equivalent to the annual salaries of the entire staff of 12 at the Geneva Diabetes Treatment and Teaching Unit!

The intrusiveness of diabetes into all aspects of individual and family life makes it a disease especially deserving of patient education efforts. Work by Gilden and colleagues (1989) suggests that older, married, diabetic men may be more amenable to diabetes education programs than younger men. For example, older men reported significantly higher quality of life and decreased stress than younger men after a teaching intervention. Dunn (1986) also studied the importance of age in adjustment to diabetes by comparing a group of 300 subjects, ranging in age from young to middle-aged to elderly. They were studied from the time of diagnosis up to 2 years following. He found that the youngest and oldest patients had more problems adjusting emotionally to the diagnosis of diabetes than did the middle-aged patients. Dunn surmised that middle-aged patients have so many family and career demands that the diagnosis had little emotional impact. Thus, findings regarding the influence of age and patient educational interventions on knowledge, metabolic, and quality of life outcomes appear to be contradictory although results of a more recent meta-analysis (Brown, 1992) suggest that age does influence knowledge outcomes with older age associated with lower levels of knowledge acquisition.

Recently, patients' perspectives on diabetes education have been assessed in research studies (Duchin & Brown, 1990; Wikblad, 1991). Although it might seem self-evident that the consumers of patient education should be polled as to their specific needs, this practice has not been a part of most diabetes teaching programs. Therefore, the two studies cited are important examples of research that attempts to understand patient perceptions of their own learning needs. In general, diabetic patients desire less pathophysiology and a greater emphasis on survival skills. They also report a need for individualized patient education based on their own disease trajectory.

Patient education in the area of diabetes management has had a long and distinguished history. Early studies conducted by Etzwiler (1967) looked at the knowledge young diabetic patients and their parents had about diabetes and discovered that neither patients nor their parents had an adequate grasp of basic information about diabetes. Proper control was surmised to result from "well informed patients cooperating with interested and knowledgeable nurses, dietitians and physicians" (Etzwiler, 1967, p. 111). Patient education has become better regulated and more precise with the entry of the American Association of Diabetes Educators (AADE), a professional group established in 1969 that certifies diabetes educators through an examination and required preceptorship process. AADE has also established a foundation that supports research in the area of diabetes and patient education. The American Diabetes Association (ADA) and the National Institute of Diabetes, Digestive, and Kidney Diseases (NIDDK) are two other organizations, the first voluntary and the second federal, that underwrite research in the areas of diabetes and patient education. The ADA has also established guidelines for the certification of diabetes teaching programs that meet national standards in 15 important areas of patient education.

Research in the area of diabetes patient education has demonstrated improved outcomes in terms of better metabolic control and decreased complications. The advent of glycosylated hemoglobins has given the diabetes health care provider a "gold standard" by which to judge the long-term effects of patient education, a tool that is not replicable in the study of other chronic illnesses. The importance of including the family in diabetes management classes and in focusing on psychosocial interventions needs greater attention by researchers (Padgett, Mumford, Hynes, & Carter, 1988). Lastly, diabetes patient education research illustrates some provocative, although contradictory, findings related to age and the efficacy of diabetes patient education. Age is an important variable that should be included in studies of other chronic illnesses and patient education.

Cancer

Nursing's involvement in patient education directed toward cancer diagnosis, treatment, rehabilitation, and survival has provided impetus for a change in the manner in which cancer is viewed—it is now considered a chronic rather than a terminal illness. Patient and health care provider partnerships have replaced the previous concept of the patient being the passive recipient of information from the physician (Adams, 1991). However, various studies indicate that there are acute, unmet needs for knowledge during the diagnostic, treatment, rehabilitation, continuing care, and remission periods, and during recurrence or advanced disease (Adams, 1991; Coughlan, 1993; Corney, Everett, Howells, & Crowther, 1992).

The review by Rimer and colleagues of research relating to patient education and cancer divided patient education approaches into three categories: diagnosis, treatment, and rehabilitation and continuing care (Rimer, Keintz, & Glassman, 1985). During the *diagnostic period*, pertinent research studies (n = 9) revealed that patients wanted more information about all aspects of various treatment regimens and prognosis. Demographic characteristics such as age, educational background, and socioeconomic status were important predictors of types of information desired. Agre and colleagues studied the amount of time nurses spend teaching cancer patients in the inpatient setting (Agre, Bookbinder, Cirrincione, & Keating, 1990). They documented that in one setting each cancer patient received 16.6 minutes of instruction each day, which they calculated as a significant amount of time. However, much of the research indicates patients still do not believe they are receiving adequate information about diagnostic and treatment strategies.

Research related to patient education and *treatment of cancer* (n = 13) indicated that information related to treatment diminished side effects and decreased oral infections. Additionally, a number of studies have demonstrated the efficacy of relaxation training, hypnosis, and guided imagery in reducing anticipatory nausea and vomiting as related to chemotherapy. Studies related to compliance with treatment regimens have illustrated the usefulness of a wide variety of educational approaches and professionals in improving compliance.

Patient education directed toward *rehabilitation and continuing care* (n = 3) has been demonstrated to enhance coping strategies, improve relationships with health professionals, and increase self-concept and self-esteem (Rimer et al., 1985). Generally, there are few studies of pain control with cancer patients or other aspects of continuing care.

Rimer and colleagues noted the following weaknesses in their review of various studies of patient education and cancer: lack of multiple impact measures, absence of health outcome measures, inadequacy of process data documenting patient education, small sample size, unsatisfactory and inappropriate instruments, and inappropriate statistical tests (Rimer, Keintz, Glassman, 1985). The authors also point out that studies frequently tend to view multidimensional constructs, such as compliance, as unidimensional and tend to neglect the effects of patient education on health status or the costs of medical care.

An important impetus in the education of patients with cancer is the recognition by the American Cancer Society (ACS) and the National Cancer Institute (NCI) that patient education should be an integral part of cancer care. The "I Can Cope" program, developed by two oncology nurses in Minnesota, was adopted nationally by the ACS and implemented in 1979 (Stevenson & Crosson, 1991). Concomitant with the adoption of the "I Can Cope" program was the federally sponsored NCI program, also implemented nationally in 1979, and entitled "Coping with Cancer." The two national cancer organizations have developed programs to benefit the public although the NCI traditionally works through health care professionals such as the Oncology Nursing Society, whereas ACS focuses on the community with 3000 ACS offices spread across the country (Stevenson & Crosson, 1991). Both the ACS and the NCI sponsor research related to cancer patient education for individuals and families.

The research related to patient education and cancer is not unlike that for heart disease and diabetes. For example, patients report they do not have adequate knowledge to make treatment decisions nor are they made aware of their trajectory of illness. As in the other two major chronic illnesses reviewed in this chapter, patient teaching research has gained over the past 20 years with the injection of doctorally prepared nurses competent in conducting research in the area of cancer and patient and family education.

Coronary Heart Disease

Coronary heart disease (CHD) causes more deaths than any other single disease for both men and women (Heart Facts, 1994). Shortened hospital stays for MI make nurses and other health care providers question if patient teaching is even appropriate for the hospitalization period. Duryee's review (1992) and the meta-analysis of Mullen and colleagues (Mullen, Mains, & Velez, 1992) indicates that formal, structured education does increase patients' knowledge and positively influences blood pressure, mortality, exercise, and diet.

Duryee's analysis concentrated on the inpatient phase of patient education after MI. Although the national mean length of stay for the time period she reviewed was 7 to 11 days, now that the mean length of stay for an uncomplicated MI is 4 to 5 days, we wonder if the same knowledge outcomes would be achieved. Likewise, we question if patients are able to incorporate education that is supposed to result in life-style changes. In particular, teaching that attempts to bring about behavioral changes, such as are needed with risk factor reduction, is ineffective when provided on an inpatient basis (Waitkoff & Imburgia, 1990). Duryee's analysis indicates that most studies demonstrate life-style changes in areas of activity and smoking but less frequently in diet. A third variable studied by Duryee that is influenced by shorter hospital stays is the most beneficial time for teaching in terms of anxiety level. Most of the studies she reviewed indicate that teaching during the stay in the coronary care unit is much less efficacious than teaching 7 to 10 days after the cardiac event. Because most patients are discharged by this time, it seems that anxiety levels may be high enough during the contemporary hospitalization period that learning is not easily achievable.

Other helpful information from Duryee's and Mullen's systematic reviews involves the type of content as well as type of educational strategy needed by CHD patients. Generally, staff and patients report that information on management of symptoms and reduction of risk factors is crucial; less crucial is material relating to pathophysiology of heart disease. Length of the patient education intervention was not found to be influential. Some studies indicated that use of audiovisual materials such as slide-tape presentations were just as effective as live educators. Mullen and colleagues (1992) found that behavior-oriented interventions rather than didactic-oriented interventions were more successful in achieving the desired outcomes. The Mullen group noted that important educational principles were rarely applied. For example, attempts to educate patients to take recommended actions in the presence of symptoms or problems were uncommon. Reinforcement and feedback, important components of effective patient education, were also routinely neglected.

Because hospital stays are now so much shorter for acute cardiac events than in previous years, it may be more logical to institute patient education and life-style change programs on an outpatient basis. A good example of a useful model for inpatient and outpatient teaching is the nurse-managed smoking cessation program described by Taylor and colleagues (Taylor, Houston-Miller, Killen, & DeBusk, 1990). This program used written materials in the hospital that teach coping strategies for cessation of smoking. Before hospital discharge patients were oriented to audiotapes for progressive muscle relaxation and given written materials. After discharge, coronary care unit nurses with special training telephoned patients to provide instruc-

tion and support. Patients who were in the experimental group had significantly lower smoking rates 12 months after discharge from the hospital. This model demonstrates a low-cost, low-technology patient education intervention for life-style changes.

Patient education and research in the field of patient teaching and heart disease have been given impetus by two national organizations, the American Heart Association (AHA), a voluntary organization, and the National Heart, Lung, and Blood Institute. Like the ADA, most of the research funding within the AHA has been oriented toward physicians although this has changed somewhat over the past 15 years through the strong nursing involvement in the AHA's Cardiovascular Nursing section. Perhaps because patient education in the area of heart disease is less focused than in diabetes owing to the diverse presentation and treatment of heart disease (e.g., hypertension, coronary artery disease, congenital cardiac lesions, and so on) and frequently has a longer period of chronicity than do the cancers, we believe that patient education has not been as well organized or as well studied by nurses as have diabetes and cancer. Studies of patient education for preventive health behaviors important to heart disease have been strong in smoking cessation, nutrition, and weight control but weak in the areas of exercise and stress management (Simons-Morton, Mullen, Mains, Tabak, & Green, 1992). Therefore, we recommend more nursing and other health professional research efforts in these areas.

Reviews of patient education directed toward cardiac patients reveal some of the same issues documented by research in diabetes patient education. Thus, it appears that the message, not the method, is important and that the message should concentrate on survival skills needed to manage a chronic condition rather than the underlying pathophysiology. Programs oriented toward changes in behavior are more efficacious than those solely focused on knowledge acquisition. Shorter hospital stays mandate outpatient education because memory and conceptualization abilities are influenced by changes in biochemical parameters.

Summary of Patient Education Research Findings

In summarizing findings from review articles, we note the emergence of pervasive themes across various diseases and as cited by health professionals in different fields. First, patient education is positively related to knowledge accrual and a number of beneficial psychosocial and physical health outcomes.

Second, a wide variety of teaching strategies including one-on-one, group, audiovisual, and psychoeducational strategies have proved useful. The combination of strategies to reinforce learning is probably more effective than a single strategy.

Third, to influence health outcomes and achieve maximal levels of adherence to medical regimen, patient education must be repetitive and reinforced at different time periods. Fourth, demographic characteristics such as age, educational background, and socioeconomic status must be considered when patient education programs are designed because they have different impacts on patient education outcomes. Although psychological factors have been frequently studied as predictors of patient education outcomes, they are more important when considered in their interaction with various teaching strategies than when examined alone.

A fifth finding involves social support as a strategy to enhance patient education. Whether social support is available as part of a group interaction technique or through inclusion of family members, the provision of social support probably interacts with the teaching intervention to increase the efficacy of patient education.

Developing Research Proposals To Study the Efficacy of Patient Education

As the discipline of nursing has become more research literate, nurses have increasingly sought methods of evaluating the efficacy of their patient education efforts. We have been involved in the generation of research proposals and the first author (Rankin) has received funding from a variety of sources including the National Center for Nursing Research (presently called the National Institute of Nursing Research), the NIDDK, and AHA. The development of a research proposal is a rather precise and tedious process that involves following the grantor's guidelines and getting necessary materials together. The most difficult aspect of designing a research proposal, however, is the conceptualization that must occur *before* the proposal is written. Indeed, the answer to the question "What do you want to know?" is the most difficult part of the process. Once the investigators have determined what it is they want to know, research texts, methodologists, and statisticians can be consulted for aspects of design, sample specification, and data analysis.

The last section of the chapter outlines the different sections involved in producing a proposal that meets the guidelines of the various institutes of the National Institutes of Health (NIH) using the U.S. Department of Health and Human Services, Public Health Service (PHS) form 398. Examples are drawn from portions of an approved but unfunded proposal submitted by Rankin to NIDDK; this proposal was chosen because the research involved patient education. The PHS format was chosen because it is one of the most rigorous and can be modified for submission to foundations or other funding sources. Form 398 is revised frequently, but the same basic elements are consistent over time in the application form.

The reader should note that whether the research planned is qualitative or quantitative research the same type of proposal format is used. Generally speaking, qualitative research seeks to generate hypotheses and deals with data that cannot be structured in a numbers format, whereas quantitative research includes data that can be structured in a numbers format or can be transposed into a numbers format (Brink & Wood, 1989). Whether research is qualitative or quantitative depends on the question being asked and the type of data available.

The longest, and most important, section of the entire proposal is the research plan. The research plan has nine different sections, six of which are covered in this chapter. The remaining three, vertebrate animals, consultants/collaborators, and consortium/contractual arrangements are well outlined in the PHS booklet and, in the case of vertebrate animals, does not apply to research regarding patient education. These same sections are found in almost all foundation and other agency proposal formats although they may be called by different titles. Many private foundations ask the investigator to summarize in lay terms how the findings will benefit the population studied. The reader is reminded that there are many different approaches to writing a research proposal and that the following section is but one approach.

Specific Aims

The specific aims section concerns the broad, long-term objectives of the proposed study. This is the first section the reviewer reads and should be a concise and articulate attempt to "grab" the reader's interest. Because the section should be approximately one page, the investigator needs to succinctly present a compelling argument for the study. Some investigators choose not to write their aims until they have developed the study in detail; in this way the aims reflect the study design and methods precisely. Specific aims should be translatable into research questions or hypotheses. The specific aims that were derived for a study to improve health outcomes for ethnic minorities with diabetes mellitus were twofold.

> The primary aim of the proposed study is: to conduct a randomized clinical trial to test the effectiveness of educational interventions (one day vs four day) and family member support (family member present or absent) on selected outcome measures (metabolic control, knowledge levels, family support, quality of life, depression, and family function) at four data collection points (before intervention, and 3, 12, and 24 months after the intervention). A

secondary aim is to describe the incidence of cardiovascular and renal complications in a sample of immigrated diabetic Chinese persons because the data are not now available.

The specific aims section also referred to a previous study funded by NIDDK that was preliminary to the randomized clinical trial and included operational definitions of important variables.

Background and Significance

The purpose of the background and significance section is to critically review the literature and document areas of existing knowledge that may be inadequate as well as specifically identifying the gaps that the study is expected to fill. The background and significance section may include a theoretical model that will be tested in the study. Theoretical linkages to extant theories should be documented so that the findings can later be interpreted within a theoretical framework. Literature that is reviewed should include recent work in the field as well as classic studies. Again, this section must be strongly stated and be able to demonstrate why the proposal is sufficiently unique and deserving of funding.

The background and significance section in the study referred to above set the stage for continued study by Rankin of Chinese immigrants with type II diabetes mellitus. The theoretical framework used was one discussed in Chapter 2 of this book, Levanthal's self-regulation model. This section included the independent variables, that is, the educational and family support interventions to enhance metabolic control as well as the dependent variables such as diabetes quality of life, depression, and glycosylated hemoglobin levels. The background and significance section concluded with the following statements:

> The importance of health education programs to teach self-care management skills to persons with diabetes has been highlighted by recent reports of the DCCT trial indicating that careful metabolic control

in insulin dependent diabetes mellitus delays the onset of complications. Health education for people with chronic illnesses, such as diabetes, is also a national priority as described in the objectives of *Healthy People 2000* (DHHS, 1990). Increasing to 40% the proportion of people with chronic illnesses receiving formal patient education as part of illness management is a national health goal. Chinese Americans with NIDDM living in the San Francisco Bay Area are a rapidly growing minority population that has not been sufficiently studied. Though educational and psychosocial interventions can enhance not only short-term control of NIDDM but also quality of life for patients and their families (Padgett et al., 1988), failure to adequately address cultural factors in the designing, implementing, and testing of these interventions can reduce their effectiveness and perpetuate current disparities in health care for minorities.

The background and significance section is an important section of the proposal because it offers the investigator an opportunity to lay the groundwork for the study of an important phenomenon. Although the investigator may believe that her proposal offers a unique chance to study patient education, it should be recognized that many proposals to study the efficacy of patient education have been funded in the past; therefore, a proposal must be exceptional to garner funding.

Preliminary Studies

The preliminary studies section allows the investigator an opportunity to report on her previous work in the same or similar areas. In this section any pilot work should be explained so that the reviewers have an opportunity to review the investigator's expertise in the field. In nonfederal applications this section may not be explicitly included. A summary of pilot work completed by Rankin included the following statements:

> This study allowed the Principle Investigator access to an important site for data collection from Chinese diabetic subjects,

critical contacts were made, and two data collection tools were translated into Chinese. This study also offered the opportunity to pilot a one-day course with the Chinese participants although there was no opportunity to compare a Chinese one-day to a four-day course during this study. Answers on the Diabetes Educational Profile (a questionnaire) indicated that diabetes mellitus was perceived as a stigmatizing illness over which this group had little control and about which they had little information. Other significant information related to the enthusiasm about doing self-blood glucose monitoring which had not been in the repertoire of this group's behaviors before; with instruction in Chinese many of the subjects began self-blood-glucose-monitoring.

A second study, also of Chinese immigrants with type II diabetes mellitus was also included in the preliminary studies section.

Research Design and Methods

The research design and methods section describes the design (e.g., experimental versus quasi-experimental) and the procedures that will be used to achieve the specific aims of the study. This section also includes the methods by which data will be gathered, analyzed, and interpreted. If statistical procedures are to be used in data analysis then they must be described in detail. A power analysis to determine sample size should also be included. If the methods are comprised solely of qualitative methods then, likewise, the procedures for analyzing qualitative data must be described. Some private foundations refer to this section simply as procedures; however, no matter how the section is titled it should be described in sufficient detail to allow the reviewers to understand how the study will be carried out and how the data will be analyzed. With increasing sophistication on the part of reviewers and less funding available, the investigator must be comprehensive and articulate in describing the research design and methods. The following portion of the proposal describes the proposed design:

A three factor, randomized clinical trial with a longitudinal, repeated measures design to test selected dependent variables is planned. The two between subjects factors are length of intervention (one day vs four day) and family support (family present or absent) and the one within subjects factor is time (before intervention, 3, 12, and 24 months after intervention). Dependent variables are biobehavioral and cognition based: metabolic control measured by glycosylated hemoglobin tests, MDRTC diabetes knowledge levels, family support, and emotion based: psychosocial impact, quality of life, depression, and family function. Data are collected before the intervention begins, and at three, twelve, and twenty-four months after the intervention.

This section also included subsections on setting, recruitment strategies, sample criteria, sample size, descriptions of the teaching interventions, and descriptions of the various data collection instruments (questionnaires) and equipment (a piece of portable medical equipment that analyzed HbA_{1c}), procedures and measurement, and data analysis. For example, the portion of the proposal that related to coding and missing data read:

> Data will be entered on a PS/2 computer using the CRUNCH interactive statistical package (CRUNCH Software Corporation). After data reduction to the appropriate subscales, analysis will proceed using CRUNCH. Two-tailed levels of significance will be set at .05. Missing data will be handled as follows: when no more than 20% of the items from a scale or subscale are missing, the mean of the scale or subscale will be substituted for that individual's missing values; however, if greater than 20% of the items are missing, the scale or subscale will be treated as missing for that individual. Descriptive statistics will be computed on demographic and medical data including data pertaining to cardiovascular and renal complications. Additionally the four groups will be compared on major covariates (e.g., age, gender, education, income, and cardiovascular and renal complications) to make certain that random assignment equally distributed the covariates.

Thus, precision and care must be part of the section titled research design and methods. We recommend that a statistician be consulted for help in terms of reading this section of the proposal. Most institutions, whether hospitals or academic settings, have consulting statisticians available for this type of assistance.

Human Subjects

Human subjects is the last section of the nine required sections in the PHS proposal format. Whether an agency requires this section or not in the formal proposal, the investigator must gain human subjects clearance before commencing a study. In addition to describing the procedures that will be used with subjects or study participants, the principle investigator must also include the plans for the recruitment of subjects, the consent process, the nature of the information to be provided to prospective participants, and the method of documenting consent. Issues regarding consent are covered in Chapter 5 of this book. The human subjects section of the proposal must include any potential risks to study participants and procedures for protecting subjects against potential risks. The purpose of obtaining human subjects clearance through an institutional review board is to protect study participants to as great an extent as possible from any physical, psychological, social, legal, or other risks. This step of the grantsmanship process is of extreme importance and must never be neglected.

In summary, the process of conceptualizing, designing, and writing a research proposal is a creative endeavor that takes approximately 3 to 6 months depending on the resources needed. We have found that proposals that are reviewed by a group of one's peers before submission to the funding agency have a much better chance of receiving favorable reviews and funding. The input of one's colleagues may save valuable time and avoid rewriting proposals in case they are not favorably reviewed. Other means of learning the proposal writing ropes include mentorship by senior nurse scientists and proposal writing workshops. Many proposals are not funded during the first submission, but are patiently reworked and resubmitted for second or even third considerations. Although the process is time consuming it is invaluable in terms of garnering funding and gaining clarity about one's own research directions.

Summary

This chapter has reviewed the state of the art regarding patient education research, reviewed research within three important chronic disease areas and the patient education research in each, and presented one approach to writing a research proposal using actual examples from a proposal. Research on patient education has become increasingly sophisticated, a fact that has helped the health care provider who needs to convince the skeptic of its efficacy. As the potential of patient education is increasingly appreciated, the research will continue to reflect the positive outcomes engendered by effective patient education.

Strategies for Critical Analysis and Application

1. If you had to convince the board of trustees in your local hospital to fund an office of patient education, which arguments based on research would you use?

2. What is the purpose of the background and significance section of a research proposal? What important points should be covered in this section if your proposal deals with prevention and detection of tuberculosis in the homeless community?

3. You have been asked to design a teaching program for adult patients with long-term epilepsy who have been prescribed anti-seizure medications. How would you measure the three levels of compliance—feasibility, adherence, and health status—outlined by Oberst?

REFERENCES

Adams, M. (1991). Information and education across the phases of cancer care. *Seminars in Oncology Nursing, 7,* 105-111.

Agre, P., Bookbinder, M., Cirrincione, C., & Keating, E. (1990). How much time do nurses spend teaching cancer patients. *Patient Education and Counseling, 16,* 29-38.

Assal, J. P., Muhlhauser, I., Pernet, A., Gfeller, R., Jorgens, V., Berger, M. (1985). Patient education as the basis for diabetes care in clinical practice and research. *Diabetologia, 28,* 602-613.

Brink, P. J., & Wood, M. J. (1989). *Advanced design in nursing research.* Newbury Park, CA: Sage.

Brown, S. A. (1990). Quality of reporting in diabetes patient education research: 1954–1986. *Research in Nursing and Health, 13,* 53-62.

Brown, S. A. (1992). Meta-analysis of diabetes patient education research: Variations in intervention effects across studies. *Research in Nursing and Health, 15,* 409-419.

Corney, R., Everett, H., Howells, A., & Crowther, M. (1992). The care of patients undergoing surgery for gynaecological cancer: The need for information, emotional support and counseling. *Journal of Advanced Nursing, 17,* 667-671.

Coughlan, M. C. (1993). Knowledge of diagnosis, treatment and its side-effects in patients receiving chemotherapy for cancer. *European Journal of Cancer Care, 2*(2), 66-71.

Delamater, A. M., Bubb, J., Davis, S. G., Smith, J.A., Schmidt, L., White, N. H., & Santiago, J. V. (1990). Randomized prospective study of self-management training with newly diagnosed diabetic children. *Diabetes Care, 13,* 492-498.

Duchin, S. P., & Brown, S. A. (1990). Patients should participate in designing diabetes educational content. *Patient Education and Counseling, 16,* 255-267.

Dunn, S. (1986). Reactions to educational techniques: Coping strategies for diabetes and learning. *Diabetic Medicine, 3,* 419-429.

Duryee, R. (1992) The efficacy of inpatient education after myocardial infarction. *Heart and Lung, 21,* 217-227.

Etzwiler, D. D. (1967). Who's teaching the diabetic? *Diabetes, 16,* 111-117.

Gilden, J. L., Hendryx, M., Casia, C., & Singh, S. P. (1989). The effectiveness of diabetes education programs for older patients and their spouses. *Journal of the American Geriatrics Society, 37,* 1023-1030.

Gortner, S. R. (1983). The history and philosophy of nursing science and research. *Advances in Nursing Science, 5:* 1-8.

Heart Facts. (1994). Dallas, TX: American Heart Association.

Holloway, R. L., Spivery, R. N., Zismer, D. K., & Withington, A. N. (1988). Aptitude X treatment interactions: Implications for patient education research. *Health Education Quarterly, 15,* 241-257.

Kim, H. S. (1993). Putting theory into practice: Problems and prospects. *Journal of Advanced Nursing, 18,* 1632-1639.

Lindeman, C. (1988). Patient education. *Annual Review of Nursing Research, G,* 29-60.

Lindeman, C., & Stetzer, R., (1973). Effect of preoperative visits by operating room nurses. *Nursing Research, 22,* 4-16.

Lindeman, C., & Van Aernam, B. (1971). Nursing intervention with the presurgical patient—the effects of structured and unstructured preoperative teaching. *Nursing Research, 20,* 319-332.

Miller, L. V., & Goldstein, J. (1972). More efficient care of diabetic patients in a county-hospital setting. *New England Journal of Medicine, 286,* 1388-1391.

Moffitt, P., Fowler, J., & Eather, G. (1979). Bed occupancy by diabetic patients. *Medical Journal of Australia, 1,* 244-245.

Muhlhauser, I., Jorgens, V., Berger, M., Graninger, W., Gürtler, W., Hornke, L., Kunz, A., Schernthaner, G., Scholz, V. & Voss, H. E. (1983). Bicentric evaluation of a teaching and treatment programme for type I (insulin-dependent) diabetic patients: Improvement of metabolic control and other measures of diabetes care for up to 22 months. *Diabetologia, 25,* 470-476.

Muhlhauser, I., Berger, M., Sonnenberg, G. E., Koch, J., Jorgens, V. Schernthaner, G., Scholz, V., & Padagogin, D. (1985). Incidence and management of severe hypoglycaemia in 434 adult patients with insulin-dependent diabetes mellitus. *Diabetes Care, 8,* 268-273.

Mullen, P. D., Mains, D. A., & Velez, R. (1992). A meta-analysis of controlled trials of cardiac patient education. *Patient Education and Counseling, 19,* 143-162.

Oberst, M. T. (1989). Perspectives on research in patient teaching. *Nursing Clinics of North America, 24,* 621-628.

Padgett, D., Mumford, E., Hynes, M., & Carter, R. (1988). Meta-analysis of the effects of educational and psychosocial interventions on management of diabetes mellitus. *Journal of Clinical Epidemiology, 41,* 1007-1030.

Rankin, S. H., & Monahan, P. (1991). Great expectations: Perceived social support in couples experiencing cardiac surgery. *Family Relations, 40,* 297-302.

Redman, B. K. (1993). Patient education at 25 years; where we have been and where we are going. *Journal of Advanced Nursing, 18,* 725-730.

Reeber, B. J. (1992). Evaluating the effects of a family education intervention. *Rehabilitation Nursing, 17,* 332-336.

Simons-Morton, D. G., Mullen, P. D., Mains, D. A., Tabak, E. R., & Green. L. W. (1992). Characteristics of controlled studies of patient education and counseling for preventive health behaviors. *Patient Education and Counseling, 19,* 175-204.

Stevenson, E., & Crosson, K. (1991). Patient education: History, development, and current directions of the American Cancer Society and the National Cancer Institute. *Seminars in Oncology Nursing, 7,* 136-142.

Taylor, C. B., Houston-Miller, N., Killen, J. D., & DeBusk, R. F. (1990). Smoking cessation after acute myocardial infarction: Effects of a nurse-managed intervention. *Annals of Internal Medicine, 113,* 118-123.

Tolsma, D. D. (1993). Patient education objectives in *Healthy People 2000*: Policy and research issues. *Patient Education and Counseling, 22,* 7-14.

U.S. Department of Health and Human Services, Public Health Service. (1990). *Healthy people 2000: National health promotion and disease prevention objectives: Full report with commentary.* (DHHS Publication No. (PHS), 91-50212). Washington, DC: U.S. Government Printing Office.

Waitkoff, B., & Imburgia, D. (1990). Patient education and continuous involvement in a phase 1 cardiac rehabilitation program. *Journal of Nursing Quality Assurance, 5,* 38-48.

Waltz C., Strickland, O., & Lenz, E. (1989). Measurement in nursing research (2nd ed.). Philadelphia: F. A. Davis.

Wikblad, K. R. (1991). Patient perspectives of diabetes care and education. *Journal of Advanced Nursing, 16,* 837-844.

Checklist for Evaluating Patient Education Materials

The following checklist is designed to be used by health professionals when they review instructional materials for use in patient education. It is adapted from The Society of Teachers of Family Medicine: *Patient Education: A Handbook for Teachers* (1979), Kansas City.

Title
Author
Publication date
Specified intended audience:
Age span: _____ to _____ (years)
Language or ethnic background
Socioeconomic group

I. Accuracy
  A. Are facts, diagrams, pictures, and other visual representations accurate?
  B. Is subject matter up to date?
II. Content
  A. Breadth or scope of coverage
    1 Does the subject matter or content presented address major areas of difficulty/functional problems experienced by many patients with the specific medical problems?
    2. Is there content (subject matter or product endorsements/advertising) included that is inappropriate for the intended audience?
  B. Balance of coverage
    1. Is the subject matter balanced in terms of emphasis on various major areas?
III. Educational Methods
  A. Organization of content
    1. Is there an organizational structure or logic that is apparent to the patient?
    2. Are major content areas set off so that material can be put into perspective?
  B. Contribution of organization of content to efficient learning
    1. Are concepts or terms introduced in an appropriate sequence?
    2. Does material start with simple concepts, then move to the more complex?
    3. Is material sequenced in a patient-friendly manner, ie. step-by-step, chronological, or topical?
    4. Is there a summary?
  C. Educational objectives or goals and methods for assessing learner achievement
    1. Are objectives explicitly stated and included in the educational material in a way that is understandable to the patient?
    2. Is it likely that patients will reach the objectives by study of the material? Is the number of objectives reasonable?
    3. Are learner-assessment methods included that help patients determine whether they have met the objectives (i.e., test questions)?
    4. Do the objectives address areas that are generally of concern *to most physicians* who treat patients with this problem?
    5. Do the objectives address areas that are generally of concern *to most patients* with the particular problem?
IV. Communication
  A. Appropriateness of the reading level for the stated audience
    1. Are other key audience characteristics specified?
    2. Whenever possible, are sentences short and simple, containing only commonly used terms, and is medical jargon avoided?
  B. Availability of feedback
    1. Are there appropriate places for the patient to practice?
    2. How will the patient obtain feedback about the mastery of facts, concepts, and principles?

Patient Education: Issues, Principles, Practices, Third Edition, by Sally H. Rankin and Karen Duffy Stallings. Lippincot–Raven Publishers, Philadelphia, © 1996.

C. Concreteness of the communication
  1. Are ideas presented clearly?
  2. Is abstract communication avoided?
D. Adequate technical quality of the material
  1. Is the print size adequate?
  2. Are spacing and layout attractive?
  3. Are pictures attractive?
  4. Are diagrams simple and clear?
E. Availability of material for the patient to take home

  1. Does the material include key information or ideas?
  2. Does the material include a step-by-step explanation of any task the patient is to perform?
VI. Cost Effectiveness/Practicality
  A. Does excessive cost of the material make it impractical?
  B. Is it possible that the same objectives can be reached by other methods?

Tool for Evaluation of Patient Education Videotapes

1. Title:
2. Beginning time:
   Ending time:
   Total running time:
3. Vocabulary: List all words with which patients may not be familiar. Are terms defined? Estimate the number of words that exceed two syllables.
4. Purpose of the film: If goals and objectives are stated, list.
5. Intended audience:
6. What type of people are portrayed in the video?
7. Questions answered by the video. Are these questions or problems commonly encountered by patients?
8. Priority areas addressed?
   What must a patient do to manage this problem?
   What decisions should patients be prepared to make?
9. Are sources suggested for further help or information?
10. Technical quality:
11. Cost:
12. Source:

Patient Education: Issues, Principles, Practices, Third Edition, by Sally H. Rankin and Karen Duffy Stallings.
Lippincott–Raven Publishers, Philadelphia, © 1996. **349**

Objectives for Prenatal Classes

Class I:
Nutrition During Pregnancy

At the close of Class I, each participant will be able to do the following:

A. Answer the following questions correctly:
1. How much weight do you plan to gain during your pregnancy?
2. Now that you are pregnant, how many more calories do you think you need: 2 times normal, 3 times normal, only 300 calories more, only 100 calories more?
3. Which of the following foods do pregnant women especially need: dairy products, sweets, fatty foods, fresh vegetables, protein foods?
4. Which of the following items might be dangerous to eat or use while you are pregnant: alcoholic beverages, salt, sugar, nicotine, caffeine?
5. In which of the following situations would a pregnant woman be wise to lose weight: if the woman were overweight before pregnancy, if the woman is diabetic and overweight, if the woman suddenly gains 10 lb that is primarily fluid?
B. List three advantages of breast-feeding.
C. State three advantages of exercise during pregnancy.
D. Choose one type of exercise and describe where and how often it will be done.

Prenatal Class II:
Physiologic and Psychological Changes of Pregnancy

By the close of Class II, each participant will be able to do the following:

A. Describe breast changes and care of the breasts during pregnancy.
B. Describe recommendations for the following during pregnancy:

1. Rest and sleep
2. Smoking and alcohol
3. Dental care
4. Travel and work
C. Name two common discomforts of pregnancy and recommended treatments.
D. State why the doctor should be consulted before *any* medication is taken during pregnancy.
E. Identify three warning signs for which the doctor should be notified immediately.
F. Demonstrate the Kegel exercise for toning pelvic musculature, demonstrate slow, deep chest breathing used during the initial stage of labor.

Prenatal Class III:
Labor and Delivery

At the close of Class III, each participant will be able to do the following:

A. Describe the work of the uterus in labor.
B. Describe the changes of the cervix in labor.
C. Describe three signs of labor.
D. Demonstrate the timing of contractions.
E. Describe how and when to contact the doctor when there has been a sign of labor.
F. Describe three stages of labor.
G. Consider own plans for labor and delivery (e.g., birthing room, rooming-in arrangements, early discharge).
H. Describe some variables that make cesarean section necessary.

Prenatal Class IV: The Newborn

At the close of Class IV, each participant/couple will be able to do the following:

A. Describe why fatigue is a problem that most new parents face.
B. Discuss two ways new parents can minimize unnecessary fatigue.

Patient Education: Issues, Principles, Practices, Third Edition, by Sally H. Rankin and Karen Duffy Stallings. Lippincott–Raven Publishers, Philadelphia, © 1996. **351**

C. Consider what "helpers" might be staying with them when they come home from the hospital and describe what they can do to help.

D. Describe three infant care problems for which the doctor should be notified.

E. Describe three needs for which babies depend on their parents.

F. Describe two issues that new parents often confront as a couple.

Prenatal Class V: The Postpartum Period

At the end of Class V, each participant will be able to do the following:

A. Identify two common postpartum discomforts and describe how to initiate relief measures.

B. Identify two symptoms or problems for which the doctor should be notified.

C. Consider a method of contraception that is acceptable to them.

D. Demonstrate the following in a mock labor and delivery:
1. Deep chest breathing
2. Shallow breathing
3. Panting
4. Pushing

NANDA APPROVED NURSING DIAGNOSES FOR 1994

Pattern 1: Exchanging

1.1.2.1	Altered Nutrition: More than body requirements
1.1.2.2	Altered Nutrition: Less than body requirements
1.1.2.3	Altered Nutrition: Potential for more than body requirements
1.2.1.1	Risk for Infection
1.2.2.1	Risk for Altered Body Temperature
1.2.2.2	Hypothermia
1.2.2.3	Hyperthermia
1.2.2.4	Ineffective Thermoregulation
1.2.3.1	Dysreflexia
1.3.1.1	Constipation
1.3.1.1.1	Perceived Constipation
1.3.1.1.2	Colonic Constipation
1.3.1.2	Diarrhea
1.3.1.3	Bowel Incontinence
1.3.2	Altered Urinary Elimination
1.3.2.1.1	Stress Incontinence
1.3.2.1.2	Reflex Incontinence
1.3.2.1.3	Urge Incontinence
1.3.2.1.4	Functional Incontinence
1.3.2.1.5	Total Incontinence
1.3.2.2	Urinary Retention
1.4.1.1	Altered (Specify Type) Tissue Perfusion (Renal, cerebral, cardiopulmonary, gastrointestinal, peripheral)
1.4.1.2.1	Fluid Volume Excess
1.4.1.2.2.1	Fluid Volume Deficit
1.4.1.2.2.2	Risk for Fluid Volume Deficit
1.4.2.1	Decreased Cardiac Output
1.5.1.1	Impaired Gas Exchange
1.5.1.2	Ineffective Airway Clearance
1.5.1.3	Ineffective Breathing Pattern
1.5.1.3.1	Inability to Sustain Spontaneous Ventilation
1.5.1.3.2	Dysfunctional Ventilatory Weaning Response (DVWR)
1.6.1	Risk for Injury
1.6.1.1	Risk for Suffocation
1.6.1.2	Risk for Poisoning
1.6.1.3	Risk for Trauma
1.6.1.4	Risk for Aspiration
1.6.1.5	Risk for Disuse Syndrome
1.6.2	Altered Protection
1.6.2.1	Impaired Tissue Integrity
1.6.2.1.1	Altered Oral Mucous Membrane
1.6.2.1.2.1	Impaired Skin Integrity
1.6.2.1.2.2	Risk for Impaired Skin Integrity
# 1.7.1	Decreased Adaptive Capacity: Intracranial
# 1.8	Energy Field Disturbance

Pattern 2: Communicating

2.1.1.1	Impaired Verbal Communication

Pattern 3: Relating

3.1.1	Impaired Social Interaction
3.1.2	Social Isolation
# 3.1.3	Risk for Loneliness
3.2.1	Altered Role Performance
3.2.1.1.1	Altered Parenting
3.2.1.1.2	Risk for Altered Parenting
# 3.2.1.1.2.1	Risk for Altered Parent/Infant/Child Attachment
3.2.1.2.1	Sexual Dysfunction
3.2.2	Altered Family Processes
3.2.2.1	Caregiver Role Strain
3.2.2.2	Risk for Caregiver Role Strain
# 3.2.2.3.1	Altered Family Process: Alcoholism
3.2.3.1	Parental Role Conflict
3.3	Altered Sexuality Pattern

Pattern 4: Valuing

4.1.1	Spiritual Distress (distress of the human spirit)
# 4.2	Potential for Enhanced Spiritual Well Being

Pattern 5: Choosing

5.1.1.1	Ineffective Individual Coping
5.1.1.1.1	Impaired Adjustment
5.1.1.1.2	Defensive Coping
5.1.1.1.3	Ineffective Denial
5.1.2.1.1	Ineffective Family Coping: Disabling
5.1.2.1.2	Ineffective Family Coping: Compromised
# 5.1.3.1	Potential for Enhanced Community Coping
# 5.1.3.2	Ineffective Community Coping
5.1.2.2	Family Coping: Potential for Growth
5.2.1	Ineffective Management of Therapeutic Regimen (Individuals)
5.2.1.1	Noncompliance (Specify)
# 5.2.2	Ineffective Management of Therapeutic Regimen: Families
# 5.2.3	Ineffective Management of Therapeutic Regimen: Community
# 5.2.4	Ineffective Management of Therapeutic Regimen: Individual
5.3.1.1	Decisional Conflict (Specify)
5.4	Health Seeking Behaviors (Specify)

Pattern 6: Moving

6.1.1.1	Impaired Physical Mobility
6.1.1.1.1	Risk for Peripheral Neurovascular Dysfunction
# 6.1.1.1.2	Risk for Perioperative Positioning Injury
6.1.1.2	Activity Intolerance
6.1.1.2.1	Fatigue
6.1.1.3	Risk for Activity Intolerance
6.2.1	Sleep Pattern Disturbance
6.3.1.1	Diversional Activity Deficit
6.4.1.1	Impaired Home Maintenance Management
6.4.2	Altered Health Maintenance
6.5.1	Feeding Self Care Deficit
6.5.1.1	Impaired Swallowing
6.5.1.2	Ineffective Breastfeeding
6.5.1.2.1	Interrupted Breastfeeding
6.5.1.3	Effective Breastfeeding
6.5.1.4	Ineffective Infant Feeding Pattern
6.5.2	Bathing/Hygiene Self Care Deficit
6.5.3	Dressing/Grooming Self Care Deficit
6.5.4	Toileting Self Care Deficit
6.6	Altered Growth and Development
6.7	Relocation Stress Syndrome
# 6.8.1	Risk of Disorganized Infant Behavior
# 6.8.2	Disorganized Infant Behavior
# 6.8.3	Potential for Enhanced Organized Infant Behavior

Pattern 7: Perceiving

7.1.1	Body Image Disturbance
7.1.2	Self Esteem Disturbance
7.1.2.1	Chronic Low Self Esteem
7.1.2.2	Situational Low Self Esteem
7.1.3	Personal Identity Disturbance
7.2	Sensory/Perceptual Alterations (Specify) (Visual, auditory, kinesthetic, gustatory, tactile, olfactory)
7.2.1.1	Unilateral Neglect
7.3.1	Hopelessness
7.3.2	Powerless

Pattern 8: Knowing

8.1.1	Knowledge Deficit (Specify)
# 8.2.1	Impaired Environmental Interpretation Syndrome
# 8.2.2	Acute Confusion
# 8.2.3	Chronic Confusion
8.3	Altered Thought Processes
# 8.3.1	Impaired Memory

Pattern 9: Feeling

9.1.1	Pain
9.1.1.1	Chronic Pain
9.2.1.1	Dysfunctional Grieving

#New diagnoses added in 1994

Index

NOTE: A *b* following a page number indicates boxed material;
a *t* following a page number indicates tabular material;
and an *f* following a page number indicates a figure.